Primary health care and psychiatric epidemiology

Edited by
Brian Cooper
and
Robin Eastwood
for
The World Psychiatric Association

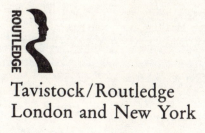

Tavistock/Routledge
London and New York

First published 1992
by Routledge
11 New Fetter Lane, London EC4P 4EE

Simultaneously published in the USA and Canada
by Routledge
a division of Routledge, Chapman and Hall, Inc.
29 West 35th Street, New York, NY 10001

© 1992 The World Psychiatric Association

Typeset in 10/12 Times by
Falcon Typographic Art Ltd, Edinburgh & London
Printed and bound in Great Britain by
Billings & Sons Limited, Worcester

British Library Cataloguing in Publication Data
Primary health care and psychiatric epidemiology
   1. Psychiatry
   I. Cooper, Brian, *1928–*   II. Eastwood, Robin   III. World
Psychiatric Association
   616.89

Library of Congress Cataloging in Publication Data
Primary health care and psychiatric epidemiology/edited by Brian
   Cooper and Robin Eastwood for the World Psychiatric Association.
   p. cm.
   'Selected contributions to an international symposium, arranged by
   the World Psychiatric Association's Section of Epidemiology and
   Community Psychiatry and held in Toronto, in 1989' – Pref.
   Includes bibliographical references and index.
   1. Psychiatric epidemiology – Congresses.   2. Family medicine –
   Congresses.   I. Cooper, Brian, 1928–.   II. Eastwood, Michael
   Robin, 1938–.   III. World Psychiatric Association. Section of
   Epidemiology and Community Psychiatry.
   [DNLM: 1. Mental Disorders – epidemiology – congresses. 2. Mental
   Disorders – therapy – congresses. 3. Primary Health Care – congresses.
   WM 100 P9517 1989]
   RC455.2.E64P755 1991
   362.2'0422 – dc20
   DNLM/DLC
   for Library of Congress   91–662
                                                              CIP
ISBN 0–415–07073–2

Primary health care and psychiatric epidemiology

In recent years, primary health care has been gaining in significance as a setting both for research on mental illness in the general population and for the development of new preventive approaches in this field. The growing need for research has received impetus from the escalating costs of hospital-based health care, the re-structuring of health services in a number of countries, with an increased emphasis on community care and prevention, and the World Health Organization's 'Health for All' campaign, in response to which a growing number of national planning documents have been published. These developments have already stimulated a new interest in the scope for epidemiological and evaluative investigations based on general medical practice.

This book consists of selected contributions to the first international scientific meeting on the topic, held in Toronto in 1989. It is made up of five sections, dealing respectively with: the growth and development of a new research field; findings of psychiatric surveys in general practice in a number of different countries; specialist and generalist medical care for mental illness – issues of selection and referral; and specialist aspects of late-life mental disorders encountered in such research. The inclusion of reports from groups of workers in the USA, the UK, the Netherlands, Germany, Spain, Italy, Finland, Canada, Australia and other countries testifies to the rapid spread of interest in these questions.

With the exception of the first two chapters, which sketch the background of public-health and general-practice epidemiology, all the contributions are focused on general practice as a field laboratory for study of the occurrence, distribution, diagnostic composition and risk factors of psychiatric illness in unselected populations, and present data, largely unpublished, from the authors' own projects. These findings confirm the importance of research in general practice as a major growing-point of social psychiatry and provide guidelines for further progress in the years ahead.

This book will be an invaluable source of reference to all psychiatrists, psychologists, general practitioners and health care professionals concerned with mental disorders in the wider community.

The Editors: Brian Cooper is Professor of Epidemiological Psychiatry at the University of Heidelberg, and Head of Section of Epidemiological Psychiatry at the Central Institute of Mental Health, Mannheim, Germany. Robin Eastwood is Professor of Psychiatry and Preventive Medicine and Biostatics at the Clarke Institute of Psychiatry, Toronto, Canada.

Contents

List of figures and tables   viii
List of contributors   xv
Preface   xix

**Part I Psychiatric epidemiology and general practice:
the development of a research field**

1 The science of epidemiology: empirical data gathering,
  public-health action, or both?   3
  Leon Eisenberg

2 Psychiatric illness, epidemiology and the
  general practitioner   14
  Brian Cooper

3 The 'research magnificent' comes of age   32
  Michael Shepherd

4 Primary care and psychiatric epidemiology:
  the psychiatrist's perspective   44
  David Goldberg and Linda Gask

**Part II Psychiatric field surveys in the primary
health-care setting: an international
perspective**

5 Psychiatric morbidity in general practice:
  a community-wide perspective   59
  Alex Richman

6 Mental health care in primary health care:
   a case for action   69
   Morton Kramer, Eleanor Simonsick, Bruno Lima
   and Itzhak Levav

7 Psychiatric illness and services in a UK health centre   99
   Brian Jarman

8 Psychosocial complaints in general practice:
   a national survey in the Netherlands   109
   Peter F. M. Verhaak, Joke M. Bosman,
   Marleen Foets and Koos van der Velden

9 Psychiatric morbidity and physical illness among
   general practice patients in Cantabria, Spain   123
   J. L. Vázquez-Barquero

10 Mental disorders in primary care
   in a health district of Bahia, Brazil   133
   N. M. de Almeida-Filho, V. S. Santana,
   E. C. Moreira, M. G. Modesto and M. B. Oliveira

11 Use of services by homeless and disaffiliated
   individuals with severe mental disorders: a study in Melbourne   142
   Helen Herrman, Patrick McGorry, Pamela Bennett,
   Katrina Varnavides and Bruce Singh

Part III Psychiatric and general medical services:
        issues of patient selection, referral and
        treatment

12 The relationship of usual source of health
   care to the prevalence of psychiatric disorder and
   the utilization of ambulatory mental health services in
   the United States   163
   Martha L. Bruce, Gary L. Tischler and Philip J. Leaf

13 Care of mental health problems in Finland:
   selection between primary medical and psychiatric
   specialist services   178
   V. Lehtinen, M. Joukamaa, T. Jyrkinen, K. Lahtela,
   R. Raitasalo, J. Maatela and A. Aromaa

14 Psychiatric morbidity in general practice in
   Verona: the importance of parallel studies at
   the primary and specialist levels of health care   188
   M. Tansella, C. Bellantuono and P. Williams

15 Prescribing of psychotropic drugs by primary-care
physicians and psychiatrists: a study in Iceland   198
Tómas Helgason

Part IV Late-life mental disorders and primary health care

16 Late-life mental disorders and primary health care:
a review of research   213
Brian Cooper

17 Prevalence and one-year course of dementia in
an English city: an application of CAMDEX   234
Daniel W. O'Connor and Penelope A. Pollitt

18 Cognitive disorders and dementia among elderly
general-practice patients in a West German city   253
Horst Bickel

19 Dementia: case ascertainment and health service
utilization in a US rural community   277
*Mary Ganguli, Lewis H. Kuller, Steven Belle,
Graham Ratcliff, F. Jacob Huff and Katherine M. Detre*

**Part V Problems of method: case-finding,
       classification and taxonomy**

20 Identification of psychiatric cases in primary
health-care settings: the utility of two-phase
screening designs   293
Patrick E. Shrout

21 The latent structure of anxiety and depression in
treated and untreated samples of two US populations   307
William W. Eaton and Howard D. Chilcoat

22 Psychiatric syndromes among persons in contact with
general medical and psychiatric services in eastern Baltimore   319
*James C. Anthony, Alan J. Romanoski, Gerald Nestadt,
Daniel E. Ford and Morton Kramer*

23 Somatization in primary health care:
prevalence and determinants   341
K. W. Bridges and D. P. Goldberg

Index   351

Figures and tables

FIGURES

4.1 Pathways to psychiatric care in South Manchester 46
5.1 Prevalence of treated mental illness, 1975–81 61
5.2 Inception of psychiatric treatment, by age-group and setting of first contact, New Brunswick, 1977–79 64
5.3 Primary medical care for mental disorder: cumulative percentage in cohort of 18-year-olds 65
6.1 Distribution of office visits by physician specialty: United States, Jan. 1980 – Dec. 1981 (percentages) 93
7.1 Psychiatric out-patient referrals as a proportion of all out-patient referrals, 1974–86 103
7.2 Trends in referral to hospital psychiatry and to facilities within the health centre, 1971–86 104
8.1 Proportions of doctor–patient encounters having some psychiatric component, for four different patient groups 116
15.1 Comparison of the prevalence of psychotropic drug use, according to sex and age, with number of defined daily doses (DDD) per 1,000 inhabitants 201
18.1 Mean test scores on augmented Hierarchic Dementia Scale, according to severity of dementia (CAMDEX criteria 265
18.2 Mean test scores on augmented Hierarchic Dementia Scale, according to general practitioners' rating of cognitive impairment 267
18.3 Cumulative distribution of Hierarchic Dementia Scale total scores, according to severity of dementia (CAMDEX criteria) 268
20.1 Cost ratio of screen to diagnosis for which one- and two-phase designs are equally efficient for prevalence estimation when prevalence is .05 302
20.2 Cost ratio of screen to diagnosis for which one- and two-phase

designs are equally efficient for case-identification when
prevalence is .05   304

TABLES

2.1 Comparison of rates of psychiatric illness contact at different
    levels of mental health care, England, 1981   18
2.2 Efficiency of detection of psychiatric abnormality by
    general practitioners, assessed by comparison with the results
    of standardized screening methods   21
3.1 Kappa agreements for ICD/ICHPPC diagnoses   37
3.2 Proportion of psychiatric patients with each of the eight most
    common record types (× 100)   39
4.1 Comparison of the rates of psychiatric morbidity, at different
    levels of care, in three European cities   45
4.2 Two-stage surveys of psychiatric disorder in primary medical
    care: recent US studies   46
4.3 Determinants of the ability to identify psychological distress:
    findings of early research   49
4.4 Management skills of doctors with high identification indices   50
4.5 Definition of somatization   51
4.6 Improvement in re-attribution skills of GP trainees after
    exposure to focused training   53
5.1 Psychiatric resources in New Brunswick, Canada   60
5.2 Prevalence and inception rate by year and type of service
    setting, 1975–80   63
5.3 Inceptions: cases recorded during 1977–79 and not in 1975–76   63
6.1 Distribution of population 18 years of age and older by
    selected demographic characteristics   73
6.2 Distribution of persons 18 years of age and older by presence
    or absence of current DIS/DSM-III and physical disorder   74
6.3 Prevalence rates of: (a) all physical disorders; (b) physical
    disorders only; (c) physical disorders and mental disorders,
    and (d) percentage of all physical disorders with a mental disorder,
    by selected demographic characteristics   75
6.4 Prevalence rates of: (a) all mental disorders; (b) mental
    disorders only; (c) mental disorders and physical disorders;
    and (d) percentage of all mental disorders with a physical
    disorder, by selected demographic characteristics   77
6.5 Percentage of persons 18 years of age and older with a
    physical disorder who also had a specific mental disorder   80
6.6 Percentage of persons 18 years of age and older with a mental
    disorder who reported a specific physical disorder   82
6.7 Adjusted odds ratios, for the prevalence of any mental

disorder and selected disorders among persons reporting a
physical disorder   85
6.8 Prevalence odds ratios associated with household type relative
to those for married couple families, for any mental disorder
and selected disorders among persons reporting a current
physical disorder, adjusted for sex, race, age, education and
household income   87
6.9 Percentage of ambulatory health and/or mental health visits
in past six months by persons with (1) no mental or physical
disorder; (2) physical disorder only; (3) mental disorder only;
(4) both physical and mental disorder, by sex, race and age   88
7.1 Use of psychiatric hospital services in England, 1966–86   100
8.1 Three-month consulting rate for psychological complaints   112
8.2 Three-month consulting rate for conditions judged by the GP
to be 'not entirely physical'   113
8.3 Three-month consulting rates for psychiatric illness and for
selected psychiatric diagnoses   114
8.4 Three-month consulting rates for psychological complaints
and conditions judged by the GP to be 'not entirely physical',
for groups with different marital status, different educational
level and in different urban/rural areas   115
8.5 Number of patients and of doctor–patient contacts in four
sub-groups of consulting patients   117
9.1 Survey sample: contacts, refusals and non-contacts, by
sex   125
9.2 Distribution of diagnosed somatic pathology in the survey
sample, by sex   126
9.3 Psychiatric morbidity, according to selected demographic
characteristics, in respondents with somatic pathology
diagnosed by general practitioners   127
9.4 Psychiatric morbidity, according to selected social
characteristics, in respondents with somatic pathology
diagnosed by general practitioners   128
9.5 Significant joint effects of socio-demographic variables on
the frequency of psychiatric morbidity of respondents with
diagnosed somatic pathology   129
9.6 Estimated probability of psychiatric morbidity, according to
demographic profile   130
10.1 Demographic characteristics of the survey sample   135
10.2 Type of medical complaint given as main reason for
consultation, by age and gender   137
10.3 Proportions of patients with (a) neuropsychiatric diagnoses
and (b) psychopharmacological prescriptions recorded, by age
and gender   138

10.4 Weighted proportions of patients with neuropsychiatric
     diagnoses, by gender and age-group   139
10.5 Weighted proportions of patients in the main neuropsychiatric
     diagnostic categories, by gender   140
11.1 Study population and sample by type of accommodation   147
11.2 Frequency of reported treatment for emotional problems and
     hospitalization for emotional problems, by broad diagnostic
     category derived from SCID-R 'lifetime' diagnoses   150
11.3 Current psychotropic medication by type of medication and
     (a) age of respondent, (b) sex of respondent, and (c) type of
     accommodation   151
11.4 Frequency of current medication use by categories of
     DSM-III-R disorders   152
11.5 Present service use in respondents by medication use   153
11.6 Category of psychiatric disorder (DSM-III-R) by current
     service use   153
11.7 Distribution of respondents by current duration of
     homelessness   154
11.8 Apparent sequence in onset of first episode of severe mental
     disorder and homelessness, by sex   155
12.1 Distribution according to usual sources of medical care in five
     ECA communities   167
12.2 Percentages of respondents with specific socio-demographic
     and economic characteristics, according to usual source of
     health care   169
12.3 Percentage of respondents with current or recent (within
     one year) psychiatric disorder, according to usual source of
     health care   170
12.4 Percentage of respondents in contact with mental health
     specialty services, according to usual source of health care
     and psychiatric status at interview   172
12.5 Proportion of respondents using mental health specialty
     services, and frequency of visits, according to usual source of
     health care and psychiatric status at interview   173
13.1 Sex and age distribution of the sample   180
13.2 Frequency of utilization of primary or specialist mental health
     services, according to age and sex   182
13.3 Relationship of health factors with utilization of primary or
     specialist mental health services   183
13.4 Relationship of marital status with utilization of primary or
     specialist mental health services   184
13.5 Relationship of income and area of residence to utilization of
     primary or specialist mental health services   185
13.6 Use of primary mental health services among those

receiving some treatment, indicated as adjusted relative
risk ratios   186

14.1 Permeability of Filter no. 3 in South-Verona: number
and percentage of contacts referred to the South-Verona
Community Psychiatric Service by GPs in 1982–87   192

14.2 Permeability of Filter no. 3 in South-Verona: number and
percentage of first-time contacts referred to the South-Verona
Community Psychiatric Service by GPs before and after a
general practice study conducted in the area   192

14.3 Estimated one-week prevalence rates of psychiatric morbidity
in South-Verona   194

15.1 Distribution of physicians, patients and prescriptions, and
number of psychotropic drugs per prescription by specialty of
the prescribing doctor   200

15.2 Distribution of psychotropic drugs prescribed over one month, by
specialty of physicians   203

15.3 Distribution of psychotropic drugs prescribed over one month, by
physicians of different specialties   204

15.4 Prescriptions with psychotropic drugs only or combined with
other drugs, by specialty of physicians   205

15.5 Mean PDD/DDD according to ATC drug category and
specialty of prescribing physician   205

15.6 Mean PDD/DDD according to ATC drug groups and age of
prescribing physician   206

15.7 Analysis of variance of prescribed daily doses as proportion of
defined daily doses by ATC drug groups, specialty and age of
physicians   207

16.1 Prevalence of late-life dementia (severe or moderately severe)
in general-practice-based surveys, compared with estimates
from area field-survey data   215

16.2 Accuracy of general practitioners in assessing cognitive status
of elderly patients. Selected samples: comparison of two research
projects   219

16.3 Randomized controlled trials of community intervention
programmes for the elderly   223

16.4 Expected numbers of mentally ill elderly in a standard
area population of 250,000, and in a group-practice patient
population of 12,500 (severe and moderately severe
cases only)   227

17.1 Demographic characteristics of study population compared
with the whole of the same age-group in the Cambridge urban
area census   237

17.2 The prevalence of mild, moderate and severe dementia by
age-group   238

17.3 Comparison of initial and follow-up dementia severity ratings   239

17.4 Changes in mean MMSE scores of normal, minimally
demented and demented subjects over 1 year   241

17.5 Comparison of CAMDEX and Clinical Dementia Rating
severity gradings   244

18.1 Areas of functioning measured by the sub-tests of the
augmented Hierarchic Dementia Scale   258

18.2 Distribution of cognitive status ratings of elderly consulting
patients, made by the general practitioners, by age-group of
the patients   261

18.3 Drawing the interview sample   262

18.4 Distribution of interviewed patients according to cognitive
status: general practitioners' ratings compared with research
interview assessments   263

18.5 Extrapolation of severity ratings onto the whole patient
collective, by correction of the GPs' assessments   264

18.6 Correlation of augmented HDS sub-scale scores with severity
of dementia and socio-demographic characteristics   269

18.7 Influence of severity of dementia, age, sex and social class on
the augmented HDS sub-scale scores: results of analysis of
co-variance   270

19.1 MoVIES cognitive screening battery   281

19.2 Demographic composition by cognitive impairment: random
sample   283

19.3 Health-service utilization by cognitive impairment   284

19.4 Health and social-services utilization and cognitive
impairment   285

19.5 Demographics: intact, impaired and demented groups   286

19.6 Health-service utilization: intact, impaired and demented
groups   287

19.7 Health-service utilization and dementia   288

20.1 Schematic layout of expected results from a two-phase survey   296

20.2 Planning a two-phase prevalence estimation procedure: a
hypothetical numerical example   299

21.1 Use of primary health care and psychiatric specialist services:
Baltimore and Durham ECA sites   311

21.2 Latent class model with all sectors constrained to
be equal   312

21.3 Distributions of three latent classes according to utilization of
Medicare care: three-sector equality model   312

21.4 Statistics for selected latent class models   314

21.5 Latent class model with all sectors and symptoms
unconstrained   316

22.1 Selected characteristics of the Stage Two segment of the

household sample, Eastern Baltimore Mental Health
Survey, 1981   324
22.2 Estimated prevalence of PSE syndromes found in the
community and among recent users of medical and psychiatric
services: data from Stage Two of the Eastern Baltimore
Mental Health Survey, 1981   326
22.3 Estimated odds ratios showing PSE syndromes associated with
recent use of general medical services: data from the Eastern
Baltimore Mental Health Survey, 1981   329
22.4 Estimated odds ratios showing PSE syndromes associated
with recent use of specialty psychiatric services, among recent
users of general medical services; unweighted data from the
Eastern Baltimore Mental Health Survey, 1981   331
22.5 Present State Examination syndromes that were retained in
the stepwise discriminant function analyses to discriminate
recent users of general medical services from non-users and
to discriminate recent users of specialty psychiatric services
from non-users: unweighted data from the Eastern Baltimore
Mental Health Survey, 1981   332
23.1 Weighted data on a consecutive series of patients with
DSM-III psychiatric illness (excluding Adjustment Disorder)
in terms of how these were classified by the general
practitioners and by mode of presentation   345
23.2 Weighted data on patients with DSM-III illnesses in terms
of mode of presentation and presence of coexisting physical
disorder   346
23.3 Weighted data on 'hidden psychiatric morbidity' in terms
of mode of presentation and presence of coexisting physical
disorder   346
23.4 Demographic characteristics of patients in study of potential
determinants of somatization   347

Contributors

Almeida-Filho, Professor N.M. de, Federal University of Bahia, Faculty of Medicine, Department of Preventive Medicine, Salvador, Bahia, Brazil

Anthony, Professor J.C., Department of Mental Hygiene, Johns Hopkins School of Public Health, Baltimore, MD, USA

Aromaa, A., MD, Research Institute for Social Security, Social Insurance Institution, Helsinki, Finland

Bellantuono, C., MD, Department of Medical Psychology, Institute of Psychiatry, University of Verona, Italy

Belle, S., PhD, Department of Epidemiology, University of Pittsburgh, School of Public Health, Pittsburgh, PA, USA

Bennett, Dr P., Consultant Psychiatrist, Royal Park Hospital, Melbourne, Australia

Bickel, Dr H., Department of Epidemiological Psychiatry, Central Institute of Mental Health, Mannheim, Germany

Bosman, J.M., MD, Netherlands Institute of Primary Health Care (NIVEL), Utrecht, Netherlands

Bridges, Dr K.W., University of Manchester, Department of Psychiatry, Manchester Royal Infirmary, Manchester, UK

Bruce, Professor M.L., Department of Psychiatry, Yale University School of Medicine, New Haven, CT, USA

Chilcoat, H.D., MS, Department of Mental Hygiene, School of Hygiene and Public Health, Johns Hopkins University, Baltimore, MD, USA

Cooper, Professor B., Department of Epidemiological Psychiatry, Central Institute of Mental Health, Mannheim, Germany

Detre, Professor K.M., Department of Epidemiology, University of Pittsburgh, School of Public Health, Pittsburgh, PA, USA

Eastwood, Professor M.R., Clarke Institute of Psychiatry, Toronto, Canada

Eaton, Professor W.W., Department of Mental Hygiene, School of Hygiene and Public Health, Johns Hopkins University, Baltimore, MD, USA

Eisenberg, Professor L., Department of Social Medicine and Social Policy, Harvard Medical School, Boston, MA, USA

Foets, M., MD, Netherlands Institute of Primary Health Care (NIVEL), Utrecht, Netherlands

Ford, D. E., MD, Clinical Epidemiology Program and Department of Internal Medicine, Johns Hopkins University School of Medicine, Baltimore, MD, USA

Ganguli, Professor M., University of Pittsburgh, School of Medicine and School of Public Health, Western Psychiatric Institute and Clinic, Pittsburgh, PA, USA

Gask, L., University Department of Psychiatry, University Hospital of South Manchester, Withington, Manchester, UK

Goldberg, Professor D.P., University Department of Psychiatry, University Hospital of South Manchester, Withington, Manchester, UK

Helgason, Professor T., Department of Psychiatry, National University Hospital, Reykjavik, Iceland

Herrman, Dr H., Monash University, Department of Psychological Medicine, Royal Park Hospital, Melbourne, Australia

Huff, F.J., MD, Medical College of Pennsylvania and Clinical Neuroscience Research Group, Hoechst-Roussel Pharmaceuticals, Inc., Somerville, PA, USA

Jarman, Professor B., Department of General Practice, St Mary's Hospital Medical School and Lisson Grove Health Centre, London, UK

Joukamaa, M., MD, Research Institute for Social Security, Social Insurance Institution, Helsinki, Finland

Jyrkinen, T., Research Institute for Social Security, Social Insurance Institution, Helsinki, Finland

Kramer, M., ScD, Professor Emeritus, Department of Mental Hygiene, Johns Hopkins University, School of Hygiene and Public Health, Baltimore, MD, USA

Kuller, L.H., MD, DrPh, Department of Epidemiology, University of Pittsburgh School of Public Health, Pittsburgh, PA, USA

Lahtela, K., Rehabilitation Research Centre, Social Insurance Institution, Turku, Finland

Leaf, P.J., MD, Department of Psychiatry, Yale University School of Medicine, New Haven, CT, USA

Lehtinen, Professor V., MD, Rehabilitation Research Centre, Social Insurance Institution, Turku, Finland

Levav, I., MD, Regional Advisor in Mental Health, Pan American Health Organization, Washington, DC, USA

Lima, Professor B., Johns Hopkins University, Department of Psychiatry and Behavioral Sciences, School of Medicine and Department of Mental Hygiene, School of Hygiene and Public Health, Baltimore, MD, USA

Maatela, J., Rehabilitation Research Centre, Social Insurance Institution, Turku, Finland

McGorry, Dr P., Monash University Department of Psychological Medicine, Royal Park Hospital, Melbourne, Australia

Modesto, M.G., Federal University of Bahia, Faculty of Medicine, Community Health Program, Salvador, Bahia, Brazil

Moreira, E.C., Federal University of Bahia, Faculty of Medicine, Community Health Program, Salvador, Bahia, Brazil

Nestadt, G., MD, Department of Psychiatry and Behavioral Sciences, Johns Hopkins University School of Medicine, Baltimore, MD, USA

O'Connor, Professor D.W., Health Department of Victoria, Heatherton Hospital, Victoria, Australia

Oliveira, M.B., Federal University of Bahia, Faculty of Medicine, Community Health Program, Salvador, Bahia, Brazil

Pollitt, P.A., PhD, Hughes Hall Project for Later Life, Hughes Hall, Cambridge, UK

Raitasalo, R., DPh, Research Institute for Social Security, Social Insurance Institution, Helsinki, Finland

Ratcliff, Professor G., Department of Psychiatry, University of Pittsburgh School of Medicine, Pittsburgh, PA, USA

Richman, Professor A., Department of Psychiatry and Community Medicine, Dalhousie University, Halifax, Nova Scotia, Canada

Romanoski, A.J., MD, Department of Psychiatry and Behavioral Sciences, Johns Hopkins University School of Medicine, Baltimore, MD, USA

Santana, V.S., MD, Federal University of Bahia, Faculty of Medicine, Department of Preventive Medicine, Salvador, Bahia, Brazil

Shepherd, M., DM, Professor Emeritus, Institute of Psychiatry, London, UK

Shrout, Professor P.E., Columbia University School of Public Health, Division of Biostatistics, New York, NY, USA

Simonsick, E., PhD, Program of Epidemiology, Demography and Biometry, National Institute of Aging, Bethesda, MD, USA

Singh, Professor B., Department of Psychological Medicine, Royal Park Hospital, Melbourne, Australia

Tansella, Professor M., Department of Medical Psychology, Institute of Psychiatry, University of Verona, Verona, Italy

Tischler, G.L., MD, Department of Psychiatry, Yale University School of Medicine, New Haven, CT, USA

Varnavides, K., Monash University Department of Psychological Medicine, Royal Park Hospital, Melbourne, Australia

Vázquez-Barquero, Professor J.L., Cantabria Medical School, University Hospital Valdecilla, University of Cantabria, Santander, Spain

Velden, K. van der, MD, Netherlands Institute of Primary Health Care (NIVEL), Utrecht, Netherlands

Verhaak, P.F.M., MD, Netherlands Institute of Primary Care (NIVEL), Utrecht, Netherlands

Williams, Dr P., Director of Clinical Research (CNS) Glaxo, Greenford, Middlesex, UK

Preface

This volume is made up of selected contributions to an international symposium, arranged by the World Psychiatric Association's Section of Epidemiology and Community Psychiatry and held in Toronto in June 1989. The scientific programme for this meeting was planned and organized by the present editors: one (BC) as the then Chairman of the World Psychiatric Association (WPA) Section Committee, and the other (RE) as a member both of that committee and of the clinical faculty of the host institute, the Clarke Institute of Psychiatry of Toronto University.

The WPA Section of Epidemiology and Community Psychiatry has established a reputation for sponsoring international conferences on the epidemiology of mental disorders and making their proceedings widely available. Of a total of nine such meetings in the twenty years preceding the Toronto symposium, six have provided the material for publications (see the list below), each of which has maintained a sound scientific standard and been much valued by researchers in the special field of inquiry. Their most distinctive feature is that most of the contributions present findings of empirical investigation, in the form either of original research reports or critical review articles, though sometimes written in a more personal and reflective style than is nowadays usual in the specialist journals.

The present volume continues in this tradition. With the exception of the two opening chapters, which are intended to lend perspective to the whole by sketching the wider background of public health and general practice epidemiology, it is made up of reports on psychiatric research, each of which contains data derived entirely or in part from the authors' own projects. The book represents none the less a new departure in two ways. To begin with, whereas the earlier symposia all reflected contemporary progress in psychiatric epidemiology on a wide front, the Toronto meeting focused down on a single specific aspect; namely, general medical practice as a field laboratory for systematic study of the occurrence, distribution, diagnostic composition and risk factors of mental illness in unselected populations: a concentration of theme which gives cohesion to these proceedings. Secondly, whereas previous publications in the series have been of interest mainly to psychiatrists and other mental health workers, this book is aimed at a readership which includes general practitioners, public-health workers and the various professional groups engaged in community health and social services.

The scope for morbidity surveys in general practice first began to attract attention in the 1950s, most notably in the United Kingdom, where it was realized that the system of patient registration under the newly established British National Health Service presented a golden opportunity for epidemiological research. The initial large-scale survey of psychiatric illness in this setting, undertaken by Professor Michael Shepherd and his co-workers at the London Institute of Psychiatry, explored what at that time was still largely uncharted terrain. Their findings, originally published in 1966, have had a seminal influence on medical thinking about this issue, and have served both as a stimulus to psychiatric survey research in many other countries, and as a starting point for further investigation in general practice, making use of more sophisticated methods and analytical research designs.

In recent years the significance of the primary-care setting for such research, as well as for new preventive approaches, has been highlighted by the World Health Organization's 'Health for All' campaign which, commencing with the Declaration of Alma-Ata in 1978, has consistently promulgated the need for a high quality of care at community level, for physical and psychiatric ill health alike and in both developed and developing countries. The chief theoretical objection to data on psychiatric illness from general practice – that standards of case-identification and diagnosis are insufficiently reliable for scientific purposes – was never a valid argument for abandoning the field, and has gradually diminished in force with the development and application of new, standardized techniques for psychiatric screening and diagnostic assessment. A growing number of research reports have demonstrated that the use of such methods in collaborative surveys can produce real gains in epidemiological knowledge. The moment therefore seemed right for the first international symposium to signalize this progress.

The large number of countries represented here testifies to the rapid spread of interest in general practice as a research milieu. While the largest single entry came from the USA, reflecting the upsurge in psychiatric survey research that followed in the wake of President Carter's Mental Health Commission, communications were also presented from groups in the UK, the Netherlands, Germany, Italy, Spain, Finland, Iceland, Canada, Australia, Brazil and elsewhere. All those included here, though drawn from such widely differing societies and health-care systems, point to a high prevalence of mental illness and emotional distress in the patient populations; all share a common concern with the public-health consequences of these disorders, and all manifest a due regard for the requirements of scientific method, including careful statistical analysis of the research data.

This is an encouraging harvest, and helps to confirm our belief that research and co-operation in primary health care now represent one of the major growing points of social psychiatry. But it must be stressed that it is a discipline still at an early stage of development and enjoying only a very modest status in the hierarchy of academic medical priorities. An international conference on this theme would hardly have been feasible twenty, or even ten years ago. Investigations of the kind described here cannot as a rule hope to attract support and funding on a scale comparable to that commanded by high-prestige biomedical projects, or indeed even the minimum necessary to ensure continuing activity. Moreover, the research impulses have almost all come from medical clinicians; the input from teaching departments of community medicine, nursing and social work has been small, while with a few distinguished exceptions social scientists and health economists have evinced little interest in the field.

An expansion of primary care research, even though still with only limited resources, can be anticipated for the next decade, as the need for more effective and economic forms of community health care becomes ever more pressing. The most rapid progress may well be made in those countries which have recently begun to set up the necessary health-service structures, as indeed the examples of Spain and Italy suggest. Given such a basis we can hope to see a growth of longitudinal, cohort and case-control studies of the kind required to ascertain the environmental risk factors of mental disorder, investigations into the service needs of emotionally disturbed children and their families, evaluative research on community self-help initiatives and a number of other outstanding problems for whose exploration the primary care team is uniquely equipped. It is our hope that the present volume will help to point the direction for these advances and provide some guidelines along the way.

The Editors
January 1991

PUBLICATIONS FROM THE WPA SECTION OF EPIDEMIOLOGY AND COMMUNITY PSYCHIATRY

Cooper, B. (ed.) (1987) *Psychiatric Epidemiology: Progress and Prospects*, London: Croom Helm.
Cooper, B. and Helgason, T. (eds) (1989) *Epidemiology and the Prevention of Mental Disorders*, London: Routledge.
Hare, E.H. and Wing, J.K. (eds) (1970) *Psychiatric Epidemiology*, London: Oxford University Press.

Robins, L.N., Clayton, P.J., and Wing, J.K. (eds) (1980) *The Social Consequences of Psychiatric Illness*, New York: Brunner Mazel.

Wing, J.K. and Häfner, H. (eds) (1973) *Roots of Evaluation*, London: Oxford University Press.

Wing, J.K., Bebbington, P., and Robins, L.N. (eds) (1981) *What is a Case? The Problem of Definition in Psychiatric Community Surveys*, London: Grant McIntyre.

Psychiatric epidemiology and general practice: the development of a research field

Chapter 1

The science of epidemiology
Empirical data gathering, public-health action, or both?

Leon Eisenberg

The application of the methods of psychiatric epidemiology to the study of mental health problems in primary health care is a relatively recent development (Shepherd 1990). That short history made it possible for the founder of this field of investigation, Professor Michael Shepherd, to be a participant in the World Psychiatric Association Symposium reported in this volume, a symposium convened just thirty years after the publication of his first report on the topic (Shepherd *et al.* 1959). Few recognized its importance at the time; fewer still took it up. For the next several decades, psychiatric epidemiology in primary care was broadened and deepened primarily by Michael Shepherd and the Maudsley psychiatrists he helped to train and equip to explore this terrain: David Goldberg, John Cooper, Anthony Clare and Anthony Mann in Britain, Brian Cooper in Germany, Robin Eastwood in Canada, Michele Tansella in Italy, Assen Jablensky in Bulgaria and Norman Sartorius at the World Health Organization.

Despite some missionary work in the States by David Goldberg, recognition of the size of the mental health burden in general medical practice did not begin to take hold in North America until the paper by Regier and co-workers (1978) on what they called the *de facto* US mental health services system. Their account made it evident that, in the USA, just as in the UK and in the developing world (Harding *et al.* 1980), primary-care physicians are the principal, and often the only, resource for patients who are psychologically disturbed. I use the phrase 'did not begin to take hold' advisedly. Psychiatric educators and mental health policy makers in the USA continue to pay lip-service to the implications of the epidemiologic data for modifications in the organization of service delivery and in the education of generalists. The record in the UK, if still far short of the mark, is considerably better in this regard, much of that progress being due to systematic data produced by psychiatrists trained at the Maudsley.

How bizarre, now that Professor Shepherd has become Emeritus, for his General Practice Unit to have been phased out as part of the savage Thatcher retrenchment on research expenditures! In the UK, as in the USA, Tory governments have learned that epidemiologic surveillance, because it reveals gaps in service delivery, generates public pressure for additional care and, hence, additional costs (Eisenberg 1989a). With 'prevention' the new password in health policy, it is no small irony that governments are opting to prevent research; that is, the systematic gathering and release of information on the operation of the health services. The operative principle seems to be that what the public doesn't know won't hurt it ('it', in this instance, being the government!).

What makes the study of psychiatric disorders in primary care so crucial is that it asks questions which matter for patients, for front-line doctors and for health policy makers. How great is the burden of psychological ill health in the case load of primary care physicians? To what extent is that burden recognized by either patients or doctors? Does its identification lead to useful interventions? Can the diagnostic and therapeutic performance of generalists be improved? Are psychological treatments feasible within the economic and personnel constraints of primary health care? Because the answers are responsive to practical issues in health-care delivery, epidemiologic research designed to probe such matters remains grounded in clinical reality (Williams *et al.* 1989; Sartorius *et al.* 1990).

That service orientation distinguishes research on primary care from epidemiologic studies which use symptom counts and cut-off scores to tote up 'cases' without reference to disability or to care-seeking behaviour. Preoccupation with internalist criteria and with methodologic precision transmutes the means of research into its ends. Epidemiologists of the latter persuasion will take their cue from Sir William Thomson (1889), later Lord Kelvin, who wrote:

> When you can measure what you are speaking about, and express it in numbers, you know something about it, but when you cannot measure it, when you cannot express it in numbers, your knowledge is of a meagre and unsatisfactory kind; it may be the beginning of knowledge, but you have scarcely, in your thoughts, advanced to the stage of *science*, whatever the matter may be.
>
> (Thomson 1889)

Sir William's statement epitomizes the positivism (and the arrogance) of modern reductionistic science. For too many, I fear, it will suffice for a description of epidemiology, a science whose findings are, after all, 'expressed in numbers'. Indeed, as the methods of epidemiology become more precise and its mathematics more elegant, its practitioners harbour the hope that the 'real' scientists on the medical faculty (the 'basic' scientists) will accept epidemiology as a legitimate intellectual enterprise.*

---

* That such a day is not quite upon us is evident from a conversation with a distinguished biochemist (and an altogether remarkable human being). He had no objection, my colleague told me, to the first US Surgeon General's warning printed on cigarette packages to the effect that 'Smoking may be Dangerous to Your Health'. That was

But epidemiology (like all science) is far more than measurements and numbers. Recall the rejoinder by Jacob Viner, late Professor of Economics at Princeton, to Kelvin's dictum: 'When you can measure it, when you can express it in numbers, your knowledge is still of a meager and unsatisfactory kind!' His remark was not intended as a clever and cynical riposte. He went on to explain: 'It is a mistake to measure for measurement's sake and to let the possibilities of measurement be decisive as to the range of problems to be investigated.' I recount this interchange (Merton *et al.* 1984) because there is a not inconsiderable danger that the remarkable progress in the methods of psychiatric epidemiology in recent decades may lead to so narrow a preoccupation with methodologic elegance as to obscure the fundamental social purposes of the endeavour.

Some years ago I encountered a graduate student who had passed his orals but was in a quandary about choosing a suitable thesis problem. Referred to me by a colleague, he asked if I could identify a topic for him in child psychiatry. The one stricture he placed on my advice was that the study be framed in such fashion that the data collected would be suitable for analysis of variance, the only statistical technique he had mastered! ANOVA seemed quite elegant to him; he wasn't up to more advanced methods; and he hated the thought of wasting the effort he had put into learning ANOVA by not using it for his thesis!

My account is not invented; the student and his request were real. If his having so far lost the purpose of the research thesis required for his doctorate seems bizarre to you, do not condemn the hapless lad too hastily. Recall the faculty colleagues responsible for the legion of clinical studies that follow upon the availability of a new (preferably automated) method for measuring a presumptively important metabolite in blood, urine or cerebrospinal fluid. Has not psychiatric epidemiology seen its share of studies in which structured interviews and diagnostic algorithms have been pressed into use to obtain 'answers' to unasked questions? Some such investigations compute rates of 'caseness' that defy clinical judgement, unless, of course, one has as keen a diagnostic eye as the first year surgical registrar who commented, as he scanned a crowd of pedestrians: 'Look at them; they're all pre-op!'

Wade Hampton Frost (1936), in his introduction to a reprint of John Snow's work on cholera, reminded the reader:

Epidemiology at any given time is something more than the total of its established facts. It includes their orderly arrangement into chains of inference which extend more or less beyond the bounds of direct

---

fair enough. But he (though a non-smoker) was indignant at the new message which has replaced it: 'Cigarettes Cause Cancer'. He insisted that because the precise mechanism of carcinogenesis has not yet been deciphered, public health authorities have no right to say 'cause', whatever the strength of the epidemiologic evidence.

observation. Such of these chains as are well and truly laid guide investigation to the facts of the future; those that are ill-made fetter progress.

(1936: ix)

In addition to its utility in testing hypotheses about the causes of diseases, J.N. Morris (1975) highlights among the uses of epidemiology its roles as 'the intelligence service of public health' and as 'a main method of studying the social aspects of health and disease'. During the nineteenth century, epidemiologic data fuelled the social reform movement; in turn, the passion of social reformers spurred the extension of the epidemiologic paradigm into new areas of inquiry. When Rudolf Virchow inaugurated the journal *Die Medizinische Reform* in 1847, he announced that 'medical statistics will be our standard of measurement: we will weigh life for life and see where the dead lie thicker, among the workers or among the privileged' (Virchow, cited in Rosen 1947). Virchow and his friends emphasized the scientific (that is, epidemiologic) study of the social and economic conditions that influence health. The epidemiologic data base provided the rationale for social measures designed to promote health and prevent disease (Eisenberg 1984).

In London, Edwin Chadwick's 1842 *Report on the Sanitary Conditions of the Labouring Population* documented the disproportionate concentration of disease among the working classes; just eight years earlier, Chadwick had been a principal architect of the Poor Law Amendment Act (Webster 1990). He then argued that the 'profligacy' of poor relief was demoralizing to its recipients; on further study, the facts led him to conclude that it was filthy living conditions that spawned 'moral turpitude' rather than the other way round (Acheson 1990). For his data, he was largely dependent upon William Farr, the Registrar General. Just how committed Farr himself was to the movement for reform is evident from what he wrote in 1843:

Over the supply of water – the sewerage – the burial places – the width of streets – the removal of public nuisances – the poor can have no command . . . and it is precisely upon these points that the Government can interfere with most advantage. The Legislature would enact the removal of known sources of disease, and, if necessary, trench upon the liberty of the subject and the privilege of property, upon the same principle that it arrests and removes murderers, who, if left unmolested, would probably only destroy lives by hundreds, while the physical causes which have been averted to in this paper, destroy thousands – hundreds of thousands of lives.

(Farr, cited in Wohl 1983)

Similar notes sounded in America. John C. Griscom, City Inspector of the New York Board of Health, was inspired by Chadwick, as is evident from the title of his 1848 book: *The Sanitary Condition of the Laboring Population of New York*. He noted first, 'that there is an immense amount of sickness, physical disability, and premature mortality, among the poorer classes'; second, 'that these are, to a large extent, unnecessary, being in a great degree the results of causes which are removable'; third, 'that these physical evils are productive of moral evils of great magnitude and number, and which, if considered only in a pecuniary point of view should arouse the government and individuals to the consideration of the best means for their relief and prevention'; and fourth, that it was the responsibility of health officers 'to suggest the means of alleviating these evils and preventing their recurrence to so great an extent'. By analysing the associations between living conditions and expectations of survival, notable successes in achieving sanitary reforms were won, well before the germ theory of disease was established (Rosen 1958).

Then as now, public-health policy decisions reflect value judgements – informed by science but value judgements none the less; thus they are, in the final analysis, political decisions. Virchow (1848) put the matter succinctly: 'Medicine is a social science, and politics is nothing more than medicine on a large scale.' The role of political constituencies in health-policy debates is most evident in an historical instance in which neither the 'liberals' nor the 'conservatives' grasped the cause or mode of transmission of the disease they meant to control: yellow fever.

In the fall of 1793, a major epidemic of yellow fever struck Philadelphia; half the population fled the city; 10 per cent died before the epidemic remitted (Powell 1949). No public issue had higher priority than halting the spread of the fever. Philadelphia was the medical capital of the new republic, its physicians the best to be had, but the medical science of the time provided no sure grounds to distinguish between competing theories of cause. It would be another century before the mosquito was identified as the vector, and a filterable virus as the agent, of the disease.

In that context, the panic produced by the epidemic fuelled the flames of political passion incited by the French Revolution (Pernick 1978). Some physicians supported Alexander Hamilton, who despised the revolution; others followed Thomas Jefferson, for whom monarchy was the principal foe. Xenophobia had been aroused by the arrival in early August of more than 2,000 French refugees from Haiti. The Hamiltonian physicians, espousing an 'importation' theory, blamed the epidemic on the refugees still disembarking from their ships; the Jeffersonian supporters of 'localism' saw the roots of the disease in such domestic causes as miasmas from local swamps and effluvia from insanitary docks. When the Hamiltonians won control of the College of Physicians, they passed a resolution that asserted: 'No instance has ever occurred of the disease called the yellow fever, having been generated in this city, or in any other parts of the United States . . . but there have been frequent instances of its having been imported' (Pernick

1978: 243). The political implications of the competing medical theories of cause made the adoption of a single course of action by the divided city impossible. The necessity for compromise led Pennsylvania and other threatened states to undertake both quarantine and sanitary reform.

Did this episode reflect nothing more than the folly of politicized physicians at a benighted time? Are matters different now? Consider the medical response to 'black lung' in our own century. The term refers to a clinical pattern of progressive respiratory embarrassment whose prevalence and severity increases with years at work in the mines. Although observers a hundred years ago had noted the heavy burden of respiratory distress among miners, their pulmonary disability was variously attributed to 'miner's asthma', 'a norm' for the occupation, to malingering, or to emotional disorder (Smith 1981). Physicians working for the United Mine Workers Health and Welfare Fund who diagnosed pneumoconiosis rather than pulmonary tuberculosis (the routine diagnosis of company doctors) were denied local hospital staff appointments and were subject to threats as well as to shots fired at their homes by assailants the local police were 'unable' to locate. Tuberculosis, 'an act of God' according to laws governing workmen's compensation, was by definition not a compensable illness; pneumoconiosis, in contrast, represented a financial liability for the mine owners. The miners' union song asks: 'Which side are you on?' The question is no idle one. The doctors who worked for the UMW risked their lives to do so.

In 1969, pneumoconiosis was officially recognized as a medical entity and included as a compensable disease in the federal Coal Mine Health and Safety Act. None the less, medical gatekeepers limited benefits to cases with 'pathognomonic' X-ray patterns, interpreted in a very restrictive fashion. Doctors took opposing positions on just how 'real' the disorder was, despite the evidence that the extent of disability paralleled the duration of work in the mines. It was not until 1978 that US legislation was amended to confer entitlement on claimants functionally impaired after long employment in the mines. No new 'facts' had been discovered; rather, a new social judgement had been applied to the extant facts (Smith 1981).

The response to human disease and disability is not inherent in the nature of things; the meaning given to disease is a social construction in which political values are decisive both for the way 'facts' are gathered and for the way those facts are interpreted (Eisenberg 1989b). Precisely because medical statistics provide the 'standard of measurement' for social reform, well-designed epidemiologic studies identify the problems that society must address if it is to attain some measure of justice. This is as true for studies of psychiatric disorders in primary-care practice as it is for more traditional studies of pathology.

Cumulatively, the data presented in this volume and in the books by Goldberg and Huxley (1980), Shepherd et al. (1986) and Sartorius et al.

(1990) make a number of things abundantly clear. The distress and dysfunction produced by psychiatric disorder among patients in primary care is extensive; much of it is not recognized by their general practitioners. When it is diagnosed, it sometimes leads to inappropriate prescribing practices; when it is not, it may result in fruitless (and sometimes risky) medical workups. Relatively brief courses of training can improve the diagnostic ability of generalists; furthermore, general practitioners (or, at least, those who volunteer for training programmes) can be taught to provide relatively effective brief psychotherapy and thus reduce the iatrogenic hazard of drug dependence.

Recent US studies on depression and its association with functional limitations and days of disability yield similar results. Although medical patients with major depression are at higher risk for disability, even those with depressive symptoms not meeting criteria for disorder exhibit significant impairment (Wells *et al.* 1989). In a catchment area population study (Broadhead *et al.* 1990), 'minor depression' accounted for a larger total of disability days and days lost from work than did major depression, because it is so much more prevalent. In the USA, primary-care physicians provide such care as is given for about half of all patients with depression; they rely heavily on tricyclic antidepressants to treat the conditions they diagnose (Kessler *et al.* 1987); yet the effectiveness of tricyclics in treating minor depression is doubtful (Paykel *et al.* 1988).

Thus, in both the USA and the UK, epidemiologic research has demonstrated that there is a sizeable mental health burden manifested by disability as well as distress in the community. Further, it has shown that the primary-care practitioners who serve the majority of these patients lack appropriate diagnostic and therapeutic skills for the recognition and management of psychiatric disorders. Finally, it provides evidence that training schemes for physicians can improve the effectiveness of their performance. So much having been demonstrated, why has government not acted on the health-policy implications of such findings? The answer is not far to seek: it takes more time, and thus costs more, to deliver more and better services. In an era when cost control has taken precedence over improving health, the findings from epidemiologic research are an embarrassment to government.

This should come as no surprise in view of US epidemiologic data on race and health, data that call for a Chadwick Report. Life expectancy for blacks in the United States is six years less than it is for whites. The gap between whites and blacks (which had been decreasing during this century) has *increased* over the last four years (National Center for Health Statistics 1990). Factors contributing to this differential include: infant mortality rates more than twice as high for blacks; greater mortality from AIDS, blacks being at more than twice the risk for death from this disease; a homicide rate among males 15 to 24 years of age which is more than seven times higher for blacks (85.6) than it is for whites (11.2) (Fingerhut and Kleinman 1990); and higher mortality from cardiovascular disease, cirrhosis and cancer. Indeed, McCord and Freeman (1990) have calculated that black men in Harlem (a section of New York City that is 96 per cent black) are less likely to attain the age of 65 than men in Bangladesh! Liebman *et al.* (1990) report similar data for ghetto areas of Philadelphia, just as Jenkins *et al.* (1977) had done for black neighbourhoods in Boston. Mortality rates in these areas are so high as to warrant their designation as 'natural disaster areas' under US law.

Deaths are inversely related to income, as they are in the UK (Department of Health and Social Services 1980; Whitehead 1987) and are aggregated by race and by urban census tracts, the highest rates being found in the inner-city areas inhabited by ethnic minorities. Massey and Denton (1989) have evaluated US metropolitan areas on five dimensions of segregation: evenness (the degree to which the percentage of minority members within residential areas differs from the city-wide average); exposure (shared neighbourhoods); clustering (extent to which minority areas adjoin each other); centralization (degree to which minorities are settled in the central city); and concentration (amount of physical space occupied by minorities). A high index on any dimension represents isolation from the resources and opportunities which influence social and economic well-being; deleterious effects multiply with high scores across dimensions. Segregation is ubiquitous in all large metropolitan areas of the United States. The multidimensional character of black residential segregation is an important determinant of the growing social, economic and health gap between the black underclass and the rest of American society.

Mortality rates enable us, in Virchow's metaphor, to 'weigh life for life and see where the dead lie thicker'. They cannot fully convey the misery and despair that accompany life when death is so cheap. Can it be much different from life in the slum of Chadwick's London? In the Frontispiece to his treatise on public health in Victorian England, Wohl (1983) calls attention to a letter published in *The Times* of London, on Thursday, 5 July 1849. In part, it reads:

Sur, – may we beg and beseach your proteckshion and power, We are Sur, as it may be, livin in a Willderniss, so far as the rest of London knows anything of us or as the rich and great people care about. We live in muck and filthe. We aint got no priviz, no dust bins, no drains, no water-splies, and no drain or suer in the hole place. The Suer Company, in Greek St., Soho Square, all great, rich and powerful men, take no notice watsomedever of our cumplaints. The Stenche of a Gully-hole is disgustin. We all of us suffur, and numbers are ill, and if the Colera comes Lord help us . . .

Preaye Sir com and see us, for we are livin like piggs, and it aint faire we shoulde be so ill treted. We are your respeckfull servents in Church Lane, Carrier St., and the other corts.

Teusday, Juley 3, 1849

Charles Webster (1990) argues that the failures of health policy in the UK during the 1980s 'betrays many similarities with the 1830's'. The data epitomized in the preceding paragraphs tell much the same story for the USA. In both countries, the threat to public health begs for the intervention of a new generation of Virchows, Chadwicks and Farrs. It is their spirit which should – and must continue to – animate the field to which this symposium is dedicated.

Yes, epidemiology provides a scientific frame and methodology for systematic data gathering. Indeed, it rests upon an empirical base; if it did not, it would be no science at all and would contribute nothing to the improvement of health. But the choice of the data to be gathered is made precisely because of the light it can shed on the web of disease causation and, thus, enable the prevention of disease by intercepting the noxious conditions that give rise to it. What we learn from research places a responsibility on each of us individually to go public with what we know. This was stated eloquently by C. P. Snow (1961) in an address entitled 'The moral un-neutrality of Science':

> Scientists have a moral imperative to say what they know. It is going to make them unpopular in their own nation-states. It may do worse than make them unpopular. That doesn't matter. Or at least, it does matter to you and me, but it must not count in the face of the risks . . .
>
> There are going to be challenges to our intelligence and to our moral nature so long as man remains man. After all, a challenge is not . . . an excuse for slinking off and doing nothing. A challenge is something to be picked up.

REFERENCES

Acheson, E.D. (1990) 'Edwin Chadwick and the world we live in', *Lancet* ii:1482–5.

Broadhead, W.E., Blazer, D.G., George, L.K., and Tse, C.K. (1990) 'Depression, disability days, and days lost from work in a prospective epidemiologic survey', *Journal of the American Medical Association* 264:2524–8.

Department of Health and Social Services (1980) *Inequalities in health: Report of a research working group,* London.

Eisenberg, L. (1984) 'Rudolf Ludwig Karl Virchow, where are you now that we need you?', *American Journal of Medicine* 77:524–32.

Eisenberg, L. (1989a) 'The relationship between psychiatric research and public policy', in P. Williams, G. Wilkinson, and K. Rawnsley, *The Scope of Epidemiological Psychiatry: Essays in Honour of Michael Shepherd,* London: Routledge.

Eisenberg, L. (1989b) 'The social construction of mental illness', *Psychological Medicine* 18:1–19.

Fingerhut, L.A. and Kleinman, J.C. (1990) 'International and interstate comparisons of homicide among young males', *Journal of the American Medical Association* 263:3292–5.

Frost, W.H. (1936) 'Introduction' to *Snow on Cholera*, New York: Commonwealth Fund.

Goldberg, D. and Huxley, P. (1980) *Mental Illness in the Community: the Pathway to Psychiatric Care*, London: Tavistock.

Harding, T.W., Arnago, M.V., Baltazar, J., Climent, C.E., Ibrahim, H.H.A., Ignacio, L.L., Murthy, R.S., and Wig, N.N. (1980) 'Mental disorders in primary care: a study of their frequency and diagnosis in four developing countries', *Psychological Medicine* 10:231–42.

Jenkins, C.D., Tuthill, R.W., Tannenbaum, S.I., and Kirby, C.R. (1977) 'Zones of excess mortality in Massachusetts', *New England Journal of Medicine* 296:1354–6.

Kessler, L.G., Burns, B.J., Shapiro, S., Tischler, G.L., George, L.K., Hough, R.L., Bodison, D., and Miller, R.H. (1987) 'Psychiatric diagnoses of medical service users: evidence from the Epidemiologic Catchment Area Program', *American Journal of Public Health* 77:18–24.

Liebman, J., Axler, F., Kotranski, L., and Steinberg-Scribner, S. (1990) Letter to the Editor, *New England Journal of Medicine* 322:1606–7.

McCord, C. and Freeman, H.P. (1990) 'Excess mortality in Harlem', *New England Journal of Medicine* 322:173–7.

Massey, D.S. and Denton, N.A. (1989) 'Hypersegregation in US metropolitan areas: black and Hispanic segregation along five dimensions', *Demography* 26:373–91.

Merton, R.K., Sills, D.L., and Stigler, S.M. (1984) 'The Kelvin dictum and social science: an excursion into the history of an idea', *Journal of the History of the Behavioral Sciences* 20:319–31.

Morris, J.N. (1975) *Uses of Epidemiology*, Edinburgh: E. and S. Livingstone, third edn.

National Center for Health Statistics (1990) 'Advance report of final mortality statistics, 1988', *Monthly Vital Statistics Report* 39(7):1–48, Supplement, 28 Nov.

Paykel, E.S., Freeling, P., and Hollyman, J.A. (1988) 'Are tricyclic antidepressants useful for mild depression? a placebo controlled trial', *Pharmacopsychiatry* 21:15–18.

Pernick, M.S. (1978) 'Politics, parties and pestilence', in J.W. Leavitt and R.L. Numbers (eds) *Sickness and Health in America*, Madison: University of Wisconsin Press, pp. 241–56.

Powell, J.H. (1949) *Bring Out Your Dead: the Great Plague of Yellow Fever in Philadelphia in 1793*, Philadelphia: University of Pennsylvania Press.

Regier, D.A., Goldberg, I.D., and Taube, C.A. (1978) 'The de-facto US mental health services system', *Archives of General Psychiatry* 35:685–93.

Rosen, G. (1947) 'What is social medicine? a genetic analysis of the concept', *Bulletin of the History of Medicine* 21:674–733.

Rosen, G. (1958) *A History of Public Health*, New York: M.D. Publications.

Sartorius, N., Goldberg, D., De Girolamo, G., Costa e Silva, J.A., Lecrubier, Y., and Wittchen, H.U. (eds) (1990) *Psychological Disorders in General Medical Settings*, Toronto: Hogrefe and Huber.

Shepherd, M. (1990) 'The management of psychiatric disorders in the community: the research magnificent', *Journal of the Royal Society of Medicine* 83:219–22.

Shepherd, M., Fisher, N., Kessel, N., and Stein, L. (1959) 'Psychiatric morbidity in an urban practice', *Proceedings of the Royal Society of Medicine* 52:269–74.

Shepherd, M., Wilkinson, G., and Williams, P. (1986) *Mental Illness in Primary Care Settings*, London: Tavistock.

Smith, B.E. (1981) 'Black lung: the social production of disease', *International Journal of Health Services* 11:343–6.

Snow, C.P. (1961) 'The moral un-neutrality of science', *Science* 133:255–9.

Thomson, W. (1889) *Popular Lectures and Addresses*, London: Macmillan & Co.

Virchow, R. (1848) 'The charity physician', *Medical Reform*, No. 18, 3 Nov. Translated and republished in *Collected Essays on Public Health and Epidemiology*, L.J. Rather (ed.), Canton, MA: Science History Publications (1985), vol. I, p. 33.

Webster, C. (1990) *The Victorian Public Health Legacy: a Challenge to the Future*, London: The Public Health Alliance.

Wells, K.B., Stewart, A., and Hays, R.D. (1989) 'The functioning and well-being of depressed patients: results of the Medical Outcomes Study', *Journal of the American Medical Association* 262:914–19.

Whitehead, M. (1987) *The Health Divide: Inequalities in Health in the 1980s*, London: Health Education Authority.

Williams, P., Wilkinson, G., and Rawnsley, K. (1989) *The Scope of Epidemiological Psychiatry: Essays in Honour of Michael Shepherd*, London: Routledge.

Wohl, A.S. (1983) *Endangered Lives: Public Health in Victorian Britain*, Cambridge, MA: Harvard University Press.

Chapter 2

Psychiatric illness, epidemiology and the general practitioner

Brian Cooper

The emergence of the general practitioner as a personal physician is reflected in nineteenth-century literature, in the figure of the country doctor so sympathetically portrayed by Balzac, George Eliot, Chekhov and other writers of the humanist school. One might have supposed that with modern advances in scientific medicine, and the increasing specialization they have brought about, the notion of the family physician as therapist, counsellor and friend would have faded from public consciousness and disappeared from our literature. In fact this has not occurred; on the contrary, despite all progress in medical technology, and the vast political and social upheavals of the present century, the image of a personal medical adviser remains undimmed in the popular imagination. Indeed, it has received no more remarkable affirmation than in our own era and from, of all places, the Soviet Union:

> Generally speaking . . . the general practitioner is the most comforting figure in our lives, and now he's being torn up by the roots. The general practitioner is a figure without whom the family cannot exist in a developed society. He knows the needs of each member of the family, just as the mother knows their tastes. There's no shame in taking to him some trivial complaint you'd never take to the out-patients' clinic, which entails getting your appointment card and waiting your turn, and where there's a quota of nine patients an hour. And yet all neglected illnesses arise out of these trivial complaints. How many adult human beings are there now, at this minute, rushing about in mute panic wishing they could find a doctor, the kind of person to whom they can pour out the fears they have deeply concealed or even found shameful?
>
> (Solzhenitsyn 1971)

Significantly, the chapter of *Cancer Ward* containing this passage is entitled 'The Old Doctor': the speaker is an elderly man who is also a physician of the old school, practising alone and not ashamed to take cash across the table because, ironically, in a form of society which reduces the individual to a cipher, this is his only way of retaining some degree of professional freedom. Solzhenitsyn here pinpoints a deep-seated human need for a doctor who is not primarily a servant of the state; not just another agent of control, but whose first loyalty is to his patients and who is prepared when necessary to intervene on their behalf, against the socio-political pressures and adverse conditions that threaten their health, physical and mental. This is the need that keeps the idea of a personal doctor alive.

But what the great writers have intuitively grasped has been all too often ignored by the medical profession itself. With the proliferation of medical specialties and hospital departments, the general practitioner came to be regarded more and more as a sort of poor cousin, the colleague who had failed to climb the rungs of the careers ladder (Curwen 1964). Psychiatrists, in particular, have been slow to grasp the importance of good general medical services for the care of the mentally ill. In pursuing that elusive goal, 'community care', they have neglected the part played by the family doctor and his team (Shepherd 1989). Only within the past two decades has there been a quickening of interest in this topic, stimulated by the findings of epidemiological research. The high prevalence of psychiatric morbidity reported from area field studies indicates a level of need in the general population that can never be met by specialist agencies alone, however well-staffed and equipped, but only by a primary-care service capable of paying attention both to the patient's psychological state and to his family and social background. The conclusion of a British research group, that the cardinal requirement for improvement of the mental health services in that country is not a large expansion and proliferation of psychiatric agencies, but rather a strengthening of the family doctor in his therapeutic role (Shepherd *et al.* 1966), has gradually come to seem just as cogent in many other parts of the world. Thus the long-term potential of applied research as a mediator of change in medical practice has been demonstrated once again.

RESEARCH IN GENERAL PRACTICE

Clinical and epidemiological research alike have a long tradition in general practice. Major advances in medical knowledge have been contributed by practising physicians, who made good use of their opportunities both to study the natural history of disease and to test out new remedies. Among such advances may be numbered the use of foxglove extract in treating congestive heart failure (Withering 1785), the development of a vaccine against smallpox (Jenner 1798), the first clinical description of the shaking palsy (Parkinson 1817) and definition of the spread of typhoid fever (Budd 1873). Many physicians who gained fame in specialist fields began their researches while still in local medical practice: among them John Snow, who demonstrated the water-borne transmission of cholera (Thomas 1968), Robert Koch, discoverer of the tubercle bacillus (Koch

1882), the cardiologist James Mackenzie (Mair 1986) and the public-health pioneer Alfred Grotjahn (Greenwood 1946). The monograph by William Pickles (1939), with its careful accounts of infective hepatitis and epidemic myalgia, was a late blossom of the tradition of epidemiological research in country practice.

Inevitably, with the growth of specialized technology, the single-handed physician's scope for research began to diminish. But in the post-war age, two new developments have encouraged the growth of large-scale collaborative investigation. First, pre-paid health insurance schemes have served to make available defined populations for the estimation of morbidity rates. Thus in the UK, where the National Health Service has proved especially conducive to such research, 98 per cent of the population are said to be registered with general practitioners; 60 to 70 per cent of these will consult at least once in any given year, and only about 10 per cent will fail to appear within three years (Sharp and Morrell 1989). Here is a ready-made framework for epidemiological inquiry. Second, the growth of collaborative studies has been encouraged by the foundation, in a growing number of countries, of Colleges of General Practitioners or analogous bodies, whose avowed aim is to promote professional and academic standards, and to encourage scientific research. Practising physicians have been enabled once again to contribute to medical knowledge, this time by participating in national or regional surveys, applying standardized methods and adding their practice findings to the common pool. Such studies have yielded information on the prevalence and distribution of diabetes mellitus, iron-deficiency anaemia, hypertension, epilepsy and other common diseases of modern society. Reports on the health consequences of oral contraception, based on an ongoing prospective study of 46,000 women by a total of 1,400 participating GPs, provide impressive testimony to the potential for general-practice research to be found where there is high motivation and an appropriate health-service structure (Royal College of General Practitioners 1974; 1983). Comparable trends have been signalized by publications in a number of other countries, including Australia (Australian Royal College of General Practitioners 1966), Norway (Bentsen 1970) and the Netherlands (Foets et al. 1986). In recent years, the movement has gained added impetus from the formation of international bodies, such as the World Organization of National Colleges (WONCA 1979), the International Society of General Practice (Newman 1989) and the European Research Workshop (Hull 1982).

GENERAL PRACTICE RESEARCH AND
PSYCHIATRIC EPIDEMIOLOGY

These developments carry implications for the study of mental disorders. Most of our knowledge of the epidemiology of these conditions is drawn from one or other of two principal sources: either from the records of specialist mental health agencies or from area morbidity surveys. The data derived from the former source – for example, through national hospital inquiries, or from area cumulative case registers – are not as a rule difficult to interpret or to analyse; the diagnosis in each case has been recorded by a psychiatrist and clinical case-notes are available. But the diagnostic rates computed on this basis may prove seriously misleading if they are thought to give a true picture of the psychiatric morbidity to be found in the population as a whole. The material will by definition be restricted to cases selected into specialist care via medical referral or hospital admission, and the factors that influence this selective process cannot be taken into account, unless unreferred cases present in the same population can also be examined to give a basis for comparison.

In an area field survey, different problems arise. A representative sample can be drawn and the way opened to finding undeclared cases of illness, but the investigator is quite dependent on the public readiness to co-operate. Moreover, if no skilled psychiatric exploration can be made, a respondent's health complaints may be very difficult to appraise in terms of underlying psychopathology. The information obtained, usually at a single interview, may well be inadequate for making a diagnosis. These difficulties cannot be resolved by the use of standardized interviews or computer algorithms.

Data from general medical practice owe their special significance to the position they occupy in the middle ground between these contrasting approaches. A physician with responsibility for the primary medical care of a defined population is at a unique vantage point from which to observe all forms of ill health, except the trivial, which exist among its members. In addition, his advantage for detecting psychiatric illness is greatly enhanced by the qualities which he himself can bring to the care and management of the mentally ill (WHO 1973).

1 Most mentally disturbed persons are quite prepared to consult their family doctors for somatic complaints, which they themselves often do not perceive as having psychological or emotional causes.

2 Many patients, especially among the elderly, present to their doctors with a combination of physical and mental ill health. The GP is in the best position to prescribe treatment for both, while at the same time avoiding unnecessary or possibly harmful diagnostic investigations, combating any hypochondriacal tendencies in the patient, and sparing him from a fruitless peregrination through different hospital departments.

Table 2.1 Comparison of rates of psychiatric illness contact at different levels of mental health care, England, 1981 (rates per 100,000 general population, both sexes and all age-groups combined)

Level of service contact	Rate of contact for mental disorders (ICD-9 categories 290–315)
General practitioner consultations[1]	22,980
Psychiatric out-patient attendances[2]	3,532
Psychiatric day-patient attendances[2]	4,943
Psychiatric in-patient admissions[2]	397

[1] Obtained from third national morbidity survey, 1981–82 (Royal College of General Practitioners 1986)
[2] Obtained from Mental Health Enquiry for England 1981 (DHSS 1982)
Source: Sharp and Morrell (1989)

3 The GP often maintains contact with patients, at least intermittently, over a period of many years, and is thus well placed to provide the long-term care and management required by many who suffer from serious psychological difficulties. His prolonged acquaintance with patients and their families provides him with access to much background information, not so readily acquired by hospital specialists, which can be of the greatest value in judging the significance of new complaints, or of changes in the patient's pattern of behaviour.
4 Psychopharmacological treatment or psychotherapy can be administered on a less formal basis and in a setting already familiar to the patient, with less risk of 'labelling' him as a deviant, or reinforcing him in adoption of the sick role, than might be occasioned by specialist referral.

Although it is common knowledge that, in a great many medical practices today, these innate advantages are not being properly exploited, their enumeration alone goes some way towards explaining why the primary care physician is becoming accepted as a key figure, both in epidemiological inquiry and in treatment of the mentally ill (Clare and Lader 1982; Shepherd *et al.* 1986).

PSYCHIATRIC MORBIDITY IN GENERAL PRACTICE POPULATIONS

The basic descriptive statistics supplied by large-scale general morbidity surveys are already impressive. Table 2.1, drawing on the third of a series of surveys, based on general practice, which have been carried out in the UK (Royal College of General Practitioners 1986), compares consultation rates for mental illness in general practice with corresponding rates for psychiatric out-patient and day-patient attendance, and for psychiatric in-patient admission, for the same population. The practice consultation rates can be seen to outnumber those for hospital out-patient attendance by seven to one, and those for in-patient admission by nearly 60 to one (Sharp and Morrell 1989).

Studies that are focused on a particular category of disease will tend to report higher rates for that group of conditions than are supplied by general morbidity surveys, which collect data impartially on all forms of ill health. This 'halo effect' is certainly apparent for psychiatric disorder. In the survey of London practices (Shepherd et al. 1966), in which the participating doctors were asked to keep a special record of all cases with a major psychiatric component, the one-year consulting rate was 139.4 per 1,000 registered adult patients. Approximately three-quarters of these had diagnoses included in Chapter V (Mental Disorders) of the ICD, but the remaining one-quarter presented physical illness or symptoms with some associated psychological disturbance, and would not have been given a psychiatric diagnosis according to the standard classifications.

The great advantage of the British Health Service system for epidemiology resides in the fact that nearly everyone is registered with a general practitioner. Although most other countries have no such comprehensive framework of patient registration, some approach to a representative population coverage may still be feasible. In the USA, for example, membership of pre-paid health insurance plans has been used as a basis for epidemiological sampling. A study in Washington, DC, organized by the National Institute of Mental Health (Locke et al. 1966), reported psychiatric abnormality in 14.6 per cent of a sample of registered adult patients, a result closely similar to that reported from the London survey.

If no registered patient population is definable, the frequency of psychiatric illness can be estimated only among those persons who consult their doctors within a stated time period, and it will not then be justifiable to extrapolate the resulting rates onto the remainder of the population. The proportion of consulting patients falling into any given illness category may depend partly on the length of the recording period; persons with neurotic disorders, for example, tend to be over-represented in surveys of short duration, simply because they consult frequently. This source of bias must be borne in mind when comparing data from different surveys. For example, practice-based studies in Austria (Strotzka 1969), Switzerland (Agosti *et al*. 1974) and Norway (Øgar 1977) have provided prevalence estimates based on observation periods of three, two and six months, respectively, while in a German study point-prevalence ratios were computed from a two-week period of recording in each practice in turn (Zintl-Wiegand *et al*. 1980).

A more intractable problem of method arises from the wide variation in case reporting by individual GPs, which must cast some doubt on the validity of their diagnostic assessments. Thus, Shepherd *et al*. (1966) found an inter-practice variation in psychiatric one-year prevalence, ranging from 38 to 323 per 1,000 registered adult patients, despite the fact that all the doctors used the same standard proforma and guidelines. The differences could be only partly explained in socio-demographic terms, and seemed to be more closely related to diagnostic habits of the individual doctors. A more detailed study (Marks *et al*. 1979) has since suggested that the main factors involved are the GP's ability to conduct a psychiatric examination and his understanding of the links between mental state and social functioning. Yet the problem is by no means specific to mental disorder, morbidity surveys having demonstrated almost as wide a range of variation for such other diagnostic categories as respiratory and musculo-skeletal diseases.

Many studies have confirmed that the commonest forms of psychological abnormality encountered in general practice are minor affective disorders, characterized by a depressive mood-state, anxiety, fatigue, irritability, sleep disturbance, poor concentration and a number of vegetative and other somatic complaints. Because all such symptoms are widely spread in patient populations, and in terms of frequency and severity manifest a continuous distribution, the distinction between 'cases' and 'normals' is essentially an artificial one, and depends on agreement in setting the boundaries for what is to be classified as morbid. This dimensional character of the clinical phenomena is undoubtedly one major reason for the low level of diagnostic agreement found among physicians.

The development of standardized psychiatric screening techniques has been thought to offer a way out of the dilemma. They are basically complaint inventories or symptom check-lists, equipped with some simple scoring method and a recommended cut-off score to establish the required morbidity threshold. Their application to large samples can yield frequency estimates that are independent of the individual doctors' diagnostic sets, and hence free from observer error. Since the introduction of the General Health Questionnaire – GHQ – (Goldberg 1972), a number of studies have been undertaken in general practice, making use of one or other version of this instrument, or of some similar technique whose reliability

Table 2.2 Efficiency of detection of psychiatric abnormality by general
practitioners, assessed by comparison with the results of
standardized screening methods

Study	Screening instrument	Sample size	Case detection by the GPs:	
			Sensitivity	Specificity
Chancellor et al. 1977 (Australia)	GHQ–30	1,301 (15 GPs)	0.27	0.88
Marks et al. 1979 (Great Britain)	GHQ–60	4,098 (91 GPs)	0.54 (mean)*	–
Hesbacher et al. 1980 (USA)	Johns Hopkins Symptom Check-list-25	720 (6 GPs)	0.64	0.93
Brodaty et al. 1982 (Australia)	GHQ–30	185 (14 GPs)	0.49*	–
Skuse and Williams 1984 (Great Britain)	Clinical Interview Schedule	272 (1 GP)	0.51	0.90
Hennrikus et al. 1986 (Australia)	GHQ–30	1,722 (50 GPs)	0.74*	0.91*

* Corrected for the accuracy of the screening instrument

Source: Sanson-Fisher and Hennrikus (1988)

and validity in case detection are comparably high, to give an independent
check of the GPs' own clinical judgements. The results of six such studies
are summarized in Table 2.2. Although they show considerable variation, a
general trend is apparent for the practitioners to fail to identify a significant
proportion of the 'cases' picked out by the screening tests. The error is not
a random one, since few of the patients who obtain low scores on screening
are wrongly classified as 'cases' by the GPs: the overall trend is definitely
in the direction of under-diagnosis.

In discussing these findings, Sanson-Fisher and Hennrikus (1988) point
out that, before practising physicians can be expected to improve their
own techniques for eliciting psychiatric symptoms and recognizing 'hidden'
psychiatric morbidity, they must be convinced that the effort is worthwhile,
in that it can lead to effective treatment and make a difference to the
patients' state of health. Unfortunately, information on this crucial question
is still sparse and to some extent conflicting. The most encouraging study
so far, that by Johnstone and Goldberg (1976), used random allocation to
assign patients with 'hidden' psychiatric morbidity, detected at screening,
either to a treatment or to a control group. No treatment regime was

prescribed by the research design, but the GP was told only which patients had been included in the former group. The effects of case detection proved beneficial for the patients in this group, apparently because the GP, once informed, took steps to treat and help them. A change was also observed in their consulting behaviour, in that they began to present more often with overt emotional problems, and less often with somatic complaints. These intriguing findings have not proved easy to replicate in some other practice settings, perhaps because the doctors concerned were less closely involved, or less inclined to respond to the screening results with active intervention. The issue of psychiatric case detection, it seems, should not be considered in isolation, but needs to be viewed in the broader context of the structure and style of medical practice, and the interaction which takes place between patient and doctor at each consultation (cf. Goldberg and Gask, this volume).

A second obstacle to diagnostic agreement arises from the unsatisfactory nature of the existing systems of illness classification. The two most widely used standard classifications of psychiatric disorder, the International Classification of Diseases, Chapter V (Mental Disorders) (WHO 1978) and the so-called DSM-III system (American Psychiatric Association 1980), were both developed primarily to meet the requirements of hospital-based specialist practice. They are inappropriate for use in general practice, being largely devoted to an elaborate classification of the major psychoses and other severe forms of mental illness, and paying little regard to the ill-defined, relatively mild forms of disturbance which make up such a large proportion of all cases among the GP's patient clientele.

Although dissatisfaction with the standard classifications is now wide-spread, there is as yet no consensus of informed opinion as to how the situation could be improved. Jenkins, Smeeton and Shepherd (1988), who conducted a detailed study in co-operation with twenty-seven London practitioners, rightly emphasize that some form of diagnostic taxonomy is essential for research purposes, and that a purely treatment-orientated approach must in the long run prove inadequate, since it can only be as complex as the current, strictly limited, range of therapeutic options. They also conclude that the system which has been developed specifically for use in general practice, the International Classification of Health Problems in Primary Care – ICHPPC – (WONCA 1979), is itself of only limited value with respect to psychiatric disorders, since it appears that GPs are unable to apply it in a consistent manner. The solution they propose is a highly ambitious one: the construction of a multiaxial system of disease classification, which should have separate axes for physical illness, psychological disorder, personality variants and social problems. The Mental Health Division of WHO has in fact been engaged for a number of years, with support from the Rockefeller Foundation and the US National Institute of Mental Health, in constructing a system for recording health problems triaxially and conducting field trials with it in a number of countries. This system, which prudently omits the dimension of personality, involves use of the ICD or ICHPPC to record physical illness diagnoses, and tacking on an additional axis each for common psychological complaints and categories of social difficulty. Some idea of what this entails in a cross-cultural context may be gleaned from the fact that the list of relevant social problems ranges from 'insufficient food or water' to 'tension between co-wives'.

Whether in fact the use of a triaxial classification will prove feasible in the primary-care setting, even in developed industrial countries, remains open to question. There is, though, little doubt that attention must be paid to the domains of physical ill health, psychological disturbance and social dysfunction, if an adequate diagnostic formulation is to be made in each individual case. Studies in general practice have shown repeatedly that mental and emotional disorders very often present at consultation in the guise of, or in close association with, physical symptoms. To some extent, this mode of presentation is socio-culturally determined, since patients are not only conditioned to regard physical illness as more acceptable than emotional conflicts, but are also aware of what their doctors expect to hear from them in the way of complaints. In addition, however, there seems to be a true association between the distributions of physical and psychiatric morbidity in the general population (Eastwood 1975), which grows more strongly positive with advancing years.

Psychosocial stress and adverse life circumstances are also recognized as major provoking causes of psychiatric illness (Brown and Harris 1978; 1989). Those patients who manifest affective disorders or related conditions tend to be drawn disproportionally from socially disadvantaged groups of the population: women, especially the widowed, divorced and separated; those of low social status and earning power; the long-term unemployed; persons who are socially isolated, disabled or living in unsatisfactory housing. The occurrence of stressful or threatening life events, including the onset of physical illness, is a precipitating cause in many instances (Cooper and Sylph 1973). Although there are certainly large differences in personal predisposition, which go towards determining the individual's response to adversity, the pragmatic physician, in seeking the best point to intervene, can never afford to neglect either the consequences of social stress for patients, or the possibility that it might be alleviated by supportive measures.

PSYCHIATRIC SPECIALIST REFERRAL AND LIAISON

The extent to which GPs recognize the presence of mental disturbance in their patients will influence not only the numbers they refer to psychiatric agencies, but also the stage of the illness at which such referral first occurs, and hence the mean duration of illness in patients seen by psychiatric specialists. Goldberg and Huxley (1980) focused on the first of these issues in elaborating their now well-known level-and-filter model of the pathway to psychiatric care. Their quantitative analyses take into account both the prevalence of mental illness and the extent to which this is reflected in different aspects of service provision. Level 1 refers to all medically significant mental disorders present in the general population, the majority of which pass through the first filter to reach Level 2 when the affected persons consult their family doctors, for whatever reason. If the GP at this stage detects the presence of a psychological disturbance, the patient in effect passes through the second filter and arrives at Level 3, that at which his condition is recognized and he receives medical advice and treatment for it. Since a proportion of cases are not recognized (see Table 2.2), many patients do not pass through the second filter at this stage.

A small minority of patients whose disorders are detected by the GP will be referred on by him to a psychiatric agency, and thus pass through the third filter to reach Level 4. Finally, an even smaller number will pass through the last filter to reach Level 5, which represents admission to psychiatric in-patient care.

Because the relative permeability of each of these filters is modifiable in various ways, it may prove possible to improve the functioning of the different parts of the system. No very penetrating analysis is required to grasp that, in global terms, the first filter is by far the most important, or that its permeability is in the main economically determined. If an acceptable quality of basic medical care is available only to a small, affluent minority, the question of specialist referral can be of little relevance to most of the population. Only once treatment at the primary-care level becomes readily accessible does the permeability of the remaining filters assume importance for the public health.

Goldberg and Huxley (1980), working in the British Health Service, were able to concentrate their attention on the second filter and the factors that govern its operation. In the past decade, evidence has accumulated that, at least so far as the common forms of psychiatric morbidity are concerned, this filter can be made to work more efficiently by a systematic training of GPs in observational and interviewing techniques (Gask *et al.* 1988). In addition, there are some signs that the sensitivity of practitioners to the presence of psychological disorder may be increasing spontaneously, as part of a more general secular change in medical perceptions and priorities. A number of researchers have noted this tendency with respect to dementia and depression in the elderly (cf. Cooper; O'Connor and Pollitt; Bickel: this volume).

Changes which have occurred in ambulatory psychiatric care might be expected, a priori, to increase the permeability of the third filter by promoting a closer co-operation between GPs and their psychiatric colleagues, a more informal type of patient referral and a reduction in the waiting time for appointments. This trend has been perhaps most pronounced in the UK, where it has been apostrophized by Strathdee and Williams (1984) as 'the silent growth of a new service'. Their report estimated that about one in five of consultant psychiatrists in England and Wales had switched their out-patient sessions from hospital clinics to the general practice setting: a change made practicable by the growth of group practices housed in local-authority health centres. The innovation was remarkable in having occurred spontaneously, with no official policy directives and no financial rewards. Its effects have not been systematically monitored, and there are scarcely any data bearing on the comparative efficacy of hospital- and practice-based forms of service. All we have are some descriptive accounts of local arrangements, an apparent consensus of opinion among the physicians involved in such schemes that they have much to offer, and some inferential evidence that they have resulted in a reduction in the numbers of psychiatric in-patient admissions (McKechnie et al. 1981; Williams and Balestrieri 1989).

How psychiatrists and their co-workers operate in the primary-care setting appears to depend on individual preference and a process of trial and error. A number of different, overlapping forms of collaboration have been described (Strathdee and Williams 1984; Mitchell 1989).

1 In the 'shifted out-patient' model, the psychiatrist has changed his locus of operation but not his method; he attends the practice regularly, sees individual patients referred to him by the GPs and prescribes treatment for them.
2 Here again, the psychiatrist sees referred patients and assesses each case, but an agreed treatment plan is then carried out by the patient's own doctor.
3 The psychiatrist, once having developed an effective collaboration with the practice doctors, takes on a predominantly consultative role, advising on the management of many patients without the necessity of formal case referral.
4 Assessment of individual patients is undertaken jointly by psychiatrist and GP, either in the practice or in the patient's own home, along the lines of the traditional 'domiciliary visit'.
5 The psychiatrist takes part in regular team meetings, also attended by the GPs, practice and community nurses and possibly other health professionals. Individual cases are discussed and decisions taken as to which member or members of the team should take responsibility for day-to-day case management.

Although schemes incorporating one or more of these elements have grown up somewhat haphazardly, a number of models for their more systematic development have been proposed by psychiatrists who have convinced themselves of the benefits of direct collaboration. One such model, that of a 'hive' system (Tyrer 1985), places practice-based out-patient facilities in the context of a 'catchment area' population, together with day hospitals and other local service units, the whole complex to be organized from a central hospital department. Other models give greater emphasis to the role of counsellors, working closely with the practice team (cf. Jarman, this volume), or to home visiting by community psychiatric nurses. Certainly, a health centre with a registered patient population of from 10,000 to 20,000 can be regarded as an eminently practicable base both for psychiatric out-patient sessions and for the attachment of counsellors and community psychiatric nurses (Brook and Cooper 1975). To what extent services for emotionally disturbed children and adolescents, chronic alcoholics and drug addicts, dementing old persons, or other sub-groups with distinctive needs could be deployed in such health centres is still an unresolved issue. But that the disciplines within psychiatry must change, indeed are already changing, in response to the new demands, can scarcely be doubted (Shepherd 1988).

CHANGING DISCIPLINES: DOCTORS IN THE HEALTH-CARE TEAM

Are contemporary innovations in general practice itself in harmony with these developments? In terms of service structure, the answer is probably affirmative. The general practitioner in a modern urban society has to operate in some form of organizational framework, and group medical practice within a health-care team seems the appropriate solution. The doctors working together as equal partners in such a setting can provide comprehensive general medical care for a defined population. As a group they can share opportunities for continuing medical education and the pursuit of special interests, while themselves helping to train younger doctors. They can provide mutual cover for night and weekend calls and for holiday relief, so that the practice stays independent of commercialized emergency call services. Each group can work closely with attached community nurses, whose duties include domiciliary care of the chronic sick and disabled in the community, support for family care-givers and surveillance of persons believed to be at increased risk. There is growing support for the view that the team should also include a social worker, who can mobilize social forces on behalf of patients and their families, and help to guide them through the present-day maze of welfare agencies and bureaucratic regulations (Cooper 1971). Although in rural or semi-rural practices the size of the team is bound to be smaller, the main professional groupings can still be represented on it.

Greater emphasis can now be placed on prevention, or what Tudor

Hart (1990) has termed 'proactive' (in contrast to reactive) patient care: an approach that has to be deliberately encouraged by supplementary fees where medical remuneration is on an item-of-service basis, but which on the whole is more likely to flourish, and to observe the spirit not just the letter, in a system based on capitation payments for comprehensive, continuing whole-patient care. Monitoring of high-risk groups does not involve only routine blood-pressure and urine checks; it also means keeping an eye on old people who live alone, those newly discharged from hospital, persons suffering from a bereavement, children in problem families, and many more besides. How many health insurance schemes have a scale of fees for these tasks?

The technical resources for such a humane, patient-centred form of proactive care are now to hand. The first step was taken many years ago, with the introduction of age–sex registers in a few practices; but in the era of the micro-computer many more variables, including those of direct relevance for risk assessment, can be stored and retrieved in the practice setting, without breach of medical confidentiality or data-protection laws. Moreover, the scope this gives for a linkage of anonymized statistical data from individual practices, to provide pooled information on morbidity for a large defined population, will be of the greatest value for future epidemiological research.

Disciplines in general practice are undergoing change, just as surely as those in psychiatry. Awareness of these trends has led to calls for a 'new kind of doctor' (Tudor Hart 1988), who will be concerned with the health of a population, as well as with the illnesses of individual patients. It is a goal with which all protagonists of social medicine and social psychiatry can readily identify. Yet there is a strong case too for conserving what was best in the older general practice tradition and, in particular, for keeping the individual doctor–patient relationship as the focal point of the whole medico-therapeutic endeavour. To foster in primary health care a style of relatively impersonal, episodic doctor–patient transactions, based on the concept of diagnosis and treatment as a series of technological procedures, would be to recapitulate the worst errors of modern hospital medicine, or of the eastern European policlinics, fatally undermining the progress which good general practice has achieved over the past decades. Of all patients, none would suffer in consequence more than the mentally ill, for whom it is vital that the special function of primary-care physicians should continue to be that of understanding and responding to the patient's entire communication (Browne and Freeling 1967). But this can only be so if true medical authority is perceived as being vested in the doctor–patient relationship; as flowing, not downwards from government departments or service administrators, but outwards and upwards from the contacts between sick persons and the doctors and nurses in whom they have reposed their trust. All striving towards reform should start out from this basic principle, and all health-service structures be built around it.

This modern doctor's dilemma – how to create the kind of practice organization required for proactive health care of the population, without at the same time losing the essence of personal doctoring – was given poignant expression by John Berger (1967) in his portrayal of 'Sassall', a single-handed general practitioner working in a poor rural community. Whenever he tries to understand one of his patients, writes Berger, the doctor is forced to recognize his or her undeveloped potentiality.

> He can never forget the contrast. He must ask: do they deserve the lives they lead or do they deserve better? He must answer – disregarding what they themselves might reply – that they deserve better. In individual cases he must do all that he can to help them to live more fully. He must recognize that what he can do, if one considers the community as a whole, is absurdly inadequate. He must admit that what needs to be done is outside his brief as a doctor and beyond his capacity as an individual . . .
>
> It is easy to criticize him. One can criticize him for ignoring politics. If he is so concerned with the lives of his patients – in a general as well as in a medical sense – why does he not see the necessity for political action to improve or defend their lives?
>
> One can criticize him for practising alone instead of joining a group practice or working in a health centre. Is he not an outdated nineteenth-century romantic with his ideal of single personal responsibility? And in the last analysis is not this ideal a form of paternalism?
>
> He himself is aware of the implications of such criticism. 'I sometimes wonder', he says, 'how much of me is the last of the old traditional country doctor and how much of me is a doctor of the future. Can you be both?'

Only the most sanguine of men would dare answer Sassall's rhetorical question today with an unqualified 'yes, you can'. All one can say with confidence is that in the years ahead developments in primary medical care will depend, on the one hand, on the political will to create or sustain national health services based on an underlying public-health philosophy; on the other hand on a system of medical education that pays due regard throughout to the importance of both social and psychological aspects of health and disease. Contact with young doctors now emerging from the medical schools may give one some grounds for cautious optimism on this latter score.

ACKNOWLEDGEMENT

This chapter draws in part on the introductory section of a research monograph dealing with the same theme, published some years ago in the original German (Zintl-Wiegand, Cooper and Krumm 1980).

REFERENCES

Agosti, E., Agosti, F., and Ernst, K. (1974) 'Psychisch Kranke in einer Allgemein-praxis. Eine diagnostische, soziologische und therapeutische Studie', *Schweizer Medizinische Wochenschrift* 104:322–30.
American Psychiatric Association (1980) *Diagnostic and Statistical Manual for Mental Disorders*, third edn – DSM-III, Washington, DC: APA.
Australian Royal College of General Practitioners (1966) *National Morbidity Survey Report*, Feb. 1962–Jan. 1963, Canberra: National Health and Medical Research Council.
Bentsen, B.G. (1970) *Illness and General Practice*, Oslo: Universitetsvorlaget.
Berger, J. (1967) *A Fortunate Man*, London: Allen Lane (pp. 143–7).
Brodaty, H., Andrews, G., and Kehoe, L. (1982) 'Psychiatric illness in general practice. Why is it missed?', *Australian Family Physician* 11:625–31.
Brook, P. and Cooper, B. (1975) 'Community mental health care: primary team and specialist services', *Journal of the Royal College of General Practitioners* 25:93–110.
Brown, G.W. and Harris, T.O. (1978) *Social Origins of Depression*, London: Tavistock.
Brown, G.W. and Harris, T.O. (eds) (1989) *Life Events and Illness*, London: Unwin Hyman.
Browne, K. and Freeling, P. (1967) *The Doctor–Patient Relationship*, Edinburgh: Livingstone.
Budd, W. (1873) *Typhoid Fever: its Nature, Mode of Spreading, and Prevention*, London. Reprinted in 1931 by the Delta-Omega Society, New York.
Chancellor, A., Mant, A., and Andrews, G. (1977) 'The general practitioner's identification and management of emotional disorders', *Australian Family Physician* 6:1137–43.
Clare, A.W. and Lader, M. (eds) (1982) *Psychiatry and General Practice*, London: Academic Press.
Cooper, B. (1971) 'Social work in general practice: the Derby scheme', *Lancet* i:539–42.
Cooper, B. and Sylph, J. (1973) 'Life events and the onset of neurotic illness: an investigation in general practice', *Psychological Medicine* 3:421–35.
Curwen, M. (1964) 'Lord Moran's ladder', *Journal of the Royal College of General Practitioners* 7:38–65.
Department of Health and Social Security (1982) *Mental Health Enquiry for England,* London: HMSO.
Eastwood, M.R. (1975) *The Relation between Physical and Mental Illness*, Clarke Institute of Psychiatry Monograph Series No. 4, Toronto and Buffalo, NY: University of Toronto Press.
Foets, M., Velden, J. van der, and Zee, J. van der (1986) *A National Survey of Morbidity and Interventions in General Practice*, Utrecht, Netherlands: NIVEL.

Gask, L., McGrath, G., Goldberg, D., and Millar, T. (1988) 'Improving the psychiatric skills of established general practitioners: evaluation of a group teaching', *Medical Education* 22:132–8.

Goldberg, D.P. (1972) *The Detection of Psychiatric Illness by Questionnaire*, Maudsley Monograph No. 21, London: Oxford University Press.

Goldberg, D. and Huxley, P. (1980) *Mental Illness in the Community: the Pathway to Psychiatric Care*, London: Tavistock.

Greenwood, M. (1946) 'Social medicine', *British Medical Journal* i:117–19.

Hennrikus, D., Reid, A.L.A., and Sanson-Fisher, R.W. (1986) The detection of psychological disorder in general practice. Unpublished MS, University of Newcastle, NSW.

Hesbacher, P.T., Rickels, K., Morris, R.J., Newman, H., and Rosenfeld, H. (1980) 'Psychiatric illness in family practice', *Journal of Clinical Psychiatry* 41:6–10.

Hull, F.M. (1982) 'The European General Practice Research Workshop (1971–1981)', *Journal of the Royal College of General Practitioners* 32:106–8.

Jenkins, R., Smeeton, N., and Shepherd, M. (1988) *Classification of Mental Disorder in Primary Care*, Psychological Medicine Monograph Supplement 12, Cambridge: Cambridge University Press.

Jenner, E. (1798) *An Inquiry into the Causes and Effects of the Variolae Vaccinae*, London: Law.

Johnstone, A. and Goldberg, D. (1976) 'Psychiatric screening in general practice: a controlled trial', *Lancet* i:605–8.

Koch, R. (1882) 'Die Ätiologie der Tuberkulose', *Berliner Klinische Wochenschrift* 19:221. Translated and reprinted in *The Aetiology of Tuberculosis*, New York: National Tuberculosis Association, 1932.

Locke, B.Z., Krantz, G., and Kramer, M. (1966) 'Psychiatric need and demand in a prepaid group practice program', *American Journal of Public Health* 56:895–904.

McKechnie, A.A., Philip, A.E., and Ramage, J.G. (1981) 'Psychiatric services in primary care: specialized or not?, *Journal of the Royal College of General Practitioners* 31:611–14.

Mair, A. (1986) *Sir James Mackenzie, MD, 1853–1925, General Practitioner*, London: Royal College of General Practitioners.

Marks, J.N., Goldberg, D.P., and Hillier, V.F. (1979) 'Determinants of the ability of general practitioners to detect psychiatric illness', *Psychological Medicine* 9:337–53.

Mitchell, A.R.K. (1989) 'Participating in primary care: differing styles of psychiatric liaison', *Bulletin of the Royal College of Psychiatrists* 13:135–7.

Newman, L. (1989) 'The International Society of General Practice', in *Royal College of General Practitioners: Members' Reference Book 1989*, London: RCGP (pp. 384–86).

Øgar, B. (1977) *Pasienter i norsk almenpraksis* (Patients in Norwegian general practice), Oslo: Universitetsforlaget.

Parkinson, J. (1817) *An Essay on the Shaking Palsy*, London: Sherwood, Neely & Jones.

Pickles, W.N. (1939) *Epidemiology in Country Practice*, Torquay: Devonshire Press (reissued 1972).

Royal College of General Practitioners (1974) *Oral Contraceptives and Health*, London: Pitman Medical.

Royal College of General Practitioners (1981) *A Survey of Primary Care in London*, Occasional Paper 16, London: Royal College of General Practitioners.

Royal College of General Practitioners' Oral Contraception Study (1983) 'Incidence of arterial disease among oral contraceptive users', *Journal of the Royal College of General Practitioners* 33:75–82.

Royal College of General Practitioners, Office of Population Censuses and Surveys, Department of Health and Social Security (1986) *Morbidity Statistics from General Practice. Third National Study, 1981–82*, London: HMSO.

Sanson-Fisher, R.W. and Hennrikus, D.J. (1988) 'Why do primary care physicians often fail to detect psychological disturbance in their patients?', in A.S. Henderson and G. Burrows (eds) *Handbook of Social Psychiatry*, Amsterdam: Elsevier (pp. 245–56).

Sharp, D. and Morrell, D. (1989) 'The psychiatry of general practice', in P. Williams, G. Wilkinson, and K. Rawnsley (eds) *The Scope of Epidemiological Psychiatry*, London: Routledge (pp. 404–19).

Shepherd, M. (1988) 'Changing disciplines in psychiatry', *British Journal of Psychiatry* 153:493–504.

Shepherd, M. (1989) 'Primary care of patients with mental disorder in the community', *British Medical Journal* 229:666–9.

Shepherd, M., Cooper, B., Brown, A.C., and Kalton, G. (1966) *Psychiatric Illness in General Practice*, London: Oxford University Press.

Shepherd, M., Wilkinson, G., and Williams, P. (eds) (1986) *Mental Illness in a Primary Health Care Setting*, London: Tavistock.

Skuse, D. and Williams, P. (1984) 'Screening for psychiatric disorders in general practice', *Psychological Medicine* 14:365–77.

Solzhenitsyn, A. (1971) *Cancer Ward*, Harmondsworth: Penguin (pp. 454–5).

Strathdee, G. and Williams, P. (1984) 'A survey of psychiatrists in primary care: the silent growth of a new service', *Journal of the Royal College of General Practitioners* 34:615–18.

Strotzka, H. (1969) *Kleinburg: Eine sozialpsychiatrische Feldstudie*, Vienna: Österreichischer Bundesverlag für Unterricht, Wissenschaft und Kunst.

Thomas, K.B. (1968) 'John Snow, 1813–1858', *Journal of the Royal College of General Practitioners* 16:85–94.

Tudor Hart, J. (1988) *A New Kind of Doctor*, London: Merlin Press.

Tudor Hart, J. (1990) 'Reactive and proactive care: a crisis', *British Journal of General Practice* 40:4–9.

Tyrer, P. (1985) 'The hive system: a model for a psychiatric service', *British Journal of Psychiatry* 146:571–5.

Williams, P. and Balestrieri, M. (1989) 'Psychiatric clinics in general practice: do they reduce admissions?', *British Journal of Psychiatry* 154:67–71.

Withering, W. (1785) *An Account of the Foxglove and Some of its Medical Uses*, London: Robinson.

World Health Organization (1973) *Psychiatry and Primary Medical Care. Report on a Working Group*, Copenhagen: WHO Regional Office for Europe.

World Health Organization (1978) *Mental Disorders: Glossary and Guide to their Identification in Accordance with the Ninth Revision of the International Classification of Diseases*, Geneva: WHO.

WONCA (World Organization of National Colleges, Academics and Academic Associations of General Practitioners and Family Physicians) (1979) *International Classification of Health Problems in Primary Health Care*, second edn – ICHPPC-2, Oxford: Oxford University Press.

Zintl-Wiegand, A., Cooper, B., and Krumm, B. (1980) *Psychisch Kranke in der ärztlichen Allgemeinpraxis. Eine Untersuchung in der Stadt Mannheim*, Weinheim, Basel: Beltz.

Chapter 3

The 'research magnificent' cornes of age

Michael Shepherd

I should like to begin this brief review of epidemiological psychiatry in the primary-care setting by recalling that it was a general practitioner, Sir James Mackenzie, who first applied the term 'epidemiology' to non-infectious diseases (Mair 1986). Shortly afterwards a prominent British psychiatrist, Hubert Bond, in a paper entitled 'The position of psychological medicine in medicine and allied services', commented:

> It is my strong conviction that the general practitioner should, under suitable arrangements, be of the greatest possible service to the cause of psychological medicine. . . . Were he encouraged to be systematic in his observations and to adopt some method of recording them, they would be of inestimable value in collecting valuable data for that which in our work might well be called 'the research magnificent', in other words, a knowledge of the prolegomena and earliest stages of mental disorder.
>
> (Bond 1921)

Despite these pronouncements, it was some time before such work began. During the inter-war period the early epidemiological studies of mental disorder focused on the functional psychoses and mental subnormality, and little attention was paid to general practice (Shepherd 1982). World War II, however, gave an impetus to the subject by exposing the dimensions of psychiatric morbidity in both the general and the military populations. In the USA the findings acted as a spur to the bringing of mental disorder squarely into the orbit of public health, as is well reflected in the published proceedings of the meetings organized by the Milbank Memorial Fund during the immediate post-war decade. In one of these meetings, at which the central issue of case-definition was raised as an issue for discussion, the consensus of opinion was that though a 'case' of mental disorder could not be defined, a psychiatric patient was a person who consulted a psychiatrist. Though this view was broadly accepted by psychiatrists and public-health workers alike, it was challenged directly by Dr George Baehr, the director of the Health Insurance Plan of New York, who pointed out that

There are many more cases not seen by a psychiatrist than are seen by him. When it comes to the neuroses they are the concern of the personal physician of the family who has a great advantage over the psychiatrist if he will use his position as family doctor and if he understands what he sees: he sees the cases in the making.

(Baehr 1953)

Baehr then went on to make another telling point: 'unfortunately the personal physician is a vanishing species in the USA. Under our fee-for-service system of private practice, the future of family medical care is threatened, especially among the population of low and moderate income.' The absence of this infrastructure of primary care in North America undoubtedly influenced workers in the field of psychiatric epidemiology with an interest in extramural morbidity to concentrate their research efforts on the general population.

By contrast, in Britain the introduction of the National Health Service made it possible to utilize the records of general practitioners as a means of obtaining such data. Almost all of the population was registered with a family doctor, and in 1955 the situation was formally acknowledged by the setting up of a National Morbidity Survey based on general practitioner records (General Register Office 1958–62). For this survey it was necessary to modify the customary indices of morbidity, and the Statistics Sub-committee of the Registrar General's Advisory Committee on Medical Nomenclature and Statistics produced a report on the measurement of morbidity for the purpose, side-stepping the problem of case-definition:

The term 'case' of sickness is not defined because it is impracticable to give a definition which would be appropriate to all diseases. The general intention is that it should cover the whole course of one disease in one person as far as that course is relevant to the particular inquiry concerned.

(General Register Office 1954)

The Sub-committee favoured the use of spells of sickness, prevalence rates and consultation rates as more appropriate indices of morbidity, all of which featured in the structure of the first National Morbidity Survey. Yet, although this survey took account of mental disorder, the resulting data proved to be inadequate, largely because case-detection by practitioners was patchy and the diagnoses were unstandardized.

In the light of these deficiencies I felt that it would be worth mounting a more sophisticated survey targeted on psychiatric illness in general practice. The results of this study, carried out in the early 1960s, revealed a large volume of hitherto unacknowledged mental illness, and convinced me that to pursue this middle ground in psychiatric epidemiology (Shepherd and

Wilkinson 1988) offered prospects at least as inviting as the more fashionable pursuit of the elusive 'cases' in the general population by means of a battery of purpose-designed 'instruments'. For the purpose it was possible to form a small research unit, the General Practice Research Unit (GPRU), which for almost thirty years concentrated on epidemiological studies and health services research in the field of primary care. Some twenty-five books and 400 scientific papers attest to its productivity (Wilkinson 1989). Here I will highlight some aspects of the epidemiological work within the framework of the symposium.

First, I would emphasize the differences between this approach and that adopted by the workers who have concentrated on case-detection in the community at large. As Kräupl Taylor (1980) has pointed out, the concept of psychiatric morbidity depends on one or more of three criteria, namely (1) subjective distress associated with symptoms, (2) objective behaviour arousing social concern, and (3) medical help-seeking on the patient's part. The medical dimension has traditionally been most closely identified with patients in specialist mental health care, many of them in specialized institutions where anti-social behaviour accounts for admission in a substantial proportion of cases, the majority of them severely ill. By extending the definition of medical concern to incorporate general practitioners, however, it becomes theoretically possible to have the physician screen mental illness in the community and, in the process, to provide an estimate of conspicuous morbidity. For operational purposes this incorporates an individual whose symptoms, behaviour, distress or discomfort lead to a medical consultation at which a psychiatric diagnosis is made by a medically qualified participant observer.

The difference between this approach and that of the general population investigators emerged clearly at two recent meetings. In one of these, a European Symposium on Social Psychiatry, devoted to epidemiological research as basis for the organization of extramural psychiatry, a paper entitled 'The truth about psychiatric morbidity?' set out a traditional argument:

> An epidemiological survey should not be done unless the clinical syndromes have been listed beforehand, and defined properly as to their criteria for inclusion and exclusion. An assessment of 'caseness' on the assembled data is inadequate. Second, the next logical step is to steer the process of deciding in such a way that it cannot be directed by aspects of illness behaviour which are not consciously accounted for. The obvious answer is a computer programme . . .
>
> Third, it is perhaps wisest at present to screen populations only for disease entities with a circumscribed clinical picture and course, and for which circumscribed treatment programmes have been developed or are being tested. To include what Wing called the 'non-specific or

lesser psychiatric syndromes' (such as worrying or muscular tension) might result in turning away psychiatric services from their real task with the major syndromes, and prevent social and welfare services from developing their own and less expensive forms of care.

(Giel 1980)

The second symposium was organized by the WPA Section of Epidemiology and Community Psychiatry. Entitled 'What is a case?', its sub-title was, significantly, 'The problem of definition in psychiatric community surveys' (Wing, Bebbington and Robins 1981). Only two contributors made direct reference to primary care, one stating:

There are two ways in which the question of prevalence can be approached. One is the way of the clinician starting from the base of knowledge he has assembled in dealing with the patients he sees in hospital. These patients are, in effect, defined for him by referral agencies over which he has little or no control. He looks at the characteristics of these patients, specifies them by laying down some relatively objective criteria, and then applies the same criteria in the community at large. Another approach is to start at the other end of the problem and to travel in the opposite direction: to seek in the community those who are distressed and to discover what it is that leads some of these people to become psychiatric patients and others not. Most patients still come to the psychiatrist by way of the general practitioners, so first we need to ask what it is that brings psychologically distressed people to their GPs.

(Ingham 1981)

The other contributor acknowledged the case for involving the primary-care physician, only to dismiss it:

Most of the neurotically ill do not seek medical advice. The point can be reinforced with the Canberra data. It was found that of those with a PSE Index of Definition of 5 or more (threshold or definite case), 9 per cent had consulted a psychiatrist in the last month and 41 per cent had seen their general practitioner. The corresponding figures for those with specific symptoms (Index of Definition of 4) were 5 per cent and 37 per cent, and for lower values of the Index of Definition 0 per cent and 25 per cent. Clearly, psychiatrist-contacts cannot provide an adequate picture of neurosis in the community. GP contacts are certainly higher among 'cases' but many will not be presenting psychiatrically nor be recognised by their GPs as emotionally disturbed.

(Duncan-Jones 1981)

Such findings, it might be maintained, point not to the disregard of the information obtained from general practice so much as the need to improve the general practitioner's capacity for case-identification. To meet this objective the GPRU undertook a series of investigations of three types:

1 The design and standardization of a number of measuring instruments, including the General Health Questionnaire (Goldberg 1972), the Clinical Interview Schedule (Goldberg *et al.* 1970), and the Social Problems Schedule (Clare and Cairns 1978).
2 The ascertainment of 'illness behaviour', so as to identify individuals who do and do not make regular use of medical services. Murray and Corney, for example, studied two groups of individuals with equivalent psychosocial problems and have shown the differences in GP attendance to be accounted for by (a) personality and attitude variables; (b) the degree of concern with bodily function; (c) favourable or unfavourable attitudes to drugs, and (d) the presence or absence of a lay network of medically knowledgeable people (Murray and Corney 1988).
3 The more precise measurement of illness-episodes by means of health-diaries (Murray 1985).

What clinical findings emerge from this work? Several studies have now confirmed our original observation that affective disorders constitute the great bulk of mental disturbance presenting in general practice (Shepherd *et al.* 1966). Most of the morbidity detected can be loosely described as depression, anxiety or a combination of the two, with or without accompanying physical illness or social problems. The more precise classification of such illness, however, raises problems of its own.

These conditions comprise a relatively wide range of phenomena, dominated by a depressive mood, anxiety, fatigue, irritability, poor concentration and a variety of somatic complaints. Something is known about the aetiology of the minor affective disorders in terms of genetics, stress factors and lack of social support, but it is rarely possible to ascertain precisely the cause of a specific episode in the individual case. It is, therefore, not possible to construct a categorical schema of classification based on causal factors at present. None the less, it is necessary to categorize the disorders for the purposes of description, communication and treatment taking account of the extent and severity of the symptoms, their social context and extent, their consequences, their relationship to concurrent physical illness, and the patient's coping abilities.

In the sphere of diagnosis and classification a major obstacle is presented by observer variation, a phenomenon which is notoriously pronounced among general practitioners. To examine it we presented a series of videotapes and case vignettes to a sample of twenty-seven experienced practitioners (Jenkins, Smeeton and Shepherd 1988). The study was modelled along the lines of a comparable investigation of diagnostic practice among psychiatrists (Shepherd *et al.* 1968), in which the sources of observer

Table 3.1 Kappa agreements for ICD/ICHPPC diagnoses

	ICD		ICHPPC	
	Main	Subsidiary	Main	Subsidiary
Videos				
Anxiety state				
(300.0/3000)	0.01	−0.01	0.03	−0.01
Neurotic depression				
(300.4/3004)	0.06	0.01	0.09	0.06
Vignettes				
Anxiety state				
(300.0/3000)	0.04	0.01	0.10	−0.01
Neurotic depression				
(300.4/3004)	0.07	−0.02	0.21	−0.03

variation were shown to derive partly from perceived differences of the phenomena under observation, partly from differences in the interpretation of those phenomena and partly from inadequacies of the nosological schemata applied to the observations.

In our study, the participants were instructed in the use of the International Classification of Diseases (ICD) and of the International Classification of Health Problems in Primary Care (ICHPPC), an adaptation of the ICD for primary-care physicians. They were also invited to use their own preferred systems of classification. At first sight there was so little agreement between responses on the two international schemata as to suggest a tower of Babel (cf. Table 3.1).

A closer examination of the doctors' personal diagnoses, however, revealed a discernible pattern in that they tended to employ an idiosyncratic but recognizably multidimensional framework, incorporating several domains within their diagnostic formulations. Only a relatively small proportion of the practitioners used a single domain to describe a case; two-thirds or more of them used two or more domains for each case; and a substantial number employed three or even four domains. A detailed assessment of the factors which the participants included in their terminology indicated that they made use of psychological, physical, social and personality domains and that, contrary to expectation, only once did the diagnosis incorporate the notion of management.

It seems, therefore, that the difficulties lie less with the observers – who can agree in some measure on observations, inferences and prediction of outcome – and more with the classificatory schemata which they are expected to use. Further, the manner in which the participants tended to incorporate several domains into their diagnostic conclusions results in multidimensional formulations to which neither ICD nor ICHPPC lend themselves adequately. The significance of these findings extends beyond the narrow confines of nosology, for without an agreed system of nomenclature and classification there can be no effective communication to underpin collaborative research between investigators.

Any consideration of classification also leads inevitably to the question of outcome, which Kraepelin showed to be a central issue in categorizing the functional psychoses. The natural history of the non-psychotic disorders that predominate in general practice remains obscure. Duncan-Jones and others suggested that in theory there are two ways of deriving the relevant information by direct examination (Duncan-Jones *et al*. 1990). The first is to interview a random sample of the general population once, and take a detailed psychiatric history covering a defined period of time; this, however, is unlikely to provide accurate data because of memory lapses and retrospective bias. The second method is to draw a random sample of the population and assess their psychiatric health at frequent intervals over a period of time: this is ideal but impracticable.

Duncan-Jones's suggested way out of this impasse is to develop a mathematical model that could be used in conjunction with longitudinal data from community samples to estimate inception rates and the duration of episodes. He and his colleagues have exemplified this approach by rejecting the generally held way in which minor psychiatric symptoms are conceptualized. In most analyses of such symptoms it is assumed that subjects move from a 'healthy' state to an 'unhealthy' state as a result of exposure to various provoking factors. Health and illness are seen as discrete and distinguishable states. In contrast, Duncan-Jones's model assumes that each individual has a stable and characteristic level of symptomatology (which may be high or low) and that his or her levels of symptoms fluctuate around this characteristic level with changing conditions. The understanding of psychiatric symptoms therefore requires knowledge of both the individual's characteristic level of symptomatology and the factors which lead this level of symptomatology to fluctuate.

Unfortunately, the results of the large-scale study based on this approach are so remote from clinical experience that it seems necessary to consider alternative approaches to the problem and, in particular, the potential of data from general practice. These can be found in both macro and micro studies. The largest macro study to date is that provided by the British National Morbidity Surveys. The difficulties raised by such surveys have been analysed by Dunn and Smeeton (1989), with reference to the Second National Morbidity Survey, undertaken jointly by the Royal College of General Practitioners, the Office of Population Censuses and Surveys (OPCS) and the Department of Health and Social Security (DHSS). This was designed to yield information on episode and consultation patterns in a representative sample of general practices over a period of up to six years (1970–76). Sixty practices with altogether 115 practitioners took part in 1970–71, but only twenty-two contributed data for the whole six years,

Table 3.2 Proportion of psychiatric patients with each of the eight most common record types (× 100)

Practice	130	134	150	Record type* 135	146	147	126	136
A	41	13	15	20	13	7	11	0
B	63	41	2	1	16	4	0	0
C	38	33	18	9	17	10	0	4
D	39	50	3	33	13	9	0	0
E	15	51	35	32	5	8	1	6
F	68	25	2	3	20	16	0	0
G	49	32	9	19	4	7	14	8
H	35	68	8	2	2	6	1	0
I	32	22	41	13	9	4	20	18
J	35	48	12	6	7	4	2	0
K	10	21	60	17	8	17	0	0
L	52	28	11	16	7	9	0	1
M	56	48	1	1	9	7	0	0
N	57	40	8	10	23	7	2	2
O	43	31	11	16	21	12	2	2
P	25	21	36	22	19	8	5	10
Q	36	35	19	18	11	12	14	1
R	37	21	38	24	7	10	5	1
S	47	37	22	25	13	8	2	2
T	39	30	20	52	9	10	1	3
U	32	38	22	19	18	17	3	7
V	39	34	22	25	14	14	2	1
Mean	40	35	19	17	12	9	4	3
Ratio of highest to lowest	6.80	5.23	60.0	52.0	11.5	4.25	>50	>45

* Royal College Codes (in order of overall prevalence): 130, anxiety neurosis; 134, depressive neurosis; 150, unclassified symptoms; 135, physical disorders of presumably psychogenic origin; 146, insomnia; 147, tension headache; 126, affective psychosis; 136, neurasthenia

Source: From Dunn and Smeeton 1989

providing complete six-year records of about 60,000 individuals; details of psychiatric problems were provided for 42,000 persons. The data file contained records of the number of episodes of psychiatric disorders for each patient over the six consecutive years. In each episode there was at least one GP consultation at which a relevant diagnosis has been recorded. The file also contained the number of consultations at which a psychiatric diagnosis was made. Each patient contributed a single record of a particular disorder if, and only if, he or she had received a diagnosis of that disorder at least once during the six years.

As Dunn and Smeeton observe, inter-practice variation is so large that 'one is inclined to conclude that the records reveal more about the GPs than about their patients'. The reporting of a prevalence rate of depression almost twice that of the first survey indicates the validity of their comment. The most that could be concluded was that:

1 Females experience twice as many psychiatric illness-episodes as males.
2 The same sex-difference emerges from stochastic modelling of anxiety and depression.
3 Women, middle-aged persons and transients are all at increased risk for episodes of mental illness.
4 'Proneness' to depressive episodes, examined by means of the Poisson distribution (assuming equality of proneness) and a 'flexible proneness' model, the Negative Binomial Distribution (NBD), was not equally distributed.
5 Inter-practice variation can be diminished by standardizing the criteria of diagnosis, most effectively by intensive study of individual practices repeated over long periods of time.

The last of these points brings us back to the issue of outcome. One of the major findings of the study by Jenkins *et al*. (1988) was the difficulty experienced by the GPs in predicting the prognosis of the disorders under consideration, reflecting a lack of adequate information about the natural history of the disorders presenting to them. Longitudinal studies over substantial periods of time are still rare in general practice but the GPRU has mounted several such inquiries; from these it appeared that approximately three-quarters of new psychiatric illnesses recover within one year, during which time personality and social factors are crucial in determining outcome (Mann, Jenkins and Belsey 1981). By contrast, when the illness lasts for over five years the chances of recovery within the next twelve months fall to about one in thirteen. As an heuristic hypothesis to account for the data, it has been suggested that there are two broad groups of neurotic disorder encountered in general practice: one of chronic conditions occurring among a relatively unchanging section of the population, and another group of short-term reactions characterizing a continually changing population and with a good overall prognosis.

Further, thanks to the meticulous record-keeping of one practitioner (Dr John Fry) it has been possible to carry out a follow-up of twenty years on his patient population. The psychiatric diagnoses given to 1,530 patients have been tabulated and analysed, along with prescription data, referral patterns and physical status. The results show that some three-quarters of the women and one-half of the men had been seen in the practice during these two decades on at least one occasion for a problem diagnosed by the general practitioner as wholly or largely psychiatric in nature. Women not only suffered far more commonly than men from depression but it was for them a relatively chronic complaint. Approximately 70 per cent of women attended at some time during the follow-up period with a depressive episode and just over 40 per cent with an anxiety or phobic state. The figures for the men are 32 per cent and 41 per cent respectively. This study further confirms the extent to which the large pool of minor psychiatric morbidity is handled almost entirely by the GP himself. Over the twenty years only eighty-four of the 1,530 patients (5.5 per cent) were ever referred to a psychiatric out-patient clinic and only 47 (3.1 per cent) were admitted to a psychiatric hospital or department.

With regard to the future, the results of the work to date carry implications for all three groups involved; namely, epidemiologists, general practitioners and psychiatrists. For epidemiologists it has become necessary to recognize primary care as the middle ground for research into extramural mental disorder, if only because in appropriate conditions of medical care the prevalence rates of psychiatric illness in general practice approximate closely to those in the general population (Goldberg and Huxley 1980). In consequence, case-identification by the practitioners need no longer be regarded as incidental to these findings obtained by elaborate, indirect methods of mensuration. There is now a strong case for a convergence between the interests and activities of both groups of investigators.

For psychiatrists, it is apparent that they must broaden their concerns if they are to participate in the development of their discipline in its public-health perspective. In the process the current emphasis on the 're-medicalization' of psychiatry may be seen to lead not simply to an awareness of biological mechanisms but also to the neglected concepts of social medicine.

Finally, for general practitioners a more active form of collaboration is becoming imperative. Morrell (1988) has commented on the distaste of primary-care physicians for epidemiology and the need for this to be overcome if they are to realize their research potential. Nowhere is the need greater than in the sphere of mental disorder. The 'research magnificent' may have come of age, but it is unlikely to reach maturity without incorporating Sir James Mackenzie's thesis that 'the opportunities for the general practitioner are essential for the investigation of disease and the progress of medicine' (Mackenzie 1921).

REFERENCES

Baehr, G. (1953) 'Discussion: definition of a case', in *Interrelations between the Social Environment and Psychiatric Disorders*, New York: Milbank Memorial Fund, pp. 155–6.

Bond, H. (1921) 'The position of psychological medicine and allied services', *Journal of Mental Science* 67:422–3.

Clare, A.W. and Cairns, V.E. (1978) 'Design, development and use of a standardised interview to assess social maladjustment and dysfunction in community studies', *Psychological Medicine* 8:589–604.

Duncan-Jones, P. (1981) 'The natural history of neurosis: probability models', in

What is a Case?, J.K. Wing, P. Bebbington, and L.N. Robins (eds), London: Grant McIntyre, pp. 161–80.

Duncan-Jones, P., Fergusson, D.M., Ormel, J.H., and Horwood, L.J. (1990) 'A model of stability and change in minor psychiatric symptoms: results from three longitudinal studies', *Psychological Medicine Supplement* 18, Cambridge: Cambridge University Press.

Dunn, G. and Smeeton, N. (1989) 'The study of episodes of psychiatric morbidity', in *The Scope of Epidemiological Psychiatry*, P. Williams, G. Wilkinson, and K. Rawnsley (eds), London: Routledge, pp. 167–77.

General Register Office (1954) 'Studies on medical and population subjects', No. 8, *Measurement of Morbidity*, London: HMSO.

General Register Office (1958–62) 'Studies on medical and population subjects', No. 14, *Morbidity Statistics from General Practice*, vols. 1–3, London: HMSO.

Giel, R. (1980) 'The truth about psychiatric morbidity?', in *Epidemiological Research as Basis for the Organization of Extramural Psychiatry*, E. Strömgren, A. Dupont, and J.A. Nielsen (eds), *Acta Psychiatrica Scandinavica Supplementum* 285, vol. 62, Copenhagen: Munksgaard.

Goldberg, D.P. (1972) *The Detection of Psychiatric Illness by Questionnaire*, London: Oxford University Press.

Goldberg, D.P., Cooper, B., Eastwood, M.R., Kedward, H.B., and Shepherd, M. (1970) 'A standardised psychiatric interview for use in community surveys', *British Journal of Preventive and Social Medicine* 24:18–23.

Goldberg, D. and Huxley, P. (1980) *Mental Illness in the Community*, London: Tavistock Publications.

Ingham, J. (1981) 'Neurosis: disease or distress?', in *What is a Case?*, J.K. Wing, P. Bebbington, and L.N. Robins (eds), London: Grant McIntyre, pp. 12–23.

Jenkins, R., Smeeton, N., and Shepherd, M. (1988) *Classification of Mental Disorder in Primary Care*, Psychological Medicine Monograph Supplement No. 12, Cambridge: Cambridge University Press.

Kräupl Taylor, F. (1980) 'The concepts of disease', *Psychological Medicine* 10:419–24.

Mackenzie, J. (1921) 'The opportunities of the general practitioner are essential for the investigation of disease and the progress of medicine', *British Medical Journal* 1: 797–804.

Mair, H. (1986) *Sir James Mackenzie, MD, 1853–1925, General Practitioner*, London: Royal College of General Practitioners, pp. 323–5.

Mann, A.H., Jenkins, R., and Belsey, E. (1981) 'The twelve-month outcome of patients with neurotic illness in general practice', *Psychological Medicine* 11:535–50.

Morrell, D. (1988) Preface, in *Epidemiology in General Practice*, D. Morrell (ed.), Oxford: Oxford University Press.

Murray, J. (1985) 'The use of health diaries in the field of psychiatric illness in general practice', *Psychological Medicine* 15:827–40.

Murray, J. and Corney, R. (1988) 'General practice attendance in women with psychosocial problems', *Social Psychiatry and Psychiatric Epidemiology* 23:175–83.

Shepherd, M. (1982) 'Psychiatric research and primary care in Britain, past, present and future', *Psychological Medicine* 12: 493–9.

Shepherd, M., Brooke, E.M., Cooper, J.B., and Lin, T-Y. (1968) 'An experimental approach to psychiatric diagnosis', *Acta Psychiatrica Scandinavica Supplementum* 201, Copenhagen: Munksgaard.

Shepherd, M., Cooper, A.B., Brown, A.C., and Kalton, G.W. (1966) *Psychiatric Illness in General Practice*, Oxford: Oxford University Press.

Shepherd, M. and Wilkinson, G. (1988) 'Primary care as the middle ground for psychiatric epidemiology', *Psychological Medicine* 18:263–7.

Wilkinson, G. (1989) 'Research report: the General Practice Research Unit', *Psychological Medicine* 19:787–90.

Wing, J.K., Bebbington, P., and Robins, L.N. (eds) (1981) *What is a Case?* London: Grant McIntyre, pp. 12–13.

Chapter 4

Primary care and psychiatric epidemiology

The psychiatrist's perspective

David Goldberg and Linda Gask

Ten years ago our group proposed a framework for thinking about psychiatric disorder in the community, consisting of five levels, separated by four filters (Goldberg and Huxley 1980). Level 1 represents morbidity as it is found in random samples of the general population, while Level 5 corresponds to the mentally ill patients admitted to psychiatric hospitals. The centre-piece of the model consists of Levels 2 and 3, which represent respectively all cases of psychological illness or distress presenting in the primary-care physician's practice, and those which he recognizes as such. The model serves to relate mental ill health in this setting, on the one hand, to events in the community and, on the other hand, to the cases treated by specialist psychiatric services.

The data we presented at that time confirmed that the specialist services were in fact dealing with only a small proportion of psychiatric morbidity, but that most mentally disturbed persons will consult their general practitioners in the course of any one year. Moreover, the data also indicated that the practitioners failed to detect a sizeable proportion of the illnesses in question: a finding with important implications for medical training. Two other European centres, Verona (Tansella and Williams 1989) and Groningen (Giel, Koeter and Ormel 1990), have since reported data relating to all five levels of this model, which indicate that the pathways to psychiatric care both in Italy and in the Netherlands are not unlike those found in the United Kingdom (see Table 4.1).

In both the former countries, most cases of psychiatric illness are encountered in the primary-care setting, but many of them are not recognized by the doctors. The data from Verona point to an additional conclusion: if the time-frame of observation is shortened from one year to one week, the first filter (illness behaviour) becomes very much more important (Tansella and Williams 1989).

In our earlier work we were uneasily aware that not all psychiatric patients have traversed a pathway to care corresponding to a smooth transition through the four filters. With encouragement from the World Health Organization, we have since studied in greater detail the pathways

Table 4.1 Comparison of the rates of psychiatric morbidity, at different levels of care, in three European cities (rates per 1,000 adults)

Level of care	Greater Manchester[1] (annual)	Groningen[2] (annual)	Verona[3] (weekly)
1 Total in the community	250	303	227
2 Primary medical care (total)	230	224	34
3 Primary medical care (recognized by the GP)	140	94	23
4 Referred to psychiatric service	17	34	4
5 In psychiatric in-patient care	6	10	0.7

[1] Goldberg and Huxley (1980)
[2] Giel, Koeter and Ormel (1990)
[3] Tansella and Williams (1989)

to mental health care in Manchester (Gater and Goldberg 1990), and have found the picture represented in Figure 4.1.

The main pathway is shown by the heavy horizontal line going from left (the community) to right (the specialist psychiatric service). It can be seen that while about two-thirds of the patients approach directly along this pathway, another fairly large group comes via the accident room, and from medical clinics in the general hospital where our department is situated. Contrary to expectation, non-medical sources of referral are uncommon, the great majority of patients entering specialist mental health care via general practice or a hospital medical clinic. This study has been replicated in eight other countries (Gater et al. 1990), and the broad findings hold good for five of these. Indeed, the only one of these countries where primary health care is not the most important source of referral to psychiatry is Indonesia.

The findings of recent North American surveys in the primary-care setting, making use of two-stage case-finding techniques, are in conformity with those of the corresponding European studies; namely, that between one-quarter and one-third of consecutive attenders in general practice are found to have a psychiatric illness according to the diagnostic guidelines provided in the ICD-10 or the DSM-III R criteria. Data from these surveys are summarized in Table 4.2.

These findings from a number of countries with differing systems of health care suggest that the general model has validity in an international

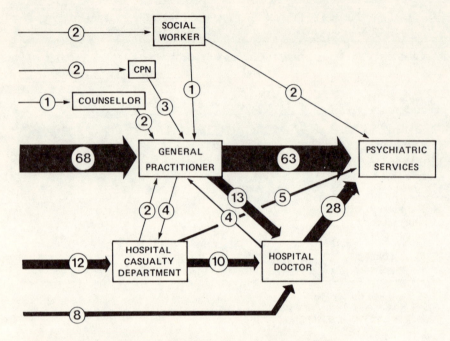

Figure 4.1 Pathways to psychiatric care in South Manchester.
Source: Gater and Goldberg 1990

Table 4.2 Two-stage surveys of psychiatric disorder in primary medical care:
recent US studies

Authors	First-stage screening method	Second-stage diagnostic assessment method	Proportion of psychiatric cases among consecutive attenders(%)
Hoeper *et al.* (1979) (Marshfield, WI)	GHQ–30	SADS-RDC	26.7
Schulberg *et al.* (1985) (Pittsburg, PA)	GHQ–30	DSM-III criteria	31.3
Von Korff *et al.* (1987) (Baltimore, MD)	GHQ–30	DIS-DSM III	25.0
Barrett *et al.* (1988) (Hanover, NH)	SCL–49	SADS-RDC	26.5

context, and that its implications for medical practice and training are of considerable importance to the quality and efficiency of mental health-care provision for many populations. The present contribution examines some of these implications and summarizes the findings of research into the question undertaken by our group, including recent studies.

IS INCREASED DETECTION WORTHWHILE?

Fifteen years ago we carried out a small project with a single-handed practitioner in Yorkshire (Johnstone and Goldberg 1976), in which patients with high scores on a screening questionnaire were assigned randomly either to an index group, about whose mental state the GP was informed, or to a control group, about whom he was not. The outcome at three months was found to be very much better for the index group than for the controls, the latter tending to improve more slowly throughout the survey year.

This project has since been replicated in different ways by Zung et al. (1983) and Rand, Badger and Coggings (1988). However, two other research groups in the USA – those of Hoeper et al. (1984) in Wisconsin and Shapiro et al. (1987) in Baltimore – were unable to confirm our findings. It seems that these workers interpreted the original study rather literally: although in our publication we had reported that the GP was informed about the screening scores of the index group, we did not suggest that this information in itself was responsible for the favourable outcome. What helped the patients was what the doctor did as a result of the information he was given. In the two US studies with negative findings, it appears that the practitioners did nothing different for the index and control groups of patients. Indeed, it would seem that they played a generally passive role in the research projects. The GP probably needs to be a willing and active participant if positive results are to be achieved.

Two further studies, using independent research assessments of depressive illness and a naturalistic, rather than a control design, have shown convincingly that cases of depression which are recognized by the GP have a better outcome than those which are not. One was a British study by Tylee and Freeling (1989) and the other a more recent study in the Netherlands by Ormel et al. (1990). The latter compared 106 patients whose depression was detected by the GP with eighty patients whose illnesses were not detected, and showed that the former group had a significantly better outcome at six months. As in the earlier study by Johnstone and Goldberg (1976), improvement was not confined to patients receiving a particular form of treatment. Although in both these studies severely depressed patients were prescribed antidepressants, it seemed that the doctor–patient transaction was modified in other ways: patients were encouraged to discuss their problems and were given counselling about

them. More recently, two controlled studies – by Thomson *et al.* (1982) in
Scotland and Hollyman *et al.* (1988) in London – have shown that depressed
patients in general practice do significantly better on antidepressants than
on placebos. Moreover, in the study by Zung *et al.* (1983), patients thought
not sufficiently depressed to require antidepressants did worse than the
more severely ill patients for whom these were prescribed. Thus the weight
of the evidence strongly suggests that improving the detection of depressive
states in general practice does help the patients.

WHAT MAKES SOME DOCTORS GOOD AT DETECTING PSYCHIATRIC ILLNESS?

Earlier preoccupation with the rate for mental illness among his patients
reported by a particular doctor has been overtaken by an interest in the
doctor's ability to detect mental disorder when it is present. This ability
was quantified by Marks, Goldberg and Hillier (1979) as an 'identification
index' which, if a two-stage screening procedure is used, is given by the
number of detected true positives divided by the expected number of true
positives. In their study, the mean identification index among ninety-one
Manchester GPs was found to be 54 per cent, which means that on average
these doctors were probably missing about 46 per cent of the psychiatric
cases among their patients.

The investigators considered factors related either to the doctor or the
patient, which might account for this variation. Doctors with high identification indices were rated by an independent observer as having greater
interest in, and concern for, the individual patient, being more interested
in psychiatry, and being more experienced in patient management; they
were also somewhat older than the average. More detailed analysis showed
that such doctors asked more questions directed to psychosocial problems,
avoided technical jargon, were more likely to be settled in their practices
and tended to have higher qualifications. Table 4.3 summarizes the features
of their behaviour in the interview situation.

These research findings led to the development of training courses for
family doctors (Gask *et al.* 1987; 1988), which involved the evaluators
in watching videotapes of interviews between family doctors, who were
about to attend our training courses, and patients who had just completed
a psychiatric screening questionnaire. It became clear that two factors were
at work in explaining how psychological disorders came to be missed. The
first, already known to us, was that some doctors do not respond to either
verbal or non-verbal cues that indicate psychological distress; the second
was that some patients do not at consultation show any evidence of
psychological disorder despite high scores on the screening questionnaire.
These observations led us to test the hypothesis that the patients' failure
to give cues indicating distress might be related to specific behaviours of

Table 4.3 Determinants of the ability to identify psychological distress: findings of early research[1]

Start of interview:
> Makes eye contact
> Clarifies nature of patient's complaint

General interview skills:
> Picks up verbal cues
> Picks up non-verbal cues
> Deals well with interruptions
> Doesn't bury himself in case-notes
> Makes supportive comments

Types of question asked:
> Directive 'psychiatric' questions
> Closed 'psychiatric' questions
> Questions about family and home situation

[1] Goldberg and Huxley (1980)

the doctors. Davenport, Goldberg and Millar (1987) were able to show that certain characteristics of the doctor did indeed influence the giving of cues by the patient. Videotaped interviews demonstrated that patients gave more such cues, particularly of a verbal or vocal nature, when talking to doctors with a high success in identifying psychiatric disorder, than did those whose doctors had a low success in case-identification.

In this experiment we used videotapes of real encounters between doctors and patients. We selected three vocational trainees with high rates of case-identification, and the three with the lowest rates. We used a nested design, so that for each of the six selected doctors we studied four interviews with patients with low GHQ scores, and four with high scores. The interviews were rated by a psychiatrist blind to the experimental design and also to the ratings and scores. The results – Davenport, Goldberg and Millar (1987) – show, in brief, that patients being interviewed by doctors with a high identification index will

 give more verbal cues;
 have more distress in their voices;
 tend to have more restless movements.

Those patients interviewed by doctors with high case detection made the diagnosis easier for the doctors by giving during the interview more cues indicating psychological distress. In an analysis of variance, significant interaction terms were found between GP and patient variables, suggesting that these doctors had effectively encouraged the patients with high GHQ scores to give expression to their distress at consultation.

Study of the videotapes showed that the successful case-detectors tended to make more eye-contact with their patients throughout the interviews.

Table 4.4 Management skills of doctors with high identification indices[1]

Giving information[2]:
> Gives explanatory information
> Gives information in a *negotiated* way
> Gives information clearly
> Checks that information is understood

Prescribing medication[2]:
> Tells name of prescribed drug
> Explains any side-effects

Advice and treatment[2]:
> Gives advice and treatment instructions clearly
> Gives advice and treatment in a *negotiated* way
> Checks that advice and instructions are understood

[1] Millar, Goldberg and Jenkins (1991)
[2] Behaviours significantly more common in dealing with all patients: low as well as high scorers on GHQ

They facilitated their patients more and asked more questions with a social content. In contrast, their less adept colleagues asked more 'closed' questions and tended to be looking in the patients' notes while speaking to them. All these differences in behaviour between the two groups of doctors were present irrespective of the patients' GHQ scores; the only difference specific for patients with high GHQ scores was that the more adept doctors tended to ask such patients directive social questions about their home life early in the interview. It therefore seems possible that the ability to detect psychosocial distress demonstrated by these doctors should be thought of as part of their generally superior communication and management skills.

We therefore turned from the 'problem-solving' part of the interview, on which attention had so far been focused, to the latter parts concerned with management skills, to discover whether this was indeed the case. It can be seen from Table 4.4 that doctors with a high identification index are indeed much better at communicating with their patients, whether they are prescribing ointment for a rash, giving advice on the management of heart failure or counselling someone who is depressed. Indeed, the only management skills they display more frequently with patients who have high GHQ scores turn out to be fairly predictable behaviours concerned with prescribing psychotropics and giving psychosocial information and advice. It thus seems likely that the ability to make accurate assessments of psychological distress is not a specific skill, but part of a generally superior ability to communicate with patients.

Table 4.5 Definition of somatization[1]

All the following four criteria must be satisfied:

A *Presentation*	the presenting complaint must be of somatic symptom(s)
B *Attribution*	the patient must regard his problem as one of physical illness
C *Mental health status*	psychiatric disorder must be identified as present, according to the Research Diagnostic Criteria (RDC)
D *Causal connection*	the investigator must be satisfied that the presenting complaints are due to the psychiatric disorder (C), or at least exacerbated by it

[1] Bridges and Goldberg (1987)

THE PROBLEM OF AFFECTIVE ILLNESS PRESENTING WITH SOMATIC COMPLAINTS

Some patients fail to express their psychological distress at consultation and present exclusively somatic complaints. Rosen, Kleinman and Katon (1982) have termed episodes of psychiatric illness which present in this form 'subacute somatization'. The criteria which must be fulfilled to justify this diagnostic label in our own work are shown in Table 4.5.

Bridges and Goldberg (1987), studying a sample of 590 general-practice patients with new episodes of illness, found that while only 5 per cent showed conspicuous psychiatric morbidity, and these had a 95 per cent chance of being recognized by the practitioners, a further 19 per cent presented with only somatic symptoms of psychological distress, but these had a less than 50 per cent chance of being detected. Whereas 57 per cent of all psychiatric diagnoses made in primary health care fulfilled the criteria set out in Table 4.5, in the presence of co-existing physical disease only one-third were detected by the GPs.

With this large sub-group in mind, we designed a videotaped teaching package for general practitioners, dealing with the management of psychological distress which presents as somatic complaints. In order to produce maximum change, we devised a two-part videotaped learning package, first showing the component parts of the package and then using micro-skills and role rehearsal (Gask and Goldberg 1989). The intervention was aimed at persuading such patients to reframe their complaints and to change the attributions which they make concerning the cause of their symptoms. The training package is concerned with the acquisition of a set of skills and makes use of videotape demonstrations followed by role-playing and micro-teaching of each individual skill. Subsequently, the practitioners on our training courses discuss with our staff their actual encounters with such patients.

One part of the training package – 'changing the agenda' – is concerned with the medical skills required during the course of interview and consists of four component parts:

1 how to communicate to a patient the results of physical examination;
2 how to convince him or her that the doctor knows his symptoms are real and not imaginary or simulated;
3 how to verbalize affective disturbance and related symptoms; and
4 how to make a patient aware of the links between his symptoms and his life situation.

It is important in this context that the GP should acquire skills in interviewing in such a way that emotional distress relevant to the patient's manifested symptoms will be elicited, that the severity of distress and the need for intervention will be correctly assessed, and that he will be able to listen with sympathy and understanding, to refrain from judgemental comments and to offer informed and helpful counselling. Models for this type of training have been proposed by Lesser (1985) and by Bensing and Sluijs (1985). Results of the first two courses held in Manchester, summarized in Table 4.6, demonstrate significant improvement in the doctors' interviewing skills.

IMPROVING COLLABORATION BETWEEN PSYCHIATRISTS AND GENERAL PRACTITIONERS

In the UK, Strathdee and Williams (1985) have shown that psychiatrists are progressively extending their extramural services into the community, most often by conducting out-patient clinics in local health centres and group practices. Although many now work regularly in this setting, the new service has developed in a haphazard and wholly unplanned way. The approaches used have been characterized by a number of different models. The 'shifted out-patients' model implies simply that the psychiatrist moves the locus of his out-patient activities from the hospital clinic to the primary-care setting, whilst keeping his mode of work largely unchanged. In this situation, he may concentrate largely on patients who have been discharged from the psychiatric hospital, rather than on advising about the management of new cases. He need not necessarily acquire any new skills or work in closer conjunction with his GP colleagues. The model is thus essentially a conservative one. The 'consultation-liaison' model implies a more radical change, since it offers opportunities for the psychiatrist to make contact with patients who would not normally be referred to him and whose day-to-day management remains with the practitioners. In this way, the psychiatrist gains experience in dealing with different

Table 4.6 Improvement in re-attribution skills of GP trainees after exposure to focused training[1]

(a) No. of doctors whose score after training is:

	increased	unchanged	decreased	Probability level
Clarification	5	13	2	NS
Picks up non-verbal cues	11	7	2	0.05
Empathy	14	2	4	0.005

(b) Changes in mean scores after training:

	Pre-training mean score	Post-training mean score	
'Helping to feel understood'			
Asks about other symptoms	8	16	0.05
Asks about social family factors	1.75	2.40	0.05
Explores health beliefs	9	13	NS
'Changing the agenda'			
Acknowledges reality of patient's symptoms	2	8	0.05
Summarizes mood symptoms	14	20	0.05
Summarizes life events	13	20	0.05
'Making the link'			
Overall ability	1.0	2.8	0.005

[1] Gask et al. (1989)

types of problem and may be able to make a positive contribution to the style and quality of patient care in those practices to which he is attached.

However psychiatrists choose to co-operate with family doctors, it is clear that they must gain a working knowledge of the range of mental health problems encountered in the primary-care setting, and that such knowledge will be acquired most readily by means of teamwork with the practitioners and other health professionals, as well as by contact with individual patients. Having gained such experience, the psychiatrist can participate in the training of family doctors, making use of audio- or videotape feedback to ensure that his teaching is effective and firmly rooted in the realities of medical practice.

FUTURE DIRECTIONS

Apart from these important public health tasks, aimed at what Shepherd *et al.* (1966) characterized as 'strengthening the family doctor in his therapeutic role', an additional major objective for the future will be to find ways of preventing further illness episodes in those patients who are at high risk of relapse. Although follow-up studies have shown that two-thirds of the patients seen in general practice who meet the criteria for a psychiatric 'case' will be back within the 'normal' range of mental health three months later, many of these remain at high risk for relapse in the future, if and when adverse life situations are encountered. Apart from the chemical prophylaxis of major psychotic and affective illness, very little is known about how to reduce the risk of relapse. Intriguing claims have been made for the use of cognitive techniques in preventing relapse in depression, for the value of 'befriending', organized by local voluntary groups, and for the teaching of 'coping skills' as a method of reducing vulnerability to stress. There is now a pressing need for studies of the feasibility and efficacy of all these approaches in the primary-care setting.

ACKNOWLEDGEMENT

The work described in this chapter was collaborative research by a team of investigators. The Pathways to Care study was carried out by Richard Gater. The work on interview skills was undertaken with Tim Millar, Sarah Davenport and Leslie Jenkins; that on somatization with Keith Bridges, and that on teaching interview skills with Francis Creed and Graeme McGrath. Dawn Black, Sylvia Kaaya and Richard Porter also assisted in the research programme.

REFERENCES

Barrett, J., Barrett, J., Oxman, T., and Gerber, P. (1988) 'The prevalence of psychiatric disorders in a primary care practice', *Archives of General Psychiatry* 45:1100–6.
Bensing, J.M. and Sluijs, E.M. (1985) 'Evaluation of an interview training course for general practitioners', *Social Science and Medicine* 20:737–44.
Bridges, K. and Goldberg, P. (1987) 'Somatic presentations of DSM-III psychiatric disorder in primary care', *Journal of Psychosomatic Research* 29:563–9.
Davenport, S., Goldberg, D., and Millar, T. (1987) 'How psychiatric disorders are missed during medical consultations', *Lancet* ii:439–41.

Gask, L. and Goldberg, D. (1989) *Teaching Techniques of Re-attribution: a Videotaped Learning Package*, Department of Psychiatry, Withington Hospital, Manchester, U.K. (available from authors).

Gask, L., Goldberg, D., Lesser, A.T., and Millar, T. (1987) 'Improving the psychiatric skills of the general practice trainee: an evaluation of a group training course', *Medical Education* 21:362–8.

Gask, L., Goldberg, D., Porter, R., and Creed, F. (1989) 'The treatment of somatization: evaluation of a teaching package with general practice trainees', *Journal of Psychosomatic Research* 33:697–703.

Gask, L., McGrath, G., Goldberg, D., and Millar, T. (1988) 'Improving the psychiatric skills of established general practitioners: evaluation of a group teaching', *Medical Education* 22:132–8.

Gater, R., de Almeida e Souza, R., Caraveo, J., Chandrasekar, C., Dhadphale, M., Goldberg, D., al Kathiri, A., de Llano, G., Mubbashar, M., Silhan, K., Thong, D., Torres, F., and Sartorius, N. (1990) 'The pathways to psychiatric care: a cross-cultural study', *Psychological Medicine*.

Gater, R. and Goldberg, D. (1990) 'Pathways to psychiatric care in South Manchester', *British Journal of Psychiatry*.

Giel, R., Koeter, M.W., and Ormel, J. (1990) 'Detection and referral of primary care patients with mental health problems', in D. Goldberg and D. Tantam (eds) *The Public Health Impact of Mental Disorders*, Basel: Hogrefe-Huber.

Goldberg, D. and Huxley, P. (1980) *Mental Illness in the Community: the Pathway to Psychiatric Care*, London: Tavistock.

Hoeper, E., Nycz, G., Cleary, P., Regier, D., and Goldberg, I. (1979) 'Estimated prevalence of RDC mental disorder in primary medical care', *International Journal of Mental Health* 8:6–15.

Hoeper, E., Nycz, G., Kessler, L., Burke, J., and Pierce, W. (1984) 'The usefulness of screening for mental illness', *Lancet* i:33–5.

Hollyman, J., Freeling, P., Paykel, E., Bhat, A., and Sedgewick, P. (1988) 'Double-blind placebo-controlled trial among depressed patients in general practice', *Journal of the Royal College of General Practitioners* 38:393–7.

Johnstone, A. and Goldberg, D.P. (1976) 'Psychiatric screening in general practice: a controlled trial', *Lancet* i:605–8.

Korff, M. von, Shapiro, S., Burke, J., Teitelbaum, M., Skinner, E., German, P., Turner, R., Klein, L., and Burns, B. (1987) 'Anxiety and depression in a primary care clinic', *Archives of General Psychiatry* 44:152–6.

Lesser, A.L. (1985) 'Problem-based interviewing in general practice: a model', *Medical Education* 19:299–304.

Marks, J., Goldberg, D., and Hillier, V. (1979) 'Determinants of the ability of general practitioners to detect psychological illness', *Psychological Medicine* 9:337–53.

Millar, T. and Goldberg, D. (1991) 'Determinants of the ability of general practitioners to manage common disorders', *British Journal of General Practice*.

Ormel, J., Koeter, H., van den Brink, W., and van de Willige, G. (1990) 'The extent of non-recognition of mental health problems in primary care and its effects on management and outcome', in D. Goldberg and D. Tantam (eds), *The Public Health Impact of Mental Disorder*, Basel: Hogrefe-Huber (in press).

Rand, E., Badger, L., and Coggings, D. (1988) 'Towards a resolution of contradictions – utility of feedback from the GHQ', *General Hospital Psychiatry* 10:189–96.

Rosen, G., Kleinman, A., and Katon, W. (1982) 'Somatisation in family practice: a biopsychosocial approach', *Journal of Family Practice* 14:427–37.

Schulberg, C., McClelland, M., Coulehan, J., Bolck, M., and Werner, G. (1986) 'Psychiatric decision-making in general practice', *General Hospital Psychiatry* 8:1–6.

Shapiro, S., German, P., Skinner, E., Korff, M. von, Turner, R., Klein, L., Teitelbaum, M., Kramer, M., Burke, J., and Burns, B. (1987) 'An experiment to change detection and management of mental morbidity in primary care', *Medical Care* 25:327–39.

Shepherd, M., Cooper, B., Brown, A.C., and Kalton, G. (1966) *Psychiatric Illness in General Practice*, London: Oxford University Press.

Strathdee, G. and Williams, P. (1985) 'Patterns of collaboration', in P. Williams, G. Wilkinson, and M. Shepherd (eds), *Mental Illness in Primary Care Settings*, London: Tavistock.

Tansella, M. and Williams, P. (1989) 'The spectrum of psychiatric morbidity in a defined geographical area', *Psychological Medicine* 19:765–79.

Thomson, J., Rankin, H., Aschcroft, G., Yates, C., McQueen, J., and Cummings, S. (1982) 'The treatment of depression in general practice: a comparison of L-tryptophan and amitryptiline with placebo', *Psychological Medicine* 12:741–51.

Tylee, A. and Freeling, P. (1989) 'The recognition, diagnosis and acknowledgement of depressive disorders by general practitioners', in E. Paykel and K. Herbst (eds), *Depression: an Integrative Approach*, London: Heinemann.

Zung, W.W., Magill, M., Moore, J.T., and George, D.T. (1983) 'Recognition and treatment of depression in a family medical practice', *Journal of Clinical Psychiatry* 44:3–6.

Part II

Psychiatric field surveys in the primary health-care setting: an international perspective

Chapter 5

Psychiatric morbidity in general practice

A community-wide perspective

Alex Richman

Many patients in general practice have some type of mental disorder. What proportion of the general population is recognized by general practitioners as having mental disorders? What is the course of further mental health care for those recognized by general practitioners? What is the overlap between the mental disorders recognized in general practice and those seen in specialized psychiatric settings? What is the cumulative probability of mental illness ever being recognized by general practitioners?

Many authors emphasize the high prevalence of mental disorder in primary care (Goldberg and Huxley 1980; Shepherd *et al.* 1981; Wilkinson 1986). The Epidemiologic Catchment Area studies in the USA show that more of the persons with mental disorders in the community visit primary-care services than specialty services (Shapiro *et al.* 1984). Most studies have found that general practitioners fail to recognize a high proportion of cases with mental disorders (Goldberg and Huxley 1980); a few, however, have found that general practitioners recognized most of the disorders identified by other means (von Korff *et al.* 1987). Primary-care physicians in office practice appear to respond with psychotropic medication or counselling more often than they record a diagnosis of mental disorder (Jencks 1985). In addition to the patients with mental disorder seen in office practice, many others treated on medical and surgical wards of general hospitals are not seen by psychiatrists (Hendryx and Bootzin 1986).

Psychiatric case registers have not included patients seen in primary-care settings (ten Horn *et al.* 1986). Wilkinson (1986) emphasized the need for research into both the short- and long-term course and outcome of mental disorders seen in primary-care settings, in order to bring hospital-based longitudinal studies into perspective. There are, so far, no reports on the interrelations of primary care with the specialist sector.

The present contribution describes a province-wide mental health data base that includes data from primary-care offices and general hospital medical and surgical wards. It is the first such study to use case-register types of data to answer questions about primary care.

Table 5.1 Psychiatric resources in New Brunswick, Canada

Type of resource	Rate per 100,000	
	Canada	New Brunswick
Mental hospital beds (under 1 year, 1975/76)	21.0	20.8
General hospital psychiatric unit beds (1975/76)	16.2	8.7
Psychiatrists (public and private practice, 1976)	9.3	4.0

BACKGROUND TO THE STUDY

Regional characteristics

New Brunswick is the third smallest province in Canada with 73,000 sq km. The population of 700,000 is evenly distributed between urban and rural areas with an average density of 9.7 persons per sq km. One-third of the population is French-speaking. During the study period (1975–81), psychiatric services were not as well developed in New Brunswick as in many other parts of Canada, as Table 5.1 indicates.

This study defines mental health-care provision as follows:

Primary mental health care:
patients with an ICD Chapter V diagnosis on a medical or surgical ward of a general hospital who were not seen by a psychiatrist;
patients who, within a two-year period, received three or more psychotherapy or counselling services from a physician who was not a psychiatrist.
Specialist mental health care:
mental hospitals, general hospital psychiatric units, mental health clinics and psychiatrists in private practice.

Source of data on psychiatric services in general practice

Universal national health insurance is available to all Canadian residents on equal terms and conditions. The programme covers hospital and private office care without any restrictions on the amount or duration of care. Patients may select their private physician. The fee-for-service system pays general practitioners for counselling and psychiatric services. There is substantial provision of psychiatric treatment and care services by general

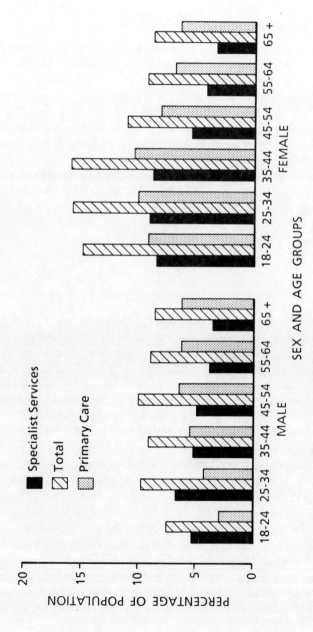

Figure 5.1 Prevalence of treated mental illness, 1975–81

practitioners, who get 40 per cent of the total Medicare payments for psychotherapy and counselling. These payments now account for 7 per cent of the general practitioner's total income from office visits (Richman and Brown 1980). The administrative data bases for payment of private physicians provided the statistical data on psychotherapy and counselling.

Linkage of statistical data from psychiatric services

In 1982 New Brunswick conducted a mental health planning survey (Cash and Richman 1982). The New Brunswick Department of Health produced a research file that collated statistical data from public psychiatric settings (mental hospitals, general hospital psychiatric units and mental health clinics), with data from general hospital medical and surgical wards and private physicians. The data for private physicians included visits to private psychiatrists as well as visits which were recorded as psychotherapy or counselling by physicians other than psychiatrists.

The mental health research data base includes over 90,000 individuals of all ages who were in contact with mental health services between January 1975 and June 1981. Further analyses of these multiple contacts (Richman and Richman 1990) show the longitudinal course of care over two years, following the definitions of the WHO study of patterns of psychiatric care (Giel *et al.* 1987).

RESULTS

Within the 78-month study period, nearly one out of nine (11.0 per cent) persons aged 18 years or over had one or more contacts with the health services in respect of a recorded mental disturbance. Five per cent of adults were in contact *only* with the primary health services. Treated prevalence according to age and sex is shown in Figure 5.1.

The next step was to look at the distribution of new cases during the survey period. These were defined as cases reported during 1977–79 who had no record of mental health contacts during 1975 or 1976. These 'inceptions' are not necessarily first-ever episodes of care, but simply cases reported for the first time during a defined time-period (Last 1983). Table 5.2 shows the distributions for all and for new cases during the years 1975–80.

Most of the inception cases which entered specialist care did so without prior psychiatric contact with primary-care physicians. Few of the specialist cases were recorded later in primary care (Table 5.3). Among the cases first recorded by a general practitioner, one-tenth later came to the specialist services and another one-third had at least two more GP visits for psychotherapy or counselling. In Figure 5.2 these data are presented according to age-group and sex.

Figure 5.3 shows the cumulative probability of receiving primary medical

Table 5.2 Prevalence and inception rates by year and type of service setting, 1975–80

| | Percentage of population (18 years and over) | | | | | |
	1975	1976	1977	1978	1979	1980
Specialist psychiatric services						
Prevalence (one year)	1.0	1.9	2.7	2.8	3.0	3.5
Inceptions	1.0	1.2	1.1	1.0	0.7	0.7
Primary health care only						
Prevalence (ward or any mental health visit within the year)	0.7	1.6	3.2	3.5	3.7	3.8
Inceptions (ward or 3+ mental health visits)	0.5	0.7	0.8	1.0	0.9	0.8

care for a psychiatric disorder. The statistical method used here (Chase and Kramer 1986) converts the age–sex specific inception rates into survival probabilities (non-inceptions), then successively multiplies the survival probabilities to determine the cumulative probability of *not* entering primary care by various ages and finally converts the probabilities of survival into probabilities of receiving primary medical care for a psychiatric disorder. The projection assumes that the 1980 inception rates will remain constant in the future, irrespective of competing causes of morbidity and mortality. This is a conditional probability, referring to persons who do not die; the probability is a theoretical construct describing what would happen if the inception rates continued for a long time (Chase and Kramer 1986; Rorsman *et al*. 1990). For a cohort of 18-year-olds, 22 per cent of

Table 5.3 Inceptions: cases recorded during 1977–79 and not in 1975–76

Agency of first contact	Annual rate per 100,000 (18 years +)	Proportion with later primary psychiatric care (%)
Mental health clinic	336	5
Private psychiatrist	285	4
Psychiatric in-patient	75	7
Medical or surgical ward	447	–
General practitioner	547	–

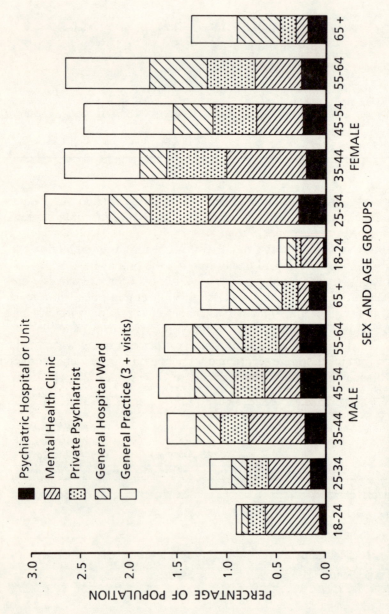

Figure 5.2 Inception of psychiatric treatment, by age-group and setting of first contact, New Brunswick, 1977–79

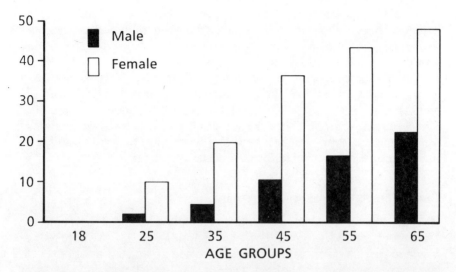

Figure 5.3 Primary medical care for mental disorder: cumulative percentage in cohort of 18-year-olds

males and 48 per cent of females would receive primary medical care for a mental disorder by the age of 65.

DISCUSSION

Recognition of mental disorders by general practitioners

There is a substantial recognition of mental disorder by general practitioners in New Brunswick. Altogether, during the period 1975–81, 7 per cent of the adult inhabitants were recorded by physicians within non-specialist settings as having a mental disorder. The proportion was lower for men (5 per cent) than for women (9 per cent). The cumulative probability of eventual contact with primary-care services for mental problems, between ages 18 and 65, is 22 per cent for men and 48 per cent for women. There is thus no support for the belief that general practitioners do not recognize a substantial amount of mental disorder in their case load.

There is a spectrum of severity and disability in mental disorders. It seems probable from the duration of contact and subsequent course that many of the disorders which received counselling or psychotherapy were mild or transient. It is not possible, however, to distinguish the type or severity of disorders in this data base. Recognition and intervention occurred early; there was little evidence of markedly increased medical costs before the initial visit for counselling or psychotherapy (Richman 1990).

There is a substantial group of patients who enter specialist mental health services without any prior contact with general practitioners. Over four-fifths of cases seen in specialist mental health services had no reported previous mental health contacts with general practitioners. The 'filter' model of illness-recognition and referral (Goldberg and Huxley 1980) does not apply, therefore, in this Canadian setting. A recent study in another region of Canada (Diaz and Richman 1990) shows that the filter model is more appropriate for the sub-group of patients with psychosocial disorders; general practitioners tend to 'psychiatrize' these cases and refer them more readily to mental health specialist settings.

Case finding in general practice settings

It is still difficult to relate data from community prevalence surveys to the kinds of service and amounts of care needed (Regier 1983). We have not yet begun to specify which 'cases' should be treated by which professional with what means at which level of care and for how long (Beigel and Sharfstein 1984; Barrett *et al.* 1988). It is not enough for programme planning that a person has a disorder to be counted; the case must be recognized as a disorder by someone (Sartorius 1985).

Further progress in psychiatric epidemiology does not require more cross-sectional prevalence studies in primary-care settings. We do not need further 'tests' of the extent to which general practitioners can use diagnostic terms derived from specialist settings. Psychiatric epidemiology needs long-term longitudinal studies that differentiate major disorders from the 'minor' disorders more frequently seen in primary care. We need to unravel the natural history of morbidity, to differentiate psychiatric prodromata, incipient disorders, sub-clinical cases, 'formes frustes' and atypical conditions. Psychiatric epidemiologists should collaborate with primary practitioners in developing a better understanding of the various forms of psychiatric morbidity which abound in primary health care, but do not fit easily into the International Classification of Diseases or the APA Diagnostic and Statistical Manual's classification. We need to identify those cases which will not recover without intervention and to determine which forms of intervention are most effective in primary-care settings (Barrett *et al.* 1988).

Patterns of psychiatric care: intersectoral studies

Until recent years there have been few systematic comparisons of different patterns of psychiatric care. The recent European multicentre comparison of patterns of care (Giel *et al.* 1987) focused on specialist psychiatric services. We need further studies of patterns of care that include also services in the primary-care sector. This contribution demonstrates that intersectoral studies of specialist and primary care are feasible and can be informative.

REFERENCES

Barrett, J.E., Oxman, T.E., and Gerber, P.D. (1988) 'The prevalence of psychiatric disorders in a primary care practice', *Archives of General Psychiatry* 45:1100–6.
Beigel, A. and Sharfstein, S.S. (1984) 'Mental health providers: not the only cause or only cure for rising costs', *American Journal of Psychiatry* 141:668–72.
Cash, L. and Richman, A. (1982) *Report of the Southern New Brunswick Mental Health Planning Committee*, St John. New Brunswick: Dept of Health.
Chase, G.A. and Kramer, M. (1986) 'The abridged census method as an estimator of lifetime risk', *Psychological Medicine* 16:865–71.
Diaz, P. and Richman, A. (1990) Psychiatrization of psychosocial predicaments in primary care: what can general practitioners do about it? Unpublished Ms. Nova Scotia: Dalhousie University.
Giel, R., Henderson, J.H., and ten Horn, G.H.M.M. (eds) (1987) *Mental Health Services in Pilot Study Areas: Report on a European Study*, Copenhagen: World Health Organization Regional Office for Europe.
Goldberg, D. and Huxley, P. (1980) *Mental Illness in the Community: the Pathway to Psychiatric Care*, London: Tavistock.
Hendryx, M. and Bootzin, R.R. (1986) 'Psychiatric episodes in general hospitals without psychiatric units', *Hospital and Community Psychiatry* 37:1025–9.
Jencks, S.F. (1985) 'Recognition of mental distress and diagnosis of mental disorder in primary care', *Journal of the American Medical Association* 253:1903–7.
Korff, M. von, Shapiro, S., Burke, J.D., Teitelbaum, M., Skinner, E.A., German, P., Turner, R.W., Klein, L., and Burns, B. (1987) 'Anxiety and depression in a primary care clinic', *Archives of General Psychiatry* 44:152–8.
Last, J.M. (ed.) (1983) *A Dictionary of Epidemiology*, New York: Oxford University Press.
Regier, D. (1983) 'Epidemiological information for mental health programs', in E.M. Laska, W.H. Gulbinat, and D.A. Regier (eds) *Information Support to Mental Health Programs*, New York: Human Sciences Press.
Richman, A. (1990) 'Do psychiatric services from general practitioners reduce the cost of medical care?', *General Hospital Psychiatry* 12:19–22.
Richman, A. and Brown, M.G. (1980) 'Reimbursement by Medicare for mental health services by general practitioners', in *Mental Health Services in Primary Care Settings: Report of a Conference*, 2–3 April 1979, Washington, DC: US Govt Printing Office.
Richman, E.M. and Richman, A. (1990) 'Converting divergent administrative data bases to person-based summaries', in *Proceedings of the Record Linkage Sessions and Workshop*, Canadian Epidemiology Research Conference, 1989, Ottawa: Select Printing Inc.
Rorsman, B., Grasbeck, A., Hagnell, O., Lanke, J., Ohman, R., Öjesjö, L., and Otterbeck, L. (1990) 'A prospective study of first incidence depression: the Lundby study, 1957–72', *British Journal of Psychiatry* 156:336–42.
Sartorius, N. (1985) 'The epidemiology of mental health disorders and public health policy', in *Research Findings Significant to Priority Setting for Mental Health Services*, Ottawa: Minister of Supply and Services, Canada.
Shapiro, S., Skinner, E., Kessler, L.G., Korff, M.R. von, German, P.S., Tischler,

G.L., Leaf, P.J., Bentham, L., Cottler, L., and Regier, D. (1984) 'Utilization of health and mental health services', *Archives of General Psychiatry* 41:971–82.

Shepherd, M., Cooper, B., Brown, A.C., and Kalton, G. (1981) *Psychiatric Illness in General Practice*, second edn, New York: Oxford University Press.

ten Horn, G.H.M.M., Giel, R., Gulbinat, W.H., and Henderson, J.H. (1986) *Psychiatric Case Registers in Public Health: a World-wide Inventory 1960–1985*, Amsterdam: Elsevier.

Wilkinson, G. (1986) *Overview of Mental Health Practices in Primary Care Settings*, National Institute of Mental Health Series DN No. 7, DHHS Publication No. (ADM) 86–1467, Washington, DC: US Govt Printing Office.

Chapter 6

The epidemiological basis for mental health care in primary health care

A case for action

Morton Kramer, Eleanor Simonsick, Bruno Lima and Itzhak Levav

A considerable number of studies have repeatedly demonstrated a strong association between physical and psychiatric disorders in the general population (Shepherd *et al.* 1981; Eastwood 1989; Wells *et al.* 1988; 1989). This chapter reports data, collected in a population-based survey of the prevalence of mental disorders in a defined area of Baltimore, Maryland, USA, that also demonstrate this association and goes further. Information was also collected from each survey subject on the presence or absence of selected physical disorders and on his or her use of health services. As a result it was possible to determine the prevalence rates of mental and physical disorders, either singly or in combination, for the survey population as well as the rates at which its members, with and without these disorders, utilized health services.

These prevalence and utilization data provide the background for a discussion of the extent to which the general and mental health agencies of the USA provide services to persons with mental disorder and suggest possible actions to improve the situation.

MATERIAL AND METHODS

1 The Eastern Baltimore Mental Health Survey

The Eastern Baltimore Mental Health Survey was carried out as part of the Epidemiologic Catchment Area programme of the National Institute of Mental Health (NIMH) (Regier *et al.* 1984). The survey area consists of three mental health catchment areas of Eastern Baltimore, each with different demographic characteristics. One area, that of the Johns Hopkins Hospital, has a high proportion of black residents and of families below the poverty level. A second area, that of the Baltimore City Hospital, is predominantly white working class with many ethnic neighbourhoods. The third area, Harbel, is predominantly white middle class. In 1980 the total population census count of the three areas combined was 241,196, of whom 176,353 (72 per cent) were 18 years or older. About 38 per cent of the population were black and 22 per cent were living below the poverty level.

2 Survey design

The survey design consisted of a multistage area probability sample of 3,817 households, about 4.5 per cent of all households in the area. Trained interviewers visited these households and obtained rosters of the members for 95 per cent. In each household, one member aged 18–64 years was chosen at random for interview and any members aged 65 years or over were also designated for interview. Of the 4,238 designated respondents, 3,481 (82 per cent) were interviewed.

3 The interview instrument

The interview instrument includes the Diagnostic Interview Schedule (DIS) (Robins *et al*. 1981), the Mini Mental Status Examination (MMSE) adapted for field research (Folstein *et al*. 1975), a series of questions related to physical disorders and an array of questions on demographic, social and economic variables and utilization of mental health, general health and other human services.

DIS/DSM-III mental disorders

The presence or absence of a DIS/DSM-III disorder is determined from responses to the Diagnostic Interview Schedule (DIS), a fully structured questionnaire, designed for use by lay interviewers, to obtain data for assessing whether or not a subject fulfils DSM-III criteria for selected mental disorders. The responses are analysed by a computer program with algorithms for the following diagnoses: (1) alcohol use disorder (alcohol abuse/dependence); (2) drug use disorder (drug abuse/dependence); (3) schizophrenic disorders (schizophrenic and schizophreniform disorders); (4) major affective disorders, including major depressive episode, bipolar disorder and dysthymia (lifetime); (5) anxiety and related disorders, including phobic disorders, panic disorder, obsessive compulsive disorder and somatization disorder; and (6) anti-social personality.

The DIS also includes severe cognitive impairment, defined as persons who scored less than 17 on the adapted MMSE.

It is important to note that the DIS does not cover all DSM-III diagnostic categories, but only those listed above. Thus, some persons classified as not meeting criteria for a DIS disorder may have had psychiatric conditions or symptoms not covered by the DIS.

The DIS produces DSM-III diagnoses with reference to several discrete time periods preceding interview: two weeks, one month, six months, one year and the entire lifetime. In this chapter, the presence of an active episode of a DIS/DSM-III disorder in the six months prior to interview is used. These episodes will be referred to as *recent*.

In the text and tables that follow the term 'mental disorder(s)' is used in lieu of the term 'DIS/DSM-III Disorder(s)'.

Physical disorders

Questions were included in the survey instrument to determine whether a respondent fulfilled criteria for a DIS/DSM-III diagnosis and whether he or she reported one or more of the following conditions: asthma; high blood sugar or diabetes; heart trouble; high blood pressure; breathing trouble (apart from asthma or heart trouble); arthritis or rheumatism; stroke; cancer.

The questions related to each condition were as follows:

1 Have you ever had_____?   ____Yes ____No
2 Do you have (the condition) now?   ____Yes ____No
3 Are you receiving regular care from a health professional such as a
  doctor or nurse practitioner for this condition?   ____Yes ____No

The responses to questions (2) and (3) for each of the above conditions were used in the analyses presented here. Responses to the questions relating to stroke and cancer were too few in number to be used in the detailed analyses but they are included in the totals for persons having any physical disorder.

The data on presence or absence of a physical disorder may not be fully reliable since they are based on self-reports, not on the results of a physical examination by a physician. Nevertheless, they provide a basis for obtaining an estimate of the extent to which persons with a recent DIS/DSM-III disorder report a specified physical disorder and, vice versa, the extent to which persons reporting a physical disorder fulfilled criteria for a recent DIS/DSM-III disorder.

Mental health and general medical services

The utilization data concern visits to ambulatory health services in the six months prior to interview by all members of the survey sample 'to get help for problems with emotions, nerves, drugs, alcohol or their mental health', and how these visits are divided between the general medical and specialty mental health agencies. The six-month period is the same as that used to estimate prevalence rates for DIS/DSM-III disorders (Shapiro *et al.* 1984). The types of resources included under the categories of specialty mental health and general medical agencies are those used by Shapiro and colleagues; namely:

Specialty mental health agencies: Psychiatrists, psychologists, psychiatric social workers, mental health counsellors in private practice or in health plans or family clinics; mental health centres; psychiatric out-patient clinics at general or Veterans Administration hospitals; out-patient clinics at psychiatric hospitals; drug treatment clinics; alcohol treatment clinics.

General medical agencies: Medical practitioners (other than psychiatrists) to whom out-patient visits were made for any health problem, including emotional or mental health problems.

4 Method of analyses

The results reported here are from the following types of analyses: (1) prevalence rates of mental and physical disorders, singly and in combination; (2) odds ratios for the prevalence of selected mental disorders among persons reporting a physical disorder by selected demographic variables and vice versa; (3) prevalence of the combined occurrence of selected mental and physical disorders; (4) percentage of persons utilizing health services within six months prior to interview who have: (a) no physical or mental disorder; (b) physical disorder only; (c) mental disorder only; (d) both physical and mental disorder.

Prevalence rates and percentage distributions are based on weighted data. The weights take into account response rates, sample selection probabilities and adjustments to 1980 census totals for Eastern Baltimore by age, sex and race (Eaton and Kessler 1985). The weighted data were used to determine the distribution of the population 18 years and over by various demographic factors and to compute the corresponding prevalence rates.

RESULTS

1 Demographic characteristics of the survey population

The distribution of the sample population aged 18 and over by the demographic variables used in this chapter and their weighted percentage distributions are given in Table 6.1.

The variables selected are known indicators of high risk for various physical and mental disorders and utilization of health and related services. They reflect the life style, behaviours, value systems, educational and socio-economic status of members of these sub-groups, and also barriers members of such groups are likely to encounter in seeking and obtaining health services. To illustrate, two of the demographic variables are years

Table 6.1 Distribution of population 18 years of age and older by selected demographic characteristics; sample frequencies and weighted per cent distributions: Baltimore ECA, 1980

Demographic characteristics	Sample size	Per cent (weighted)
Total	3,481	100.0
Gender		
Male	1,322	45.4
Female	2,159	54.6
Race		
White	2,193	65.0
Non-white	1,288	35.0
Age-group		
18 to 34	1,294	40.3
35 to 64	1,264	41.9
65 and older	923	17.8
Education		
less than high school	1,886	52.0
high school	948	28.8
more than high school	646	19.2
Marital status		
never married	793	25.2
married	1,474	48.4
separated/divorced	643	14.5
widowed	570	11.9
Household income		
less than $10,000	1,213	31.7
$10,000–$19,999	918	30.7
$20,000 and above	862	37.6
Household type		
Family		
married couple	1,592	56.5
male householder	119	4.0
female householder	768	19.1
Non-family	917	20.4
single person	712	13.6
2 or more persons	205	6.8

of school completed and type of household (family or non-family). In the USA half of all poor family householders* aged 25 years and over had not graduated from high school. About 34 per cent of all female householder

*'Householder' is the term used by the US Bureau of the Census to designate the head of a household

Table 6.2 Distribution of persons 18 years of age and older by presence or
absence of current DIS/DSM-III and physical disorder:
Baltimore ECA, 1980 (weighted)

		DIS/DSM-III disorder		
Reported physical disorder		Present	Absent	Total
Present		20,281	52,783	73,064
Absent		20,765	81,382	102,147
Total		41,046	134,165	175,211
		Per cent of total		
Present		11.6	30.1	41.7
Absent		11.9	46.4	58.3
Total		23.5	76.5	100.0

families (that is, families headed by a woman with no spouse present)
had incomes below the poverty level and 46 per cent of such families
with children were below the poverty level. Persons living alone or with
non-relatives accounted for about 21 per cent of the poor (US Bureau of
the Census 1989). Persons in these categories are at high risk for mental
and neurological disorders, engaging in health damaging behaviours and
developing somatic symptoms resulting from psychosocial stress (WHO
1986). Many of these persons are in need of health and mental health
services (Shapiro *et al*. 1985).

2 Prevalence of physical and psychiatric morbidity

Table 6.2 provides a four-fold distribution of the catchment area population
by the presence or absence of at least one of the eight previously mentioned physical disorders and the presence or absence of a recent mental
disorder.

Overall, 23.5 per cent of the population had at least one mental disorder
and 41.7 per cent at least one physical disorder; 11.6 per cent had both a
mental disorder and a physical disorder; 11.9 per cent had a mental disorder
but no physical disorder; 30.1 per cent had a physical disorder but no mental
disorder and 46.4 per cent had neither a mental nor physical disorder. Thus,
53.6 per cent of the population aged 18 and over of the Baltimore ECA
catchment area had either a mental or physical disorder.

Table 6.3 shows the percentage of persons 18 years of age and older,
in selected demographic groups, with: (a) a physical disorder; (b) the

Table 6.3 Prevalence rates (%) of: (a) all physical disorders; (b) physical disorders only; (c) physical disorders and mental disorders, and (d) percentage of all physical disorders with a mental disorder by selected demographic characteristics* (persons 18 years and older): Baltimore ECA, 1980

Demographic group	All physical disorders	Physical disorders only	Physical disorders and mental disorders	Percentage of all physical disorders with a mental disorder
(1)	(2)=(3)+(4)	(3)	(4)	(5)=(4)/(2)
All persons 18+	41.7	30.1	11.6	27.8
Gender				
Male	37.1	27.3	9.8	26.4
Female	44.6	32.5	13.1	29.3
Race				
White	42.0	31.9	10.1	24.0
Non-white	41.2	26.9	14.3	34.7
Age				
18–34	18.1	9.4	8.7	48.1
35–64	51.8	38.0	38.8	26.6
65+	71.2	58.5	12.7	17.8
Education				
Less than high school	53.6	38.4	15.2	28.4
High school	30.9	22.8	8.1	26.2
More than high school	20.5	13.6	6.9	33.7
Marital status				
Never married	23.0	13.3	9.7	42.2
Married	43.8	34.6	9.2	21.0
Separated/Divorced	45.6	26.4	19.2	42.1
Widowed	68.7	52.4	16.3	23.7
Household income				
Less than $10,000	55.5	38.0	17.5	31.5
$10,000–$19,000	38.5	27.5	12.0	30.0
$20,000 and above	30.6	24.4	6.2	20.2
Household type				
Family				
Married couple	41.2	32.1	9.1	22.1
Male householder	26.0	14.8	11.2	43.1
Female householder	39.5	25.1	14.4	36.4
Non-family				
Single person	56.6	41.3	15.3	27.0
2 or more persons	38.4	20.4	18.0	46.9

* Diagnosis of mental disorders based on the DIS/DSM-III interview (see text)

percentage of the persons with these disorders who also had a mental disorder; and Table 6.4 shows the percentage of persons with: (a) a mental disorder and (b) the percentage of the persons with these disorders who also had a physical disorder. In the text that follows demographic groups are highlighted in which the specified morbidity rate was considerably higher (at least 20 per cent higher) than the corresponding mean morbidity rate for the entire Baltimore ECA population.

Prevalence of physical disorders

The proportion of persons reporting a physical disorder was 41.7 per cent. This percentage increased sharply with advancing age, from 18.1 per cent for persons 18–34, to 71.2 per cent for those 65 and over. The demographic groups with rates considerably higher than average were: persons with less than high school education (53.6 per cent); the widowed (68.7 per cent); the persons with less than $10,000 household income (55.5 per cent) and persons living alone (56.6 per cent).

Percentage of persons with a reported physical disorder who also had a mental disorder

The proportion of persons with a physical disorder who also had a mental disorder was 27.8 per cent (column 5 of Table 6.3). This percentage decreased markedly with advancing age, from 48.1 per cent for persons 18–34 years to 17.8 per cent for persons aged 65 or over. The groups with percentages considerably higher than average were: non-whites (34.7 per cent); the never married (42.2 per cent); the separated and divorced (42.1 per cent); persons living in male and female household families (43.1 per cent and 36.4 per cent, respectively); and those living in non-family households of two or more persons (46.9 per cent).

Prevalence of mental disorders

The proportion of persons 18 years and over who were found to have a mental disorder was 23.5 per cent (Table 6.4). This rate decreased with advancing age, from 27.1 per cent for persons 18–34 to 17.3 per cent for persons 65 years and over. The groups with rates considerably higher than average were: the separated and divorced (34.0 per cent); persons living in female householder families (31.1 per cent) and those living in non-family households of two or more persons (36.8 per cent).

Table 6.4 Prevalence rates (%) of: (a) all mental disorders*; (b) mental disorders only; (c) mental disorders and physical disorders; and (d) percentage of all mental disorders with a physical disorder by selected demographic characteristics (persons 18 years and older): Baltimore ECA, 1980

Demographic group	All mental disorders	Mental disorders only	Mental disorders and physical disorders	Percentage of all mental disorders with a physical disorder
(1)	(2)=(3)+(4)	(3)	(4)	(5)=(4)/(2)
All persons 18+	23.5	11.9	11.6	49.4
Gender				
Male	21.4	11.6	9.8	45.8
Female	25.1	12.0	13.1	52.2
Race				
White	21.3	11.2	10.1	47.4
Non-white	27.3	13.0	14.3	52.4
Age				
18–34	27.1	18.4	8.7	32.1
35–64	22.5	8.7	13.8	61.3
65+	17.3	4.6	12.7	73.4
Education				
Less than high school	25.7	10.6	15.2	59.1
High school	21.0	12.3	8.1	38.6
More than high school	20.5	13.6	6.9	48.4
Marital status				
Never married	26.5	16.8	9.7	36.6
Married	19.0	9.8	9.2	48.4
Separated/Divorced	34.0	14.8	19.2	56.5
Widowed	22.3	6.0	16.3	73.1
Household income				
Less than $10,000	28.0	10.5	17.5	62.5
$10,000–$19,000	25.5	13.5	12.0	47.1
$20,000 and above	18.4	12.2	6.2	33.6
Household type				
Family				
Married couple	19.2	10.1	9.1	47.3
Male householder	22.2	11.0	11.2	50.4
Female householder	31.1	16.7	14.4	46.3
Non-family				
Single person	24.8	9.5	15.3	61.7
2 or more persons	36.8	18.8	18.0	48.9

* Diagnosis of mental disorder based on the results of the DIS/DSM-III interview (see text)

Percentage of persons with a mental disorder who also had a physical disorder

Almost 50 per cent of persons with a mental disorder also had a physical disorder (column 5 of Table 6.4). This percentage increased markedly with age, from 32.1 per cent of persons 18–34 years to 73.4 per cent for persons 65 years or over. The following demographic groups experienced rates considerably higher than average: those with less than high school education (59.1 per cent); the separated and divorced (56.5 per cent); widowed (73.1 per cent); households with income less than $10,000 per year (62.5 per cent); and those living alone (61.7 per cent).

3 Prevalence of specific mental disorders among persons reporting a current physical disorder.

The prevalence of specific mental disorders among persons reporting a physical disorder range from a low of 0.6 per cent for anti-social personality to a high of 18 per cent for anxiety disorders (Table 6.5). Intermediate rates are those for schizophrenic disorders (1.4 per cent), drug use (1.9 per cent), severe cognitive impairment (1.9 per cent), affective disorders (6.0 per cent) and alcohol use (6.9 per cent).

Persons in the youngest age-group with a physical disorder have high prevalence rates of alcohol and drug-use disorders, schizophrenic disorders, affective and anxiety disorders and anti-social personality disorders. Males show a considerable excess of alcohol and drug use and anti-social personality disorders relative to females, who have higher rates of affective and anxiety disorders. Persons separated or divorced have high rates of alcohol-use, affective and anxiety disorders.

4 Prevalence rates of specific physical disorders among persons with a mental disorder

The rates of specific physical disorders among persons with a mental disorder range from 5.2 per cent for diabetes to 26.1 per cent for arthritis (Table 6.6). Intermediate are the rates for asthma (5.7 per cent), heart trouble (10.2 per cent), trouble with breathing (14.2 per cent) and hypertension (19.2 per cent).

In general, the age-specific prevalence rates of each type of physical disorder among persons with a mental disorder increase with advancing age. The following demographic groups were found to have particularly high prevalence rates:

Heart trouble: persons 65 and over; those with less than high-school education; the separated and divorced; the widowed; members of male householder families; persons living alone, and persons living in non-family households of two or more persons.

Arthritis: persons 65 or older; those with less than high-school education; the widowed; those with less than $10,000 household income; members of male householder families and persons living alone.

Hypertension: non-whites; persons 35 years and over; those with less than high-school education; those with low household income; the widowed, and persons living alone.

5 Prevalence rates of specific physical disorders among persons with a specific mental disorder*

Comparison of the prevalence rates of specific physical disorders among persons with a specific mental disorder with the corresponding rates of persons without such disorders demonstrated that persons with:

Drug-use disorder reported heart trouble, hypertension and arthritis much less frequently, a difference most likely attributable to the relatively young age of persons with this mental disorder;

Alcohol-use disorder reported each of the physical disorders about as frequently. An exception was breathing trouble, which was considerably higher for persons with this disorder;

Schizophrenic disorders reported higher prevalence rates of heart trouble but lower rates of hypertension and arthritis;

Affective disorders reported higher prevalence rates of asthma and arthritis;

Anti-social personality reported no diabetes or heart trouble, but a higher rate of asthma and a lower rate of arthritis;

Severe cognitive impairment reported considerably higher rates of each specific physical disorder with the exception of breathing trouble.

6 Prevalence rates of specific mental disorders among persons with a specific physical disorder

Comparison of the prevalence rates of specific mental disorders among persons with a physical disorder with the rates in persons without such a disorder demonstrated that persons with:

Breathing trouble have consistently higher rates of each mental disorder;

Asthma have consistently higher rates of each mental disorder except for alcohol-use disorder for which the rates were about the same.

*The tables on which this and the next section are based are available from the authors.

Table 6.5 Percentage of persons 18 years of age and older with a physical disorder who also had a specific mental disorder[1] by selected demographic characteristics: Baltimore ECA, 1980 (weighted)

Demographic characteristic	*Type of mental disorder*							
	Any disorder	*Alcohol use*	*Drug use*	*Schizophrenic*	*Affective*[2]	*Anxiety*[3]	*Anti-social personality*	*Cognitive impairment*
Sample size	838	158	67	46	175	530	21	60
Weighted total	41,046	9,543	3,785	2,006	7,860	25,350	1,138	2,246
	Persons with a specified mental disorder (weighted)(%)							
All persons 18 +	27.8	6.9	1.9	1.4	6.0	18.2	0.6	1.9
Gender								
Male	26.4	13.7	3.0	0.7	4.3	12.2	1.2	2.4
Female	28.7	2.3	1.2	1.9	7.1	22.3	0.2	1.6
Race								
White	24.1	4.9	1.5	1.2	5.1	16.6	0.5	1.4
Non-white	34.7	10.6	2.8	1.8	7.6	21.2	0.7	2.8
Age-group								
18–34	48.2	13.5	8.7	4.7	12.9	29.9	2.1	1.2
35–64	26.7	7.9	0.8	1.1	5.5	17.5	0.4	0.6
65 and older	17.9	1.2	0.0	0.1	2.6	12.5	0.0	4.8
Education								
Less than high school	28.4	7.2	1.7	1.7	6.3	19.0	0.6	2.7
High school	26.3	5.3	1.9	0.5	4.8	17.7	0.8	0.2
More than high school	27.0	7.6	3.3	1.2	5.9	14.0	0.0	0.4
Marital status								
Never married	42.0	13.1	7.1	2.2	9.9	29.8	2.2	1.3
Married	21.0	3.7	1.2	1.1	3.7	14.1	0.2	1.0
Separated/Divorced	42.0	15.4	2.2	3.4	11.0	23.9	1.1	2.7
Widowed	23.7	3.4	0.0	0.0	4.9	15.8	0.0	4.2

Household income							
Less than $10,000	31.6	8.3	1.0	1.8	7.1	21.1	0.6	2.7
$10,000–$19,999	30.5	6.7	2.1	1.8	7.3	21.7	0.8	1.3
$20,000 and above	20.2	5.9	3.5	0.9	4.0	11.0	0.0	0.2
Household type							
Family							
Married couple	22.2	4.4	2.2	1.5	4.8	14.9	0.4	0.9
Male householder	43.0	15.6	1.7	1.6	12.4	25.9	1.9	4.1
Female householder	36.5	8.4	2.3	2.2	6.7	26.7	1.2	2.7
Non-family							
Single person	32.1	10.5	1.0	0.6	7.3	18.4	0.4	3.2
	27.0	7.0	0.7	0.4	6.9	15.9	0.0	3.7
2 or more persons	46.9	21.2	1.7	1.1	8.5	25.9	1.6	1.5

[1] Diagnosis of mental disorder based on results of the DIS/DSM-III interview (see text)
[2] Includes dysthymia
[3] Includes phobic, panic, obsessive compulsive and somatization disorders

Table 6.6 Percentage of persons 18 years of age and older with a mental disorder* who reported a specific physical disorder by selected demographic characteristics: Baltimore ECA, 1980 (weighted)

Demographic characteristics	Any physical disorder	Type of physical disorder					
		Asthma	Diabetes	Heart trouble	Hypertension	Arthritis	Breathing trouble
Sample size	1,574	151	199	346	657	926	282
Weighted total	73,064	6,565	8,986	14,880	30,134	41,049	13,215
		Persons with specified physical disorder (weighted)(%)					
All persons 18 +	49.4	5.7	5.2	10.2	19.2	26.1	14.2
Gender							
Male	45.8	6.0	5.2	10.4	16.6	23.8	15.2
Female	52.2	5.5	5.2	9.9	21.1	27.7	13.5
Race							
White	47.4	5.8	4.9	9.3	15.4	28.4	14.1
Non-white	52.4	5.5	5.6	11.3	24.7	22.7	14.4
Age-group							
18–34	32.1	4.1	1.0	4.1	7.2	10.7	12.6
35–64	61.3	7.1	8.4	12.1	28.4	35.8	16.0
65 and older	73.4	7.0	10.2	25.8	33.4	50.6	14.5
Education							
Less than high school	59.1	6.8	6.6	13.8	25.4	32.1	17.8
High school	38.6	5.5	3.0	4.8	12.7	17.8	10.4
More than high school	33.7	2.4	3.8	5.7	8.3	18.0	7.8
Marital status							
Never married	36.6	5.2	0.8	7.1	9.8	15.7	12.6
Married	48.4	3.9	6.4	8.6	18.4	24.6	10.7
Separated/Divorced	56.5	9.0	6.5	13.3	23.6	30.9	21.8
Widowed	71.3	7.0	9.6	17.1	37.7	48.6	16.2

Household income						
Less than $10,000	62.5	6.8	5.2	12.5	29.2	33.5	20.5
$10,000–$19,999	47.0	4.7	4.2	10.2	15.9	25.0	11.5
$20,000 and above	33.6	5.7	5.3	5.7	10.2	13.1	10.3
Household type						
Family						
Married couple	47.3	5.3	5.0	8.0	17.1	24.0	12.4
Male householder	50.4	2.3	6.2	15.1	22.7	40.7	21.7
Female householder	46.3	6.5	5.0	8.9	18.0	17.9	14.8
Non-family	56.2	6.1	5.5	14.7	24.2	35.6	15.9
Single person	61.7	7.0	6.8	14.5	30.5	40.6	20.1
2 or more persons	48.9	4.8	3.8	14.9	15.7	29.0	10.2

* Diagnoses of mental disorder based on results of DIS/DSM-III interview (see text)

Persons reporting diabetes, heart trouble, hypertension and arthritis have rates of specific mental disorders similar to those of other members of the survey population.

7 Odds ratios for persons with a physical disorder having a mental disorder by demographic variables

In the preceding sections prevalence rates of mental disorders among persons with a physical disorder were presented for each of a set of demographic variables: sex, race, age, education, marital status, annual household income and type of household. To disentangle the interrelationships among these variables a logistic regression was carried out in which each variable was dichotomized and the odds ratio (that is, the ratio of the prevalence rates of each of the two subdivisions of the variable) determined.

The reference categories for the demographic variables are: *sex*: males; *race*: whites; *age*: persons 35 and older; *education*: persons with more than high-school education; *marital status*: married; *income*: persons in households with income of $20,000 or more; *household type*: married couple family.

The results for each demographic variable and selected mental disorders are presented in Table 6.7. Those for household type are presented in Table 6.8.

Odds ratios of specific mental disorder

Odds ratios for persons with a physical disorder having a mental disorder are significantly higher for: persons 18–34 years (3.31, p <.001); unmarried (1.55, p<.01); and persons with household income of less than $20,000 (1.54, p <.01). The odds ratios were somewhat higher for non-whites and for persons with less than high-school education, but the differences were not significant. The odds ratio for females was only slightly less than that of males (Table 6.7).

The odds ratio for persons with a physical disorder having an alcohol-use disorder was significantly lower for females (0.13, p<.001). The corresponding ratios are significantly higher for non-whites (2.02, p<.01), persons aged 18–34 years (2.34, p<.001), and the unmarried (2.92, p<.001). The ratio for persons with household income less than $20,000 was higher than that for persons with higher income but not significantly so. The reciprocal of the odds ratio for females yields an extraordinarily high odds ratio for males – the odds of a male with a physical disorder having an alcohol-use disorder is nine times that of a female.

The odds ratios for persons with a physical disorder having an affective

Table 6.7 Adjusted odds ratios,[1,2] for the prevalence of any mental disorder[3] and selected disorders among persons reporting a physical disorder: Baltimore ECA, 1980 (unweighted)

| Demographic characteristics[4] | Any mental disorder | Type of mental disorder | | |
		Alcohol use disorder	Affective disorders	Anxiety disorders
Female	0.99 (0.76, 1.30)	0.13*** (0.08, 0.22)	1.44 (0.85, 2.46)	1.80*** (1.30, 2.51)
Non-white	1.20 (0.92, 1.55)	2.02** (1.23, 3.29)	1.00 (0.63, 1.60)	1.14 (0.84, 1.54)
Age 18–34	3.31*** (2.39, 4.62)	2.34** (1.30, 4.22)	2.86*** (1.68, 4.85)	2.61** (1.82, 3.74)
Less than high-school education	1.19 (0.89, 1.58)	1.43 (0.79, 2.59)	0.99 (0.59, 1.65)	1.27 (0.92, 1.77)
Unmarried	1.55** (1.19, 2.03)	2.92*** (1.67, 5.10)	2.08** (1.22, 3.53)	1.31 (0.96, 1.79)
Household income less than $20,000	1.54* (1.07, 2.20)	1.45 (0.73, 2.86)	1.30 (0.67, 2.51)	1.68* (1.09, 2.60)

[1] Odds ratios are based on unweighted sample data. They are adjusted to show the association of each demographic characteristic independent of the others with the odds of a person with a physical disorder having a specific DIS/DSM-III disorder. Values greater than *one* indicate that a disorder is more prevalent in that demographic group than in its reference category

[2] The asterisks after an odds ratio designate the level of the significance of the difference between the odds ratio for a characteristic and its reference category: *, $p<.05$; **, $p<.01$; ***, $p<.001$

[3] The diagnosis of mental disorder is based on the results of the DIS/DSM-III interview (see text)

[4] The ratios for each demographic group are: females/males; age 18–34/age 35 and over; unmarried/married; less than high-school education/more than high-school education; household income less than $20,000/household income more than $20,000

disorder are significantly higher for persons aged 18–34 years (2.86, $p<.001$), and the unmarried (2.08, $p<.01$). The corresponding ratios for females and for persons with household income less than $20,000 are somewhat higher than those of their reference categories, but the differences are not statistically significant. The ratios for non-whites and for persons with less than high-school education are about the same as those of their respective reference categories.

The odds ratios for anxiety disorders are significantly higher for females (1.80, $p<.001$), persons aged 18–34 years (2.61, $p<.01$) and those with household incomes less than $20,000 (1.68, $p<.05$). The ratios for non-whites, persons with less than high-school education and the unmarried are higher than those of their reference categories, but the differences are not significant.

Odds ratios by household type

The odds that persons with a physical disorder also have a mental disorder were significantly higher for persons living in female householder families and in each type of non-family household than for persons living in married couple families. However, the differences were significant only for the following specific disorders and household types (Table 6.8):

Alcohol use disorder: female householder families (2.94, p<.05); persons living alone (2.58, p<.01) and persons living in non-family households of two or more persons (3.82, p<.01);
Affective disorders: persons living alone (2.24, p<.01).

8 Odds ratios for persons with a mental disorder having a physical disorder by demographic variables.*

Odds ratios for having a physical disorder among persons with a mental disorder are significantly lower for persons 18–34 years of age (0.26, p<.001). The corresponding ratios are significantly higher for persons with less than high-school education (1.82, p <.001), and for those with less than $20,000 household income (1.93, p <.01). The ratios are higher for non-whites and unmarried but not significantly so, while that for females was about the same as that for males.

For *arthritis* the odds ratios were significantly lower for persons 18–34 years (.19, p <.001) and significantly higher for persons with less than high-school education (1.62, p<.05) and persons with household income less than $20,000 (2.10, p<.01).

For *hypertension*, the ratios were significantly higher for non-whites (2.21, p<.001), persons 35 years and older (4.76, p<.001), persons with less than high-school education (1.86, p<.01) and persons with household income less than $20,000 (2.08, p<.05).

For *heart trouble*, finally, the odds ratios were significantly higher for persons 35 and over (3.57, p<.001) and persons with less than high-school education (1.94, p<.05). The analyses by household type yielded no significant differences.

9 Utilization of health and mental health agencies

Table 6.9 presents the proportion of subjects who made any health or mental health visit during the six months prior to interview for: (1) all

*The table for these analyses is available from the authors.

Table 6.8 Prevalence odds ratios[1] associated with household type relative to those for married couple families for any mental disorder and selected disorders among persons reporting a current physical disorder, adjusted for sex, race, age, education and household income: Baltimore ECA, 1980

Household type[3]	Any mental disorder	Type of mental disorder[2] Alcohol-use disorder	Affective disorders	Anxiety disorders
Family				
Male householder	1.70 (0.73, 3.94)	1.02 (0.21, 4.96)	1.77 (0.38, 8.32)	2.03 (0.76, 5.42)
Female householder	1.58* (1.08, 2.29)	2.94* (1.26, 6.89)	1.46 (0.75, 2.84)	1.48 (0.99, 2.22)
Non-family				
Single person	1.43* (1.04, 1.97)	2.58** (1.36, 4.90)	2.24** (1.22, 4.11)	1.08 (0.75, 1.57)
2 or more persons	2.45** (1.36, 4.41)	3.82** (1.55, 9.39)	1.97 (0.74, 5.28)	1.55 (0.78, 3.08)

[1] These ratios are based on unweighted sample data
[2] The asterisks after an odds ratio designate the level of the significance of the difference between the odds ratio for its characteristic and that of the married couple family
[3] The reference category for each household type is married couple family

subjects; (2) subjects with no physical or mental disorder; (3) subjects with a physical disorder only; (4) subjects with a mental disorder only; (5) subjects with both a physical and mental disorder. It also presents the proportion of subjects in each of these five categories who made an out-patient mental health visit according to whether the visit was to a general medical or to a mental health agency.*

Contacts with a health agency

Of all adults 58.4 per cent made a general health or mental health visit during the six months prior to the interview. The utilization rate was lowest for persons with no physical or mental disorder (46.0 per cent) and highest for persons with both mental and physical disorders (76.0 per cent). The rates for persons with mental disorder only and physical disorder only were intermediate – 58.2 per cent and 70.8 per cent, respectively. This pattern of low utilization rates for persons with neither condition, high rates for those persons with both a physical and mental disorder and intermediate rates

*Table 6.9 presents utilization rates by sex, race and age only. The rates for the other demographic variables are available from the authors.

Table 6.9 Percentage of ambulatory health and/or mental health visits in past six months by persons with: (1) no mental or physical disorder; (2) physical disorder only; (3) mental disorder only; (4) both physical and mental disorder, by sex, race and age: Baltimore ECA, 1980 (weighted)*

| | | Persons with | | | |
	All persons	No mental or physical disorder	Physical disorder only	Mental disorder only	Physical and mental disorder
All persons					
Any health or mental health visit	58.4	46.0	70.8	58.2	76.0
Any mental health visit	7.1	3.6	6.0	11.7	19.5
General medical provider only	3.7	1.8	3.9	5.0	10.0
Mental health specialist	3.4	1.8	2.2	6.7	9.4
Males					
Any health or mental health visit	51.6	39.6	69.4	46.7	70.8
Any mental health visit	6.2	2.7	6.0	9.9	20.8
General medical provider only	2.9	1.1	4.0	3.8	8.7
Mental health specialist	3.3	1.6	2.0	6.1	12.1
Females					
Any health or mental health visit	64.0	52.5	71.8	67.5	79.3
Any mental health visit	7.9	4.5	6.0	13.2	18.6
General medical provider only	4.4	2.4	3.8	6.0	10.9
Mental health specialist	3.5	2.1	2.2	7.2	7.7
Whites					
Any health or mental health visit	57.2	44.8	72.6	57.9	76.5
Any mental health visit	6.0	3.5	6.1	12.8	20.0
General medical provider only	4.1	2.1	4.1	6.5	10.7
Mental health specialist	1.9	1.4	2.0	6.3	9.3
Non-whites					
Any health or mental health visit	58.6	48.4	66.9	58.7	75.4
Any mental health visit	7.3	3.7	6.0	10.0	18.8
General medical provider only	3.0	1.0	3.4	2.6	9.2
Mental health specialist	4.3	2.7	2.6	7.4	9.6
Age 18–34					
Any health or mental health visit	58.1	53.1	68.2	60.8	77.6
Any mental health visit	7.4	4.2	9.3	9.4	24.6
General medical provider only	2.7	1.9	4.5	3.6	5.1
Mental health specialist	4.7	2.3	4.8	5.8	19.5
Age 35–64					
Any health or mental health visit	57.7	38.8	71.7	56.4	74.3
Any mental health visit	8.7	3.5	6.9	19.1	21.6
General medical provider only	5.2	1.9	4.1	9.0	14.9
Mental health specialist	3.5	1.6	2.8	10.1	6.7
Age 65 and over					
Any health or mental health visit	61.0	31.7	70.4	43.0	77.9
Any mental health visit	3.2	0.4	3.5	0.0	6.1
General medical provider only	2.7	0.4	3.3	0.0	5.3
Mental health specialist	0.5	0.0	0.2	0.0	0.8

*The tables which present the visit rates for persons in the other demographic groups are available from the authors for persons with a mental disorder only and those with a physical disorder only was consistent over all demographic groups.

Contacts with mental health resources

Only 7 per cent of all adults made an out-patient visit related to a mental health problem (Shapiro *et al.* 1984). Half of these visits were to general medical agencies and the other half to mental health agencies. Again the mental health visit rate was lowest for persons with physical disorder only (6 per cent), twice as high for persons with a mental disorder only (11.7 per cent), and more than three times as high as the lowest rate for persons with both physical and mental disorders (19.5 per cent). The percentage of mental health visits made to general medical agencies varied by disorder category, being 50 per cent for persons with no physical or mental disorder, 67 per cent for persons with physical disorder only, 43 per cent for persons with a mental disorder only and 51 per cent for persons with both disorders.

Of particular interest are the differences in the rate of out-patient mental health visits to general medical agencies made by members of the different demographic categories. An index was created to demonstrate this variation; namely the number and percentage of the twenty-two demographic categories listed in Table 6.1 in which the percentage of mental health visits to a general medical agency was 50 per cent or more of the total mental health visits. The percentages for each of the several classes of subjects are as follows:

All subjects	13/22 = 59%
Subjects with:	
No mental or physical disorder	11/22 = 50%
Physical disorder only	17/22 = 77%
Mental disorder only	5/22 = 23%
Both mental and physical disorders	12/22 = 55%

The demographic categories with high percentages of mental health visits to a *general medical agency* were: females, whites, persons 35–64 and 65 and over, persons with less than high-school education, the married, the widowed, persons in households with incomes of $10,000 or more, persons in married couple families, and those in female householder families.

The demographic categories with high percentage of visits to a *mental health agency* were: males, non-whites, persons in age-group 18–34, persons with high-school and post-high-school education, the never married, persons in households with incomes of less than $10,000, persons living alone and those in non-family households of two or more persons.

DISCUSSION

This chapter reports the prevalence rates of mental and physical disorders, singly and in combination, among persons 18 years of age and over resident in the Baltimore ECA area, and the rates of utilization of health and mental health services by persons with and without these disorders specific for age, sex, race, marital status, level of education, household income and type of family and non-family households in which persons live.

Overall, 42 per cent of the survey population reported a physical disorder and 23 per cent were found to have a recent mental disorder. More than one quarter (27 per cent) of persons with a physical disorder also had a mental disorder and about half (49 per cent) of persons with a mental disorder also reported a physical disorder.

The prevalence rates of mental disorder among persons with physical disorder and of physical disorders among persons with mental disorder specific for the above-mentioned demographic variables demonstrate the complexity of co-morbidity phenomena. Odds ratio analyses, carried out to disentangle the interrelationships among these demographic variables, demonstrated the strong associations between the prevalence of mental disorder among persons with a physical disorder and a single demographic variable.

To illustrate, co-morbidity rates are particularly high for persons in demographic groups at high risk of having a mental disorder. A striking example is the significantly high odds ratios for persons with a physical disorder having alcohol use disorder. For males the ratio is nine times that for females; for non-whites, twice that for whites; for persons 18–34 years of age, more than twice that for older persons; and for the unmarried, three times that for the married.

Persons with a physical disorder living in female householder families, living alone or in non-family households, are also at a significantly high risk of having alcohol-use disorder. The respective odds are, 2.9, 2.6 and 3.8 times that of persons living in married couple families.

To unravel the reasons for the differences observed in the prevalence of the various combinations of mental and physical disorders requires an intensive multidisciplinary research effort designed to determine the role of a specific physical disorder in placing members of a specific demographic group or living arrangement with that disorder at higher risk of having a specific mental disorder and vice versa.

Studies are also needed to complete the clinical picture of persons with combined disorders (Morris 1975); that is, to determine their physical, mental and functional status at various points in time following onset of each disorder and their mortality rates. Such studies must take into account the treatments patients receive, demographic variables, other variables that characterize the subjects' life style, socio-economic status and degree of social support, as well as factors that influence their pathways to medical and psychiatric care.

As indicated earlier, the data on the prevalence of physical disorders are based on respondents' answers to questions as to whether they had one or more of the following conditions: diabetes, heart trouble, high blood pressure, trouble with breathing, arthritis and rheumatism, stroke or cancer. Accordingly, the prevalence rates reported here may be unreliable. Nevertheless, they serve to emphasize the high levels of co-morbidity likely to exist in the general population. This lack of reliability of the diagnosis of physical disorders underscores the need to include in future population-based surveys a carefully structured physical examination administered by well-trained physicians.

The diagnosis of mental disorder is based on computer analysis of responses to a carefully structured interview that operationalized DSM-III diagnostic criteria (Robins *et al.* 1981) and was administered by well-trained lay interviewers. However, the evidence is mixed as to how well diagnoses so obtained compare to diagnoses made by psychiatrists using standardized clinical examinations (Anthony *et al.* 1985; Helzer *et al.* 1985). Problems such as these underscore the need to improve case-finding techniques for detecting co-morbidity in population surveys.

This chapter also highlights several major problems related to utilization of general health and mental health services:

1 Substantial proportions of persons with physical or mental disorders or combinations of these disorders did *not* utilize a health service within six months prior to interview: 29 per cent of persons with physical disorder only; 42 per cent of persons with mental disorder only and 24 per cent for persons with both disorders.
2 Only a small proportion of persons (7.1 per cent) made a visit to either a general medical or mental health agency for a mental health problem.
3 A substantial proportion (50 per cent) of all mental health visits are made to general medical agencies.
4 Persons with both mental and physical disorders had higher rates of mental health visits (20 per cent) than did persons with mental disorder only (12 per cent) or physical disorder only (6 per cent).

The foregoing rates of morbidity and health services utilization highlight the seriousness of problems facing health officers and primary health care physicians.

Health officers must plan, develop and implement programmes to protect and promote the health of their communities. Such programmes must influence and educate persons to develop and lead healthier life styles. The health officials must identify groups needing special attention and constantly seek and develop new methods for monitoring the community's health (Morris 1975). They must collaborate with other governmental and non-governmental agencies in the development of programmes to reduce levels of poverty, illiteracy, unemployment, and other adverse socio-economic conditions associated with high prevalence rates of disease and disability and, particularly, to remove barriers to obtaining health care. With respect to the latter, the major barrier for a large segment of the non-institutional population of the USA is that they are without health insurance. Over 37 million, about 15.5 per cent of the population of the USA, were uninsured at the beginning of 1987 'with no signs of the problem disappearing' (Short *et al*. 1989). The proportion of uninsured is much higher for population groups shown to have high prevalence rates of mental and physical disorders, either singly or in combination: blacks, Hispanics, the never married, and the divorced and separated.

The data on the utilization of the general health-care agencies by persons with both mental and physical disorders highlight the many problems that must be solved in relation to these service providers. Major efforts have been under way to make primary-care physicians more aware of concurrent mental health problems in the management of their patients and to take into account their psychosocial characteristics in the diagnostic process and in their formulation of treatment plans (Parron and Solomon 1980). We would like to view this effort in the light of the findings of the present study and the distribution of office visits to physicians in the USA, classified by their specialty. These data put into perspective the overwhelming dimensions of the effort that is required to accomplish this objective.

Figure 6.1 shows the percentage distribution of office visits according to medical specialty for the two years January 1980 to December 1981 (National Center for Health Statistics 1984). During this period, there was a total of 1.16 billion visits or 580 million annually. The distribution of these visits by specialty was as follows:

Specialty	Percentage
General and family practice	32.9
Internal medicine	12.4
Paediatrics	11.1
Obstetrics and gynaecology	9.4
General surgery	5.3
Other surgical specialties	16.0
Other medical specialties	7.5
Psychiatry	2.7
All other specialties	2.7

The percentage of all office visits made by males and females with symptoms referable to psychological and mental disorder, reported by their physicians as the principal reason for the visit, was very small, as demonstrated by the following (National Center for Health Statistics 1981):

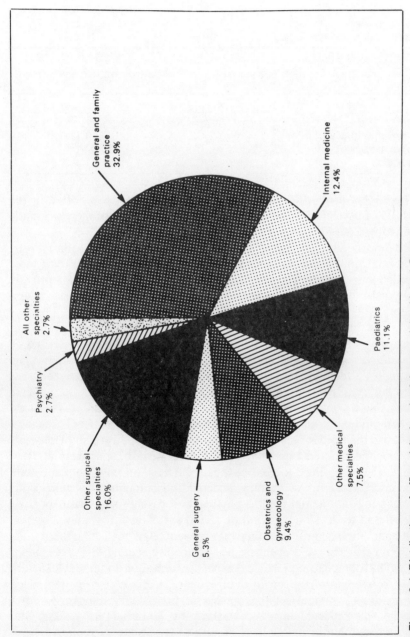

Figure 6.1 Distribution of office visits by physician specialty: United States, Jan. 1980–Dec. 1981 (percentages)
Source: National Center for Health Statistics, 1984

Specialty	Males (%)	Females (%)
General and family practice	1.4	2.0
Internal medicine	1.7	2.6
Paediatrics	0.5	0.4
General surgery	0.7	0.9
Obstetrics and gynaecology	–	0.4

The percentage of visits for social problem counselling was even lower:

	Males	Females
General and family practice	0.1	0.1
Internal medicine	0.1	0.1
Paediatrics	0.2	0.1

The largest proportion of social counselling visits was reported in the province of psychiatrists, who accounted for 87 per cent of the visits made to any physician for this purpose.

The above data are based on the principal reasons for office visits. Additional analyses are needed of the principal and other diagnoses recorded on patients' records. Also, these survey data do not provide information on the content of the interactions between physician and patient.

A major focus of this chapter is on the need for primary care physicians to be aware of the mental health and psychosocial problems presented by their patients and to take appropriate action in dealing with them. The data reported demonstrate that a parallel problem exists for psychiatrists and other personnel of mental health agencies. About half the patients visiting these agencies had both mental and physical disorders. In some demographic sub-groups this proportion is considerably higher. These facts emphasize the need for mental health specialists to be aware of the physical problems their patients may have and to deal with them appropriately.

All of the foregoing underscores the urgent need for physicians currently in practice, residents in training and medical students to acquire skills for assessing the mental health, physical and psychosocial status of their patients and to develop appropriate treatment plans for whatever mental health and physical problems they may present. Accomplishing these tasks will be no easy matter. Recent studies by Shapiro *et al.* (1987) and Hoeper *et al.* (1984) demonstrated that, even when information about mental health status of patients was given to their primary health-care providers, such information did not affect the management of their patients. Another problem was reported in a recent study by Jenkins *et al.* (1988), who found a disappointingly low level of agreement among a group of British general practitioners in arriving at a psychiatric diagnosis in their evaluation of case histories and videotapes of general practice consultations.

A major effort to improve the current situation is needed by governmental and non-governmental agencies, the certifying boards of the various specialties, medical schools, and the physicians themselves. Changes in current methods of financing primary health care through Medicare, Medicaid and private insurance are also needed to provide physicians incentives to take the time needed to deal with their patients' mental health problems (Hamburg *et al*. 1981).

But changes in the methods of financing *per se* will not solve the problem. As stated in a report of the Institute of Medicine (IOM) of the US National Academy of Sciences (Hamburg *et al*. 1981):

> With the primary care sector playing a major role in caring for much of the adult and child population with discernible mental illness, a concerted effort must be made to improve communication between mental health and general health services.

To accomplish this the IOM proposed the following research agenda, based on conceptual issues raised at its conference on Mental Health Services in General Health Care (Parron and Solomon 1980), that especially emphasizes improved collaboration and co-operation:

> development of more precise mental health criteria for use by primary care practitioners;
> development of more clearly outlined treatment patterns for particular mental health disorders;
> development of clear-cut referral criteria for use by primary care practitioners;
> development of guidelines for appropriate drug intervention across the gamut of mental health disorders;
> rigorous tests of efficacy aimed at identifying which therapies work best, for what kinds of patients, and under what conditions;
> tests of alternative strategies for providing integrated mental health care in primary health care settings; and
> investigations of the relative effectiveness of various manpower categories in dealing with differentiated problems in various treatment settings.

The recent enactment of a new public law by the US Congress should serve to advance efforts such as these and others needed to design and implement outcome and effectiveness research mentioned earlier. Under this law a new agency has been established within the US Public Health Service – the Agency for Health Care Policy and Research (Public Law 101–239, 1989). Its mandate is:

to enhance the quality, appropriateness, and effectiveness of health care services and access to such services, through the establishment of a broad base of scientific research and through the promotion of improvements in clinical practice and in the organization, financing, and delivery of health care services.

We return to the end of the title of this chapter – *A Case for Action*! The community-based epidemiological and health services data that have been presented underscore the urgent need for action. While research is needed to solve many of the problems highlighted by these data, progress towards their solution is determined to a large extent by social and political policies that lie outside the health sector (WHO 1987), and removal of barriers created by such policies is a slow process. But it cannot be emphasized too strongly that we are dealing with a dynamic situation because of the expected increase in the population of the United States in the last decade of the twentieth century. If the age-specific prevalence rates for mental disorders in the East Baltimore Mental Health Survey were to apply to the projected age distribution of the population of the USA for 1990 and that for the year 2000, the expected number of cases of mental disorders would increase from about 43 million to 46 million, and half of these cases would have an associated physical disorder. If the age-specific prevalence rates of physical disorders were to apply to the projected populations of 1990 and 2000, the expected number of cases of these physical disorders would increase from 59 million to 66 million, and about 28 per cent of these cases would have an associated mental disorder. The need for an integrated system of health care is, indeed, urgent.

ACKNOWLEDGEMENT

This project was supported by Grant Numbers MH41908 and MH14592 from the National Institute of Mental Health.

REFERENCES

Anthony, J.C., Folstein, M.F., Romanoski, A., von Korff, M.R., Nestadt, G., Chahal, R., Merchant, A., Brown, C.H., Shapiro, S., Kramer, M., and Gruenberg, E.M. (1985) 'Comparison of the lay Diagnostic Interview Schedule and standardized diagnoses: experience in eastern Baltimore', *Archives of General Psychiatry* 42:667–75.

Eastwood, R. (1989) 'The relationship between physical and psychological morbidity', in P. Williams, G. Wilkinson, and K. Rawnsley (eds) *The Scope of Epidemiological Psychiatry*, Routledge: London, pp. 210–21.

Eaton, W.W. and Kessler, L.G. (eds) (1985) 'Epidemiologic field methods in psychiatry', *The NIMH Epidemiologic Catchment Area Program*, Academic Press: New York.

Folstein, M.F., Folstein, S.E., and McHugh, P.R. (1975) 'A practical method for grading the cognitive state of patients for clinical research', *Journal of Psychiatric Research* 12: 971–8.

Hamburg, D.A., Elliot, G.R., and Parron, D.L. (eds) (1981) *Health and Behavior: Frontiers of Research in the Behavioral Sciences*, National Academy Press: Washington, DC, p. 288.

Helzer, J.E., Robins, L.N., McEvoy, L., Spitznagel, E.L., Stolzman, R., Farmer, A., and Brockington, I.F. (1985) 'A comparison of clinical diagnostic interview diagnoses: physical re-examination of lay-interviewed cases in the general population', *Archives of General Psychiatry* 42:657–66.

Hoeper, E.W., Nycz, G.R., Kessler, L.G., Burke, J., and Pierce, W. (1984) 'The usefulness of screening for mental illness', *Lancet* 1:33–5.

Jenkins, R., Smeeton, N., and Shepherd, M. (1988) 'Classification of mental disorder in primary care', *Psychological Medicine Monograph Supplement* 12:1–59.

Kessler, L.G., Tessler, R.C., and Nycz, G.R. (1983) 'Co-occurrence of psychiatric and medical morbidity in primary care', *Journal of Family Practice* 16 (2):319–24.

Morris, J. (1975) *Uses of Epidemiology*, third edn, Churchill Livingstone: Edinburgh.

National Center for Health Statistics, B.K. Cypress (1981) *Patients' Reasons for Visiting Physicians*, The National Ambulatory Medical Care Survey, United States 1977–1978. Vital and Health Statistics, Series 13, No. 56. DHHS Publication No. (PHS) 82–1717, US Government Printing Office: Washington, DC.

National Center for Health Statistics, B.K. Cypress (1984) *Patterns of Ambulatory Medical Care in Internal Medicine*, The National Ambulatory Medical Care Survey, United States, January 1980–December 1981. Vital and Health Statistics, Series 13, No. 80. DHHS Publication No. (PHS) 84–1741, US Government Printing Office: Washington, DC.

Parron, D.L. and Solomon, F. (eds) (1980) *Mental Health Services in Primary Care Settings: Report of a Conference, April 2–3, 1979*, DHHS Publication No. (ADM) 80–995, US Government Printing Office: Washington, DC.

Public Law 101–239 (1989) The Omnibus Budget Reconciliation Act of 1989, *Title IX-Agency for Health Care Policy and Research*. Document Room, US House of Representatives: Washington, DC.

Regier, D.A., Myers, J.K., Kramer, M., Robins, L.N., Blazer, D.G., Hough, R.L., Eaton, W.W., and Locke, B.Z. (1984) 'The NIMH Epidemiologic Catchment Area (ECA) Program: historical context, major objectives and study population characteristics', *Archives of General Psychiatry* 41:934–41.

Robins, L.N., Helzer, J.E., Croughan, J., and Ratcliff, K.S. (1981) 'National Institute of Mental Health Diagnostic Interview Schedule: its history, characteristics and validity', *Archives of General Psychiatry* 38:381–9.

Shapiro, S., Skinner, E.A., Kessler, L.G., von Korff, M., German, P., Tischler, G.L., Leaf, P.J., Benham, L., Cottler, L., and Regier, D.A. (1984) 'Utilization of health and mental health services: three Epidemiologic Catchment Area sites', *Archives of General Psychiatry* 41:971–8.

Shapiro, S., Skinner, E.A., Kramer, M., Steinwachs, D.M., and Regier, D.A. (1985) 'Measuring need for mental health services in a general population', *Medical Care* 23:1033–43.

Shapiro, S., German, P.S., Skinner, E.A., von Korff, M., Turner, R.W., Klein, L.E., Teitelbaum, M.L., Kramer, M., Burke, J.D., and Burns, B.J. (1987) 'An experiment to change detection and management of mental morbidity and primary care', *Medical Care* 25:237–339.

Shepherd, M., Cooper, B., Brown, A.C., and Kalton, G. (1981) 'The relationship between physical and psychiatric illness' (chap. 11:128–38); and 'The Family Health Study' (chap. 12:138–46), in *Psychiatric Illness in General Practice*, second edn, London: Oxford University Press.

Short, P.F., Monheit, A., and Beauregard, K. (1989) *Uninsured Americans*: *a 1987 Profile*, National Center for Health Services Research and Health Care Technology Assessment, Rockville, MD.

US Bureau of the Census (1989) *Poverty in the United States: 1987*, Current Population Reports, Series P-60, No. 163, US Government Printing Office: Washington, DC.

Wells, K.B., Golding, J.M., and Burnham, M.A. (1988) 'Psychiatric disorder in a sample of the general population with and without chronic medical conditions', *American Journal of Psychiatry* 145:976–81.

Wells, K.B., Golding, J.M., and Burnham, M.A. (1989) 'Chronic medical conditions in a sample of the general population with anxiety, affective and substance use disorders', *American Journal of Psychiatry* 146:1440–6.

World Health Organization (1986) 'Mental, neurologic and psychosocial disorders', *World Health Statistics Annual,* pp. 24–8, Geneva: WHO.

World Health Organization (1987) *Evaluation of the Strategy for Health for All by the Year 2000: Seventh Report on the World Health Situation,* Vol.1, *Global Review,* Geneva: WHO.

Chapter 7

Psychiatric illness and services in a UK health centre

Brian Jarman

In the UK, patients are normally registered from birth with a general practitioner, or else register when they enter the country. About 98 per cent of the population is so registered. Their medical records are transferred from doctor to doctor when they move house. Around 30 per cent of general practitioners now work in health centres, which are provided by the local health authorities, and the rest in premises which they themselves own or rent. Most general practitioners (about 72 per cent in 1986) work in primary-care teams, with groups of three or more doctors. The other professionals in these teams are usually district nurses, health visitors (nurses who specialize in preventive care), community psychiatric nurses, receptionists, social workers, physiotherapists and speech therapists. There is a very even distribution of general practitioners across the country, the average number of patients registered with each doctor varying by only plus or minus 120 around an average of 2,000 in the 190 health districts of England. This evenness is a result of the activities of the Medical Practices Committee, which is responsible for the distribution of general practitioners.

In the UK, as in other countries, there has been a reduction in the length of time which mentally ill patients spend in psychiatric hospitals and a partial transfer of responsibility for their care to community services provided by district health authorities and by general practitioners. However, in England over the past twenty years there has been almost no change in the numbers of new out-patient referrals by general practitioners to psychiatrists, and even a slight increase in the numbers of psychiatric admissions to (or deaths and discharges from) psychiatric hospitals. What has changed dramatically has been the average duration of stay in the psychiatric hospitals, which fell from 361 days in 1966 to 139 days in 1986: a reduction of over 60 per cent in twenty years. This has resulted in a steady reduction in the number of psychiatric beds occupied daily, from 174,000 to 96,000 over the same period. The peak of psychiatric bed occupancy was in 1954–55, the year in which chlorpromazine treatment was introduced. Since then there has been a

Table 7.1 Use of psychiatric hospital services in England, 1966–86[1]

Index of utilization		Year	
	1966	1976	1986
Deaths and discharges (000s)	176	198	252
Average length of stay (days)	361	245	139
Beds occupied daily (000s)	174	133	96
Day-case attendances (000s)	–	15	10
New out-patients (000s)	201	200	205

[1]Source: Department of Health and Social Security (1988)

steady reduction, which is still continuing. The trends are summarized in Table 7.1.

Although the movement of psychiatric care away from the long-term institutional setting which has occurred gradually over the past thirty-five years has been well documented, the provision of mental health services in the community has not been studied in any detail, at any rate at the general practice level. Most persons with mental health problems are dealt with entirely by their general practitioners (Goldberg and Huxley 1980; Shepherd *et al.* 1981). The modes of treatment open to the practitioners are as follows:

1 counselling by the practitioners themselves, the nature of which depends upon the individual practitioner's training, experience and personal skills;
2 prescribing of various psychotropic drugs;
3 interventions aimed at improving the patient's social conditions (such as help with a rehousing application or support for social security welfare benefits);
4 referral to one or more of a number of medical or social agencies.

In many areas, mental health agencies have followed the general trend from being based mainly in psychiatric hospitals to being based in general hospitals or in the community. In a health centre, the referral facilities available to the general practitioner may include attached psychiatrists or psychologists who attend the centre regularly, counsellors, community psychiatric nurses and social workers.

EXPERIENCE IN ONE METROPOLITAN GENERAL PRACTICE

The aim of this contribution is to document the change in provision of mental health services in one group general practice since 1972, and to pinpoint those changes which have occurred since the practice moved into a health centre. The Lisson Grove Health Centre is situated in north-west

London, and was opened on 1 April 1978. The three practices which moved into the centre had previously been in separate premises in the vicinity and could trace their history back to the 1930s or earlier. The extra space which became available with the move into the health centre, and the presence of para-medical workers in the same building, permitted us to refer patients with mental illness for treatment within the centre, instead of sending them to hospital psychiatric departments. The shift of the locus of treatment from hospital to health centre was particularly marked for psychiatric illness: more so, indeed, than for any other specialty. This report traces the evolution of new service patterns and procedures, and discusses the advantages and drawbacks of such a change.

Research method

There were 12,000 patients registered with the three health centre practices in 1978 and there are now (in 1989) over 20,000. Data are available for one of the three practices, which initially had some 5,000 patients and now has 8,500. This practice has had either three or four general practitioners and one GP trainee throughout the whole period, and for the past eight years has also had a GP house officer in a rotation scheme with St Mary's Hospital, Paddington, a nearby teaching hospital.

Details of all consultations have been recorded on a computer in the practice since 1 October 1971, and the total is now over 250,000. The present report is based on an analysis of data for the period 1971–88, covering a total of 227,000 consultations. It includes a period of seven years when the practice was still being conducted in smaller premises nearby, and had a much smaller team. The available data are of two main types:

those to do with patient characteristics: the so-called registration data file, which includes the patient's age, sex, marital status, social class, data of registration, etc;
those to do with the consultation: which doctor was seen, the date and place of consultation, diagnoses, referrals, investigations, prescriptions, etc.

Data on all contacts are recorded by receptionists and doctors, and are coded. Only those involving face-to-face contact between doctor and patient are reported here. The data analysis is done using a main frame computer, while sub-sets of the data are also analysed on a micro-computer (currently a Toshiba T5200). A validation study of 500 randomly selected cases showed close agreement between the computerized records and the medical notes, only 0.5 per cent of consultations being unrecorded in one or the other. The main discrepancies were found: (a) in the coding of social class (5 per cent disagreement); (b) between doctors in the decision as to what to record as the main diagnosis (20 per cent disagreement), and

(c) in an under-recording of hospital admissions when these had not been arranged by the practice.

Research findings

1   Mental health problems within context of general practice

Each year, 14 to 16 per cent of all consultations receive a main diagnosis as a mental health problem according to Chapter V of the International Classification of Diseases, Eighth Revision (ICD-8). Following introduction of the Ninth Revision (ICD-9), the proportion of mental illness diagnoses was reduced to about 10 per cent, but some diagnoses included in the mental illness section of ICD-8 were now coded elsewhere, in the supplementary classification of 'factors influencing health status and contact with health services'. This group of conditions includes items such as psychological trauma, family, housing and economic problems, and other psychosocial difficulties. The total for mental illness and these 'supplementary' conditions combined remained steady at about 15 per cent of all consultations. The fact that the corresponding proportion found in the 1981–82 National Morbidity Survey, based on 100 practices in England (Royal College of General Practitioners 1986), was only about 10 per cent can be related to the special features of practice in an inner city area with high social pathology. The estimate of 15 per cent is increased to about 20 per cent if all those consultations are also included at which a psychiatric condition is recorded, but only as a subsidiary diagnosis. Probably more mental health problems would be recorded as subsidiary diagnoses if our coding system were more sophisticated.

Of all patients with mental illness diagnoses recorded from 1971 to 1977, from 2.5 per cent to 3.0 per cent were referred to psychiatric out-patient clinics. Following the provision of mental health-care facilities in the health centre itself, the rate of referral to these clinics began to fall, and by 1986 was as low as 1 per cent of all patients with a main diagnosis of mental illness. During the same period, the overall out-patient referral rate for all diagnoses remained fairly constant at from 5 per cent to 6 per cent of consultations. It is clear, therefore, that: (a) the proportion of patients with psychiatric diagnoses referred to hospital out-patient departments was lower than the average for other, non-psychiatric diagnoses, and (b) this proportion has declined to an even lower level since mental health-care facilities were provided in the centre itself: from half down to only about one-fifth of the overall rate of referral. The decline in psychiatric referrals as a proportion of all specialist referrals is shown graphically in Figure 7.1.

Coincident with this marked drop in hospital referrals, which has continued to the present, there has been a corresponding increase in referrals to counsellors and Psychiatric Community Nurses (CPNs) within the

% of all referrals

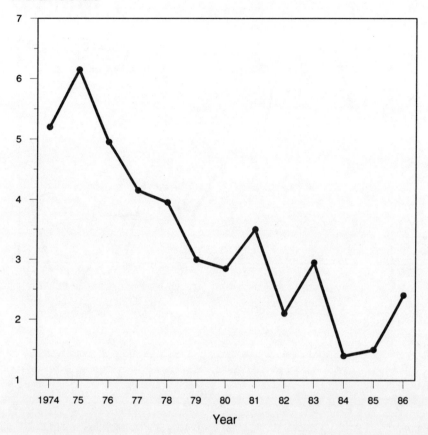

Figure 7.1 Psychiatric out-patient referrals as a proportion of all out-patient referrals, 1974–86

centre. The opposing trends are depicted in Figure 7.2. The internal referrals commenced with the introduction of this facility in the practice in 1975, and actually declined in number temporarily with the move into the new health centre three years later, but have since returned to the level reached before then. The drop in numbers of psychiatric hospital referrals was completely compensated for by the increase in referrals to counsellors and CPNs in the centre. The trends shown in Figure 7.2 provide a comparison of the numbers of psychiatric referrals (one-sixth of which are now to psychiatric day hospitals) with those to the facilities in the centre (counsellor or CPN). The small numbers of patients referred for psychoanalytic or other specific forms of psychotherapy, or for sex therapy, are not included in these analyses.

Referrals per 1.000 consultations

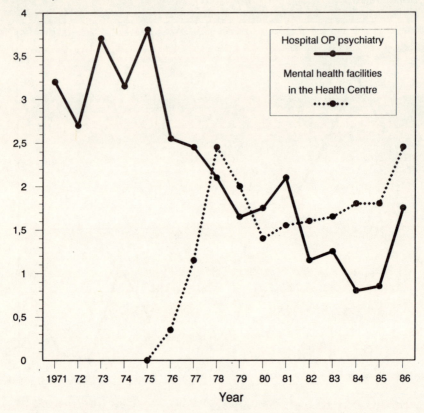

Figure 7.2 Trends in referral to hospital psychiatry and to facilities within the health centre, 1971–86

2   *Mental health services in the health centre*

All the general practitioners have taken part in 'Balint groups' (Balint 1957), which are intended to help doctors deal with the emotional problems of their patients, and some of them have developed an interest in mental health issues during the course of their practice. In 1976, not long before the move into the health centre, the Marriage Guidance Council offered to attach one of their counsellors to the practice. They pay part of the costs, and the patients themselves make whatever contributions they can afford. The first counsellor has been with the practice since 1976, and has recently been joined by a second one. In addition, a third counsellor has set up a group which meets once a week. The counsellors have a room in the health centre, and one of them is available for consultation there most of the time.

The next development was the attachment of a Community Psychiatric Nurse by the district health authority, initially on an informal basis and later more formally attached to the practice. She attends the weekly practice meetings and works in close liaison with the practice team, while remaining under the managerial responsibility of the district mental health unit. This unit is helpful in providing training, and also holiday and sickness cover, for the CPN. For a few years, the district authority provided a sex therapist for one session weekly, to give advice to the general practitioners about patients, rather than to treat the latter directly. This facility, however, has had to be withdrawn as a result of recent financial constraints.

The local authority has also appointed a social worker to be based full-time in the health centre. She also attends practice meetings and works closely with the two attached Health Visitors as well as with the CPN and counsellors. Much of her time is spent in work which is on the borderline of psychiatry; for example, dealing with problems of child sexual abuse. The weekly practice meetings provide a forum in which complex problems, overlapping the work of different professionals, can be discussed, and a key worker nominated to deal with each problem.

Finally, the practice has been enabled to advise on social security welfare benefits, by using a computer program which works out patients' benefit entitlements under the state social security rules. For four years from 1983, the Department of Health and Social Security attached an information officer to work with this program, and since then a welfare rights adviser has been employed in the centre part-time.

3   Mental health problems and their management in the health centre

In all, about 20 per cent of patients consulting at some time in the year will receive at least one diagnosis in either the mental illness classification or the 'supplementary' list of psychosocial diagnoses included in ICD-9. Mental illness consultation ratios for the years 1974–81 were examined after indirect standardization for age and sex, using the whole practice population as the standard of reference. The consultation rates were higher for females than for males, and higher among the widowed, divorced and separated patients (the latter groups increasingly so) than among those who were either single or married. The distribution by social class showed a gradual increase in the rate from Class I (professional and managerial groups) to Class V (unskilled workers).

Younger patients were more likely to have been referred to a psychiatric agency for specialist treatment, whereas older patients were more likely to have been prescribed psychotropic drugs. There has been, however, a reduction over the years in prescribing of benzodiazepines for all age-groups. Patients from social Classes I and II were more likely to have been referred for counselling or psychotherapy and those from Classes III, IV and V to have been referred to out-patient psychiatry or a psychiatric day hospital.

No attempt was made to assess outcome by means of standardized measures. Some 500 referrals between 1971 and 1988 have been followed up individually to ascertain if the patients in fact received treatment and how long they continued in treatment, following their referral. The only significant difference between the groups referred to different agencies was that those seen by counsellors in the health centre were less likely to have been rejected as unsuitable for treatment than were those seen by the external services. Indeed, the follow-up of 500 referrals showed that no single patient referred to the counsellors had been rejected as unsuitable for their help. Psychiatric hospital admission rates appeared to have declined slightly in frequency over the study period, but there are some reservations about the accuracy of the admission data.

DISCUSSION

There are a number of advantages for both patients and general practitioners in having mental health problems treated and managed in the health-centre setting.

1 Access to treatment is easier for the patient and can be facilitated by having the general practitioner, whom the patients will have known on average for some ten years, introduce them to the therapist or nurse.
2 The setting reduces any possible danger of 'labelling' associated with being seen by a psychiatrist; treatment by the therapist and by the general practitioner take place in the same building, in an environment with which the patient is already familiar.
3 Communication between the professionals concerned is much easier: the counsellors and CPNs meet together with the practitioners regularly, at least once each week.
4 The patient can be seen earlier: often on the same day if there is a crisis, and usually within a week or so for non-urgent referrals. This contrasts very favourably with a waiting time of several weeks for the psychiatric out-patient department, or possibly several months for out-patient psychotherapy.
5 The availability of other services in the health centre, such as those provided by health visitors and a social worker, together with the ease of communication between the different professionals, enables other contributory problems related to mental illness to be dealt with on the spot.

Possible disadvantages of the system could arise if too great a reliance were to be placed on the management of mental disorders in the health centre itself. There might be a lack of the expert advice which only a psychiatrist can provide, and which can lead to more effective treatment and a more favourable outcome. General practitioners or other non-psychiatric professional workers might miss the diagnosis in a condition which is potentially amenable to treatment. There is also a danger that families or other care-givers may be expected to bear too much of the burden of looking after their mentally sick relatives when they could be afforded relief by, for example, referral of the patient to a psychiatric day hospital. These possible drawbacks serve to underline the need for careful assessment of each individual case.

There has been a gradual, and at times faltering, growth of attachment schemes for psychiatrists, psychologists, social workers and CPNs to general practices in the UK since the early 1970s, and particularly in the past ten years (Gilchrist *et al.* 1978; Strathdee and Williams 1984; Tyrer 1985; Wilkinson 1988). When questioned, patients have usually expressed preference for mental health services provided in health centres or other group-practice settings to the hospital-based psychiatric services (Tyrer *et al.* 1984). Patients, general practitioners and psychiatrists alike have commented on the advantages of the former type of service, listed above. The perceived disadvantages of such schemes appear to be mostly those arising from administrative difficulties, such as the increased travelling time for the professionals, and a shortage of secretarial staff in the centres, rather than any possible drawbacks due to a lack of psychiatrist specialist expertise.

The statistical analysis presented in this chapter has been made possible by the availability of detailed records of practice activities over a period of eighteen years. This has enabled me to report in some detail the actual changes that have taken place in one group practice during the introduction of a range of mental health-care facilities.

REFERENCES

Balint, M. (1957) *The Doctor, his Patient and the Illness*, London: Pitman.

Department of Health and Social Security (1988) *Health and Personal Social Service Statistics for England: 1988 edition*, London: HMSO.

Gilchrist, I.C., Gough, J.B., Horsfall-Turner, Y.R., Ineston, E.M., Keele, G., Marks, B., and Scott, H.J. (1978) 'Social work in general practice', *Journal of the Royal College of General Practitioners* 28:675–86.

Goldberg, D. and Huxley, P. (1980) *Mental Illness in the Community: the Pathway to Psychiatric Care*, London: Tavistock.

Royal College of General Practitioners, Office of Population Censuses and Surveys, Department of Health and Social Security (1986) *Morbidity Statistics from General Practice. Third National Survey, 1981–82*, Series MB 5, no. 1, London: HMSO.

Shepherd, M., Cooper, B., Brown, A.C., and Kalton, G. (1981) *Psychiatric Illness in General Practice*, second edn, Oxford: Oxford University Press.

Strathdee, G. and Williams, P. (1984) 'A survey of psychiatrists in primary care: the silent growth of a new service', *Journal of the Royal College of General Practitioners* 34:615–18.

Tyrer, P. (1985) 'The hive system: a model for psychiatric services', *British Journal of Psychiatry* 146:571–5.

Tyrer, P., Seivewright, N., and Wollerton, S. (1984) 'General practice psychiatric clinics: impact on psychiatric services', *British Journal of Psychiatry* 145:15–19.

Wilkinson, G. (1988) 'I don't want you to see a psychiatrist', *British Medical Journal* 297:1144–5.

Chapter 8

Psychosocial complaints in general practice

A national survey in the Netherlands

Peter F. M. Verhaak, Joke M. Bosman, Marleen Foets and Koos van der Velden

Goldberg and Huxley (1980) charted the pathway to psychiatric care. They estimated the prevalence of psychiatric illness in the community (Level 1), the number of people seeking help for their distress in primary medical care (Level 2), the number of people recognized by general practitioners (GPs) as suffering from a mental illness (Level 3), and the number of patients referred by GPs to specialist mental health agencies (Levels 4 and 5). Between each level they postulated a filter that had to be passed to reach the next level: the patient's decision to seek help (between Levels 1 and 2), the doctor's recognition of the nature of the condition (between Levels 2 and 3) and his decision to refer the patient rather than to undertake the treatment himself (between Level 3 and Levels 4 and 5).

This chapter is restricted to consideration of the second and third levels, together with the filter between them. What psychosocial problems are presented to the general practitioner? With what complaints do patients in mental distress come to their GP? In which cases does he arrive at the diagnosis of a mental illness?

The commonest approach to the question of identification of psychosocial problems by the general practitioner is to assess patients' symptoms or problems (Level 2) by a standardized technique and to compare this assessment with the GP's own clinical judgement. Many recent studies have used the General Health Questionnaire (Goldberg and Blackwell 1970; Goldberg and Bridges 1987; Wright and Perini 1987) or the Center for Epidemiological Studies Depression Scale (Schulberg *et al.* 1985), sometimes in combination with a standard interview technique, to assess the patient's mental health status. The clinical judgement of the GP is in most studies obtained by approximation: some studies have restricted themselves to assessing position on a scale from 'entirely somatic' to 'entirely psychiatric', with intermediate stages such as 'physical illness with associated psychiatric symptoms'. The studies of Goldberg and his colleagues, cited above, provide examples. Other studies (Jencks 1985; Whitehouse 1987; Shepherd *et al.* 1981) have required the participating

GPs to use a standard diagnostic classification, which may lead to under-reporting of the cases of psychological disturbance which present with somatic symptoms (Crombie 1986).

Comparison between a standardized questionnaire score and the GP's clinical assessment of the patient's condition usually suggests a large measure of under-reporting by the practitioner. Some important objections can, however, be made to this approach. A clinical judgement, which is primarily the result of a request for help put forward at a specific moment (the 'demand'), is being compared with a quasi-objective assessment of the individual's health status. Moreover, the score obtained relates to the health status at a point in time, while the individual's problem and need for help have usually developed over a period.

An important goal of epidemiological research is to achieve a better knowledge of the prevalence of mental illness, in order to relate estimates of the need for services in the population to the existing level of provision. We consider the discrepancies between standardized assessments at Level 2 and clinical judgements at Level 3 to be partly a result of comparing 'needs' (as defined by the presence of morbidity) with 'demand' (as expressed in the patients' help-seeking behaviour). That such a discrepancy represents true disagreement should not be taken for granted without further investigation of the situation at these two levels. The data should be examined more closely, to see if an integration of the two types of assessment can be achieved at a higher level of abstraction.

Additional information is required about the character of the patient's complaints presented to the GP (the demand) and the development of their symptoms over time. Comparison of the demand with the GP's clinical judgement and diagnosis might help towards a better understanding of the factors which determine the pathway to psychiatric care. We postulate that between Level 2 (the complaint) and Level 3 (the diagnosis), an assessment is made by the GP which incorporates any suspicion of psychiatric morbidity at the time of consultation. His diagnosis, on the other hand, will usually be the outcome of a number of doctor–patient contacts. The present contribution examines this model in relation to the symptoms and complaints presented by patients in a large general-practice population over a three-month period.

RESEARCH METHOD

Data were obtained from the Dutch National Study of Morbidity and Interventions in General Practice (Foets, van der Velden and van der Zee 1986), in which all doctor–patient contacts were recorded for three months. Among the data recorded at these contacts were the reason for the encounter, as stated by the patient, and an assessment by the GP of any psychosocial component. 'Reason for encounter' was defined as the complaints, symptoms, requests, and so on, put forward by the patient as the reason for consulting. In this text, the terms 'complaint' and 'symptom' can be regarded as virtually synonymous with it. An episode is defined as an illness or health-related problem which results in a spell of medical care, from first to last contact. The diagnosis included in the data analysis is that reached by the end of the illness-episode in question.

Both 'reason for encounter' and diagnosis were classified according to the International Classification of Primary Care – ICPC (Lamberts and Woods 1987). The diagnostic classification is derived from the International Classification of Health Problems in Primary Care, which in turn is compatible with the International Classification of Diseases, Ninth Revision – ICD-9. The ICPC is arranged in chapters, most of which refer to organ systems: digestive system, nervous system, blood and circulation, and so on. Two of these chapters are concerned with non-organic problems: the psychological and the social. For the purpose of classification a choice has to be made for each reason for consulting and each illness-diagnosis, according to the nature of the complaint. Thus, headache will be classified as 'neurological', peptic ulcer under 'digestive system' and depressive mood under 'psychological disorder'. This can cause problems in cases in which a patient presents somatic manifestations of psychological distress. In order to overcome such difficulties, a second measure was added: the GP's assessment of each complaint on a five-point scale ranging from 'entirely physical' to 'entirely psychosocial' (cf. Crombie 1963).

All statistical data refer to individual patients and are unduplicated, to avoid possible confusion arising between diagnosis, consultation, 'reason for encounter' and illness-episode. Accordingly, the numerator consists in each instance of the number of patients with a psychiatric diagnosis, or at least one psychosocial 'reason for encounter', who presented during the three-month period of the survey, while the denominator is based on the whole practice population. In the Netherlands, GPs have registered-patient lists. To obtain reliable information on the population at risk, including its distribution by sex, age, marital status, social class and educational level, a census has been taken and basic data collected for the entire population.

SURVEY FINDINGS

In the three-month period, approximately 38 per cent of the population at risk consulted their general practitioners. Of this proportion, 59 per cent were female and 9 per cent (or 3.4 per cent of the practice population) consulted at least once with psychological symptoms. As can be seen from Table 8.1, this latter proportion rises with increasing age of the patients.

The most frequent 'psychological' reasons for consultation were complaints of depression and anxiety, sleep disorders, acute psychosocial stress and repeat prescribing of psychotropic drugs. In addition to these overtly

Table 8.1 Three-month consulting rate (persons per 1,000 population) for
psychological complaints (ICPC chapter P)

Age-group (yr)	Males per 1,000 popn	Females per 1,000 popn	Both sexes per 1,000 popn
0– 9	6.6	9.1	7.8
10–19	5.2	10.4	7.8
20–29	17.2	30.5	24.3
30–39	26.7	43.9	35.5
40–49	36.4	55.9	46.1
50–59	44.5	67.1	56.0
60–69	37.7	78.2	59.7
70–79	49.3	82.9	69.5
80 or over	47.6	62.4	57.2
All ages	24.4	42.5	33.8
No. of persons	77,944	83,668	161,612

psychological complaints, however, many cases presenting with somatic
symptoms were judged by the GPs to be not entirely physical in nature.
Hence, far more patients were assessed as having psychosocial problems
than could be estimated from the number of overtly psychological disturbances alone.

In the three-month period, 32 per cent of consulting patients (amounting
to 12 per cent of the practice population) presented on at least one occasion
with a complaint assessed as not entirely physical in nature. The complaints
and symptoms most frequently allocated to this group were general weak-
ness, headache, backache and related complaints, generalized abdominal
pain and requests for blood-pressure checks. None of these reasons was
specific to the group, but all of them – with the single exception of
blood-pressure checks – occurred more frequently within it than among
patients assessed as 'entirely physical' cases. In this context, the age
distribution differed somewhat from that shown in Table 8.1. Table 8.2
shows that the assessment 'not entirely physical' occurred most often in
the age-range from 40 to 60 years.

Altogether, 347 per 1,000 consulting patients (corresponding to 131 per
1,000 practice population) presented at least once in the three-month period
with complaints judged to be entirely or partly psychological in origin.

We now turn to Level 3 of the Goldberg–Huxley model: psychiatric diagnosis by the GP. Out of a total of 61,182 consulting patients, 2,004 (32.8 per
1,000) received a psychiatric diagnosis for at least one illness-episode. This
number corresponds to 12.3 per 1,000 population at risk. The total number
of episodes with a psychiatric diagnosis was 3,137, which corresponds to
51.0 per 1,000 consulting patients, or 19.4 per 1,000 population at risk.

Table 8.2 Three-month consulting rate (persons per 1,000 population) for conditions judged by the GP to be 'not entirely physical'

Age-group (yr)	Males per 1,000 popn	Females per 1,000 popn	Both sexes per 1,000 popn
0– 9	47.4	50.7	49.0
10–19	49.7	96.7	73.0
20–29	88.9	163.7	128.5
30–39	109.4	167.5	139.0
40–49	120.8	186.3	153.3
50–59	135.8	198.0	167.4
60–69	109.0	170.5	142.5
70–79	111.3	154.5	137.2
80 and above	66.8	68.8	68.8
All ages	85.4	144.2	118.9
No. of persons	77,944	83,668	161,612

The proportion among these patients who presented with a new psychiatric illness-episode was 35 per cent, which means a three-month incidence rate of 4.3 per 1,000 population at risk. The most frequent diagnosis in this sub-group was neurotic depression, which accounted for 38 per cent of psychiatric diagnoses. Second in rank order was the related group of 'neurasthenia', which made up an additional 17 per cent of the cases.

Table 8.3 gives the age–sex distribution for all illness-episodes. In contrast to the earlier tables, all episodes are counted, so that the same patient may be included more than once.

More psychiatric illness episodes are reported for women than for men. Generally the proportion rises with age, though this is not the case for anxiety disorders and neurasthenia, both of which peak in the age-range 40 to 59 years. The reader should bear in mind that only episodes with a firm diagnosis of mental illness are included here: the rates given in Table 8.3 would increase considerably if episodes with a symptomatic diagnosis of 'anxiety' or 'overstrain' were also included. The symptomatic diagnosis 'depressive feelings', however, was recorded less often than the diagnosis of depressive neurosis.

In Table 8.4 the findings are presented according to marital status, educational background (an indication of socio-economic status) and urban or rural area of residence. Patients who are widowed, those who completed only primary education and those resident in Amsterdam or Rotterdam all carried a higher risk of presenting psychological complaints or being assessed as a case of mental illness by the GP. The low rates for unmarried persons, however, should be regarded as a consequence of the over-representation of persons below 20 years in this sub-group. When

Table 8.3 Three-month consulting rates (episodes per 1,000 population) for psychiatric illness and for selected psychiatric diagnoses

Age-group (yr)	Males per 1,000 popn	Females per 1,000 popn	Both sexes per 1,000 popn
3.1 All psychiatric diagnoses			
0–19	1.5	2.9	2.2
20–39	11.6	20.8	16.4
40–59	20.0	32.3	26.2
60 and over	27.9	57.0	44.8
All ages	13.0	25.4	19.4
3.2 Psychotic disorders (incl. dementia)			
0–19	0.2	0.1	0.2
20–39	1.7	2.2	2.0
40–59	2.6	3.5	3.1
60 and over	8.9	12.8	11.1
All ages	2.5	3.9	3.2
3.3 Anxiety disorders (incl. phobias)			
0–19	0.7	1.1	0.9
20–39	2.2	4.5	3.4
40–59	3.7	5.2	4.5
60 and over	2.8	4.6	3.8
All ages	2.2	3.8	3.0
3.4 Depressive neuroses			
0–19	0.1	0.5	0.3
20–39	3.5	7.8	5.7
40–59	7.6	15.3	11.5
60 and over	8.4	23.4	17.1
All ages	4.2	10.4	7.4
3.5 Neurasthenia			
0–19	0.1	0.7	0.4
20–39	3.8	5.1	4.5
40–59	4.8	6.0	5.4
60 and over	2.3	3.3	2.9
All ages	2.7	3.8	3.3
No. of persons	77,944	83,668	161,612

controlled for age, married and unmarried persons showed similar rates of psychiatric illness.

There is a large disparity between the number of patients with a psychiatric diagnosis and the number presenting with complaints that were either entirely or partly psychological in nature. To gain a better understanding of this disparity, an analysis was undertaken, based on four sub-groups of patients:

Table 8.4 Three-month consulting rates (persons per 1,000 population) for psychological complaints and conditions judged by the GP to be 'not entirely physical' for groups with a different marital status, different education level and for different urban/rural areas

Background variables	No.	Psychological complaints	'Not entirely physical conditions'
Marital status			
Unmarried	62,002	16.5	82.9
Married	69,290	41.6	142.9
Divorced	3,670	80.1	216.1
Widowed	7,775	80.5	150.0
Unknown	20,256	–	–
Educational level			
Primary	27,403	62.6	176.4
Secondary	61,356	36.9	143.8
University	11,259	28.2	99.9
Unknown or still at school	62,975	–	–
Area of residence			
Rural	70,163	30.2	123.4
Suburban	64,390	35.2	108.8
Urban	20,395	35.4	110.9
Amsterdam/ Rotterdam	8,045	45.5	175.3

I   those with at least one psychiatric illness-episode in the three-month period;

II   those who presented with overtly psychological complaints, but were not given a psychiatric diagnosis;

III those who presented at least once with complaints judged to be not entirely physical in origin, but without overt psychological disturbance;

IV   those who presented only somatic complaints, and whose conditions were considered by the GPs to be entirely physical in origin.

These four groups are mutually exclusive. Table 8.5 sets out their numbers and their mean numbers of contacts with the GPs.

It can be seen that the patients in the first two groups – those with a psychiatric diagnosis or overt psychological disturbance – attended their GPs' consulting sessions more frequently, on average, than those in the third and fourth groups.

In Figure 8.1 the total of doctor–patient contacts for each of the four sub-groups is shown in proportion, together with the distribution according to the different 'reasons for encounter' in each sub-group. That is to say, while group I is made up of patients with at least one psychiatric

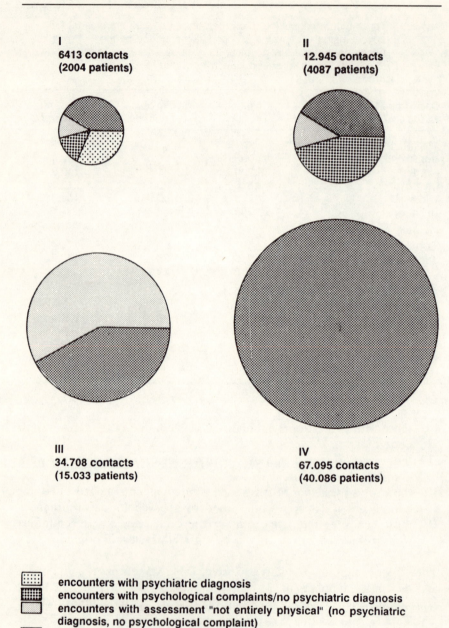

I
6413 contacts
(2004 patients)

II
12.945 contacts
(4087 patients)

III
34.708 contacts
(15.033 patients)

IV
67.095 contacts
(40.086 patients)

encounters with psychiatric diagnosis
encounters with psychological complaints/no psychiatric diagnosis
encounters with assessment "not entirely physical" (no psychiatric diagnosis, no psychological complaint)
encounters with merely physical complaints

Figure 8.1 Proportions of doctor–patient encounters having some psychiatric component, for four different patient groups (cf. Table 8.5)

Table 8.5 Number of patients and of doctor–patient contacts in four sub-groups of consulting patients

Patient group	No. of patients	Total no. of contacts in 3 months	Mean no. of contacts
I At least one psychiatric illness-episode	2,004	6,413	3.2
II At least one psychological reason for encounter	4,087	12,945	3.2
III At least one complaint assessed as 'not entirely physical'	15,033	34,708	2.3
IV Physical illness only	40,086	76,095	1.7

illness-episode, the members of these groups could also consult during the three months with any type of somatic complaint. The diagram displays the mix of possible types of contact: four for group I, three for group II, two for group III, and only one (purely physical complaints) for group IV. It appears that one-third of the consultations by group I patients and nearly half those made by group II patients were for complaints judged by the GP to be entirely physical.

Finally, a number of patients who consulted were suspected of having a mental or emotional disturbance, but could not be given a psychiatric diagnosis, did not present with any overt psychological complaints during the three-month period, and indeed did not report any symptoms that could not be adequately explained in terms of physical pathology. If in fact mental ill health was present in these cases, it could not be identified within the three-month limits of a cross-sectional survey (Verhaak et al. 1990).

DISCUSSION

How do these survey findings fit with existing evidence on psychiatric illness in primary-care settings? The relatively low proportion of psychiatric diagnoses recorded in our study is roughly in accordance with the findings reported by those general-practice surveys which relied upon the ICD classification. Jencks (1985) reported 56 psychiatric diagnoses per, 1,000 patient consultations in the NAMC survey in the United States, and Whitehouse (1987) 76 per 1,000 consultations in a study in Manchester, UK. The fact that both these authors used the number of consultations, rather than of consulting patients, as the numerator in computing diagnostic rates may account for the fact that these are somewhat higher than the 51 per 1,000 found in our study. Shepherd *et al.* (1981) found a psychiatric diagnosis rate of 102 per 1,000 for consulting patients.

The rate for depression of 14 per 1,000 consulting patients, obtained in our study, is lower than that of 21 per 1,000, reported by Whitehouse in Manchester. Our rate of seven anxiety disorders per 1,000 consulting patients is also much lower than the corresponding rate of 25 per 1,000 in Whitehouse's survey. A partial explanation for these differences lies in the fact that we included in the count only those cases with a mental-illness diagnosis; contacts resulting in a so-called 'symptom diagnosis' (IPC codes P-01 and P-29) were counted as psychological complaints in Table 8.1, but not included as formal psychiatric diagnosis. As explained above, some 10 per cent of the patients in our survey presented at least once with a psychological complaint, without receiving a diagnosis.

The total frequency of patients with non-somatic symptoms – 347 per 1,000 consulting patients and 131 per thousand population at risk – is of a comparable order of magnitude to the estimates for 'problem behaviour' reported in earlier Dutch general-practice surveys. Lamberts and Hartman (1982), for example, reported that 135 per 1,000 patients presented with psychological complaints which could not be explained in terms of somatic pathology. These estimates are also comparable to the figures obtained by applying standardized screening instruments in general practice. The General Health Questionnaire has yielded rates for probable psychiatric cases ranging from 26 per cent (Finlay-Jones and Burvill 1978) up to figures of 45 or 50 per cent (Goldberg and Blackwell 1970; Goldberg and Bridges 1987; Wright and Perini 1987). A US study which used the Schedule for Affective Disorders and Schizophrenia, SADS and Research Diagnostic Criteria, reported psychiatric diagnoses in 27 per cent of the patients surveyed (Hoeper *et al.* 1979), while Kessler *et al.* (1987) found 21.7 per cent of medical-service users in the Epidemiologic Catchment Area survey to be current psychiatric cases according to the Diagnostic Interview Schedule criteria. However, as has already been emphasized, a diagnosis based on clinical judgement cannot be equated with a score above the cut-off on a standardized instrument.

The following broad conclusions can be drawn from our research findings:

- many patients consult during a three-month period with ill health considered by the GP to be not entirely physical in origin;
- most of these, however, reported only somatic complaints during the recording period;
- only a small proportion of the 'not entirely physical' cases were allocated a psychiatric diagnosis by the GP;
- both patients given a psychiatric diagnosis and others who came with overt psychological complaints also presented a great number of purely somatic complaints, which were assessed by the GPs as entirely physical in nature.

In terms of the Goldberg–Huxley model, the filter between Levels 2 and 3 will be assessed as more or less permeable, according to the criteria which are employed in deciding whether the GP has recognized the presence of psychiatric disturbance. In the present study, whereas only 3.2 per cent of the consulting patients were given a psychiatric diagnosis, 10.0 per cent in all were recognized to have presented psychological complaints, and in all 34.5 per cent to have presented complaints that could not be accounted for in purely physical terms. It is important, therefore, to decide which of these various groups should be accepted as having passed through the filter; namely, as having been 'recognized' by the GPs. It can be argued that Level 2 should not be restricted to patients who express their distress in overt psychological terms, nor indeed Level 3 to those who are given a formal psychiatric diagnosis. Our dimensional approach makes it possible to demonstrate the importance of psychosocial problems in the patient clientele of primary-care physicians, without, however, leading to an over-estimation of the prevalence of 'recognized mental illness' in this population.

The association of psychiatric disorder with somatic illness is also reported by Kramer et al. and by Bridges and Goldberg in this volume. Though undoubtedly a general finding in epidemiological surveys of this type, its interpretation is far from simple. If the inquiry is focused on the patient's psychological status, his presentation of somatic complaints may be construed as a defence mechanism, which serves to conceal the true nature of his problems. On the other hand, if the patient's presenting complaints are regarded as constituting his request for help (or 'demand' for care), and hence as the basis of the doctor–patient transaction, they must be accepted as valid; the patient himself has in effect defined his complaint as somatic.

Probably the most useful approach lies somewhere between these two extremes. Though we are not able to indicate the correct position more precisely, our data provide two pointers. First, many patients with overt psychological disturbance consult for somatic complaints which do not appear to be causally linked to their psychological problems. In the present survey, one-third of the consultations by patients with manifest psychiatric disturbance were of this nature. Second, in a high proportion of contacts, patients presented with somatic complaints which the doctors could not account for in terms of physical illness. It is chiefly this group which gives rise to the suspicion that there is an 'iceberg' of concealed or inconspicuous psychiatric morbidity in the practice population. Most of the patients concerned have revealed no signs of deviant illness behaviour during the three-month survey period. A large majority (four-fifths) of them have come with such 'psychosomatic' symptoms on only a single occasion during this period. The group as a whole has a lower frequency of consultation than do those patients who present with overt psychological disturbance.

From these observations, we conclude that many persons who periodically suffer from psychological distress tend to transmute it into somatic complaints and to seek medical help for these, but that the underlying psychological distress is seldom put forward as the reason for consulting. A question has to be posed, therefore, as to how appropriate detection of all this hidden distress would be, and to what extent medical treatment for it would be beneficial. Copeland (1981) commented that a 'case' is 'a chimera, existing only in the mind of the investigator. Rather than regard the concept as a sort of Platonic ideal . . . the investigator should ask – "a case for what?"' On this point Goldberg (1982), in a thoughtful paper on the concept of a psychiatric 'case' in general practice, has suggested that one should also ask – 'a case for whom?' – in other words, for generalist or specialist – and has distinguished between three kinds of label a general practitioner might usefully apply:

1 Major psychiatric illnesses, for which there is a medical treatment of established value, and which can benefit from medical help whether or not the patient's coping strategies have already broken down.
2 Psychological stress not requiring specific intervention. Here four subgroups should be distinguished:
patients whose distress is 'subclinical' in intensity;
patients with transient, self-limiting reactions to some external events;
patients whose distress turns out to be unrelated to the problem for which help is being sought;
patients whose distress is well established and is in understandable relationship to an external situation which cannot be modified.
3 Psychological stress requiring intervention, of which the single largest group, according to Goldberg, is made up of patients with symptoms of both anxiety and depression accompanied by various neurasthenic symptoms, such as anergia, fatigue, lack of concentration and irritability.

Adopting this classification, we suggest that a large number of persons in the second category – psychological distress not requiring specific intervention – may be found among the patients in our survey who presented unexplained somatic symptoms. Most of these will probably never come forward with a health problem formulated in psychological terms. It cannot be said that none of them want to discuss such problems: no doubt many GPs do not offer their patients an easy opportunity to do so. However, in many instances the patient's reticence to talk about such problems should be respected and the doctor's treatment be focused – at any rate for the time being – on the presenting symptoms. A partial explanation of the discrepancy between standardized screening measures and illness behaviour, as registered in our survey, may be found in the fact that the number of people experiencing temporary psychological distress greatly exceeds the number who seek or expect medical help for it.

In conclusion, a standardized approach may well provide the most reliable estimate of the frequency of psychological disturbance, but will by its very nature tend to over-estimate the requirement for mental health care. Because such standardized techniques are usually applied in cross-sectional studies, they will also tend to over-estimate the prevalence of clinically significant psychiatric illness in the general-practice population, by including in the count a proportion of transient, self-limiting problems which the use of more precise and detailed case criteria would probably exclude. These tendencies, combined with the fact that mentally ill people have their due share of unrelated physical disorders, may account for the fact that many more patients are picked out by standardized screening procedures than are assessed by GPs as cases in need of treatment or other intervention.

To return in conclusion to the Goldberg–Huxley model: it would be useful to carry out assessments of the perceived needs of patients at Level 2, and of the extent to which these are met by the GPs themselves or, alternately, by means of psychiatric specialist referral. Only in this way could a more accurate picture be obtained of what the GPs are missing or erroneously neglecting: information which would be of great help in trying to attune need, demand and supply in primary health care.

REFERENCES

Bridges, K.W. and Goldberg, D.P. (1991) 'Somatisation in primary health care: prevalence and determinants' (this volume, pp. 341–50).

Copeland, J.R.M. (1981) 'What is a case? – a case for what?', in J.K. Wing, P. Bebbington, and L.N. Robins (eds), *What is a Case? The Problems of Definition in Community Psychiatric Surveys*, London: Grant McIntyre, pp. 7–11.

Crombie, D.L. (1963) 'The procrustean bed of medical nomenclature', *Lancet* 1:1205–6.

Crombie, D.L. (1986) 'Classification of mental illness for primary care', in M. Shepherd, G. Wilkinson, and P. Williams (eds), *Mental Illness in Primary Care Settings*, London: Tavistock, pp. 27–45.

Finlay-Jones, R.A. and Burvill, P.W. (1978) 'Contrasting demographic patterns of minor psychiatric morbidity and the community', *Psychological Medicine* 8:455–66.

Foets, M., Velden, J. van der, and Zee, J. van der (1986) *A National Survey of Morbidity and Interventions in General Practice*, Utrecht: NIVEL.

Goldberg, D. (1982) 'The concept of a psychiatric "case" in general practice', *Social Psychiatry* 17:61–5.

Goldberg, D.P. and Blackwell, B. (1970) 'Psychiatric illness in general practice: a detailed study using a new method of case identification', *British Medical Journal* ii:439–43.

Goldberg, D. and Bridges, K. (1987) 'Screening for psychiatric illness in general practice: the GP versus the General Health Questionnaire', *Journal of the Royal College of General Practitioners* 37:15–18.

Goldberg, D. and Huxley, P. (1980) *Mental illness in the Community: the Pathway to Psychiatric Care*, London: Tavistock.

Hoeper, E.W., Nycz, G.R., Cleary, P.D., Regier, D., and Goldberg, I. (1979) 'Estimated prevalence of RDC mental disorders in primary medical care', *International Journal of Mental Health* 8:6–15.

Jencks, S.I. (1985) 'Recognition of mental distress and diagnosis of mental disorder in primary care', *Journal of the American Medical Association* 253:1903–7.

Kessler, L.G., Burns, B.G., Shapiro, S., Tischler, G.L., George, L.K., Hough, R.L., Bodison, D., and Miller, R.H. (1987) 'Psychiatric diagnosis of medical service users: evidence from the epidemiologic catchment area program', *American Journal of Public Health* 77:18–24.

Kramer, M., Lima, B., Simonsick, E., and Levav, I. (1991) 'The epidemiological basis for primary health care: a case for action' (this volume, pp. 69–98).

Lamberts, H. and Hartman, B. (1982) 'Psychische en sociale problemen in de huisartspraktijk' (Psychological and social problems in general practice), *Huisarts en Wetenschap* 25:333–42.

Lamberts, H. and Woods, M. (1987) *International Classification of Primary Care*, Oxford: Oxford Medical Publications.

Schulberg, H.C., Saul, M., McClelland, M., Ganguli, M., Wallace, C., and Frank, R. (1985) 'Assessing depression in primary medical care and psychiatric practices', *Archives of General Psychiatry* 42:1164–70.

Shepherd, M., Cooper, B., Brown, A.C., and Kalton, G. (1981) *Psychiatric Illness in General Practice*, second edn, Oxford: Oxford University Press.

Verhaak, P.F.M., Wennink, H.J., and Tijhuis, M. (1990) The importance of the GHQ for general practice. *Family Practice* 7:319–24.

Whitehouse, C.R. (1987) 'A survey of the management of psychosocial illness in general practice in Manchester', *Journal of the Royal College of General Practitioners* 37:112–15.

Wright, A.F. and Perini, A.F. (1987) 'Hidden psychiatric illness: use of the General Health Questionnaire in general practice', *Journal of the Royal College of General Practitioners* 37:164–7.

Chapter 9

Psychiatric morbidity and physical illness among general practice patients in Cantabria, Spain

J. L. Vázquez-Barquero

The way in which illness is expressed is shaped to a great extent by a complex interaction between physical and psychiatric disorders. This interaction has been demonstrated in a variety of medical settings (Maguire and Granville-Grossman 1968; Ballinger 1976; Koranyi 1972; Vázquez-Barquero et al. 1985) and, in particular, in general practice populations (Shepherd et al. 1966; Bentsen 1970; Eastwood 1975). This latter group of studies is especially relevant as they provide a clearer picture of what happens in the general population, and also of the factors which influence the process of passing through the first 'filter', according to the model of care proposed by Goldberg and Huxley (1980). Despite all these findings, however, we have to conclude that the characteristics and nature of the interaction between physical and psychiatric disorders, in a general practice context, remain still in need of clarification.

Demographic factors have been found to play a relevant role in the interaction between these two types of health disorder. Of these, sex differences are the most consistently reported. Most surveys have demonstrated that the interaction is significantly stronger in females than in males (Schwab et al. 1979; Vázquez-Barquero et al. 1981; 1987; 1990). Even though the effect of age on rates of psychiatric morbidity is less pronounced (Andrews et al. 1978; Vázquez-Barquero et al. 1981), we were able to show from our community data that it can influence psychiatric consultation rates (Vázquez-Barquero et al. 1990). Furthermore, a number of surveys have reported that the association between physical and mental illness increases significantly with age (Bremer 1951; Andrews et al. 1978; Schwab et al. 1979; Vázquez-Barquero et al. 1981; 1987). The influence of marital status, on the other hand, was found to be insignificant in most surveys (Schwab et al. 1979; Vázquez-Barquero et al. 1981; 1987; 1990).

Socio-cultural factors affect the association between physical and mental illness in a complex way. Although contradictory findings have been reported, it appears that the association is stronger in the presence of certain 'negative' social conditions. This has been demonstrated, for example, by Brown and Harris with respect to a lack of family and social support, and by other authors in relation to unemployment, low social status and low educational level (Kasl *et al*. 1975; Catalano and Dooley 1977; Vázquez-Barquero *et al*. 1981; 1987; 1990).

The act of consulting a general practitioner is part of the manifestation of illness behaviour and is itself influenced by the presence either of physical or of psychiatric disorder. Thus, whereas physical illness is believed to be the best predictor of primary health-care utilization, psychiatric disorders have also emerged as a powerful determinant of the decision to seek help from the general practitioner. This has been confirmed in our community survey, in which, by calculating Levin's 'Attributable Risk' (Levin 1953), we found that 15.5 per cent of male consultations and 20.3 per cent of female consultations could be attributed to psychiatric morbidity (Vázquez-Barquero *et al*. 1990). The fact that so high a proportion of primary-care contacts is due to the presence of psychiatric illness could bias the analysis of associations between the two types of disorder. One way to overcome this difficulty is to study patients who have made contact with the doctors exclusively for some physical illness.

The aim of the present study is to explore the nature and characteristics of the association between physical and mental illness in a sample of physically ill community respondents who, in the two weeks prior to the survey, had made contact with a general practice because of somatic pathology of a non-transient nature.

SURVEY METHOD

1 Population and sampling procedure

The survey sample was drawn from the electoral register of a district of the region of Cantabria, Spain. The district has a population of 9,250 inhabitants, from which a stratified random sample of 1,223 persons (581 males and 642 females) aged 17 years or over was drawn. As shown in Table 9.1, 345 individuals (28.2 per cent) could not be interviewed, for one reason or another, including 98 (8.0 per cent) who refused to participate. Sixteen residents (1.3 per cent) were either too seriously physically ill or too mentally impaired to sustain an interview, the latter group including cases of dementia, schizophrenia and severe mental retardation. The remaining non-contacts could be ascribed either to the 'never available' group (10.1 per cent) or to deficiencies in the census-taking. All these missing individuals were replaced by others, drawn from the same stratified sample.

Respondents were interviewed in their homes using standardized medical and social interview schedules. The medical questionnaire included items related to physical health, illness behaviour and medical consultation. The respondent's reason for consulting, as well as his or her physical health

Table 9.1 Survey sample: contacts, refusals and non-contacts, by sex

Outcome of contact	Male	Female	Both sexes
Interview completed	581	642	223
Interview not completed			
(individual replaced):	197	148	345
dead	7	10	17
moved out of area	34	56	90
refused interview	60	38	98
too ill to be			
interviewed	10	6	16
could not be			
contacted	86	38	124
Total	778	790	1,568

status, was checked with the general practitioner using his medical records. The initial sample was restricted to those patients who had consulted a general practitioner in the two weeks prior to the survey, because of a physical illness. Finally, after verification by the general practitioner, only patients with a clearly diagnosed physical illness of non-transient nature were included in the further investigation and analysis. The distribution of somatic pathology in the selected sample is shown in Table 9.2.

2 Assessment and ratings

Psychiatric morbidity was rated by means of the General Health Questionnaire, 60-item version – GHQ-60 (Goldberg and Williams 1988) in its Spanish form (Vázquez-Barquero *et al.* 1986). This instrument is designed to identify and assess the degree of non-psychotic psychiatric disturbances. It has been widely used in a variety of community and medical settings. The unweighted GHQ scoring method was selected and a cut-off score of 11 applied.

For the present analysis, six socio-demographic characteristics were established and rated, each using a simple dichotomy, as follows:

Marital status was classed as either 'never married' or 'currently or formerly married'.

Age was classed as '17–44 years' or '45 years or over'.

Occupational status was classed as 'employed' or 'non-employed'. By non-employed we meant a lack of gainful occupation, whether as a result of unemployment, retirement or ill health. In the case of women, housewives with no gainful occupation were also included in this category.

Table 9.2 Distribution of diagnosed somatic pathology in the survey sample, by
     sex (N = 1,223)

Type of somatic pathology	Male (%)	Female (%)	Both sexes (%)
Single diagnoses:	15.1	22.1	18.9
cardiovascular	3.6	5.1	4.4
digestive system	0.9	1.6	1.2
rheumatic	4.3	4.7	4.5
respiratory	2.1	1.9	1.9
gynaecological	–	1.1	0.6
neurological	1.4	1.7	1.6
other	2.9	6.2	4.7
Multiple diagnoses	5.7	7.8	6.8
Total somatic pathology	20.8	29.9	25.6
No diagnosed somatic pathology	79.2	70.1	74.3
No. of persons	581	642	1,223

Educational levels were combined into two categories, called simply
   'higher' – persons with secondary school education or higher – and
   'lower' – those with primary school education only, as well as all
   illiterate individuals.
Social status, based on the respondent's own occupational class, or that
   of the father in the case of students and of the husband in the case of
   housewives, was likewise divided into 'higher' and 'lower' groups.
Area of residence was characterized as either semi-urban or rural, the
   latter group including all persons living in small villages or isolated
   farmhouses.

The effect of the socio-demographic variables on psychiatric morbidity
was explored by means of linear-logistic modelling, with a 'step-down'
procedure. For computer analysis, the GLIM program package was used
(Baker and Nelder 1987).

SURVEY FINDINGS

1 Psychiatric morbidity and socio-demographic characteristics

Table 9.3 shows associations between the GHQ score and the characteristics
sex, age and marital status. As can be seen, nearly one-third (31 per
cent) of the respondents scored above the cut-off point on the GHQ

Table 9.3 Psychiatric morbidity, according to selected demographic characteristics, in respondents with somatic pathology diagnosed by general practitioners (N = 313)

Demographic characteristic	No. of persons	High GHQ score		Estimated prevalence (%)	Statistical significance
		No.	%		
Sex:					
Male	121	26	21.5	11.9	P<0.005
Female	192	71	37.1	20.6	
Age:					
Under 45 years	70	12	17.1	9.5	P<0.005
45 years or older	243	85	35.1	19.5	
Marital status:					
Single	50	10	20.0	11.1	NS
Ever-married	263	87	33.1	18.4	
All persons	313	97	31.0	17.2	

and to that extent could be regarded as probable 'cases' of psychiatric disorder. When the validity indices of the GHQ-60 obtained by examining a Spanish community sample (Vázquez-Barquero et al. 1986) were applied to the present data, the estimated prevalence of psychiatric morbidity was found to be 17.2 per cent. The table also shows that the psychiatric prevalence was significantly higher in females than in males, and in the older than in the younger age-group. The relative excess among currently or formerly married individuals, on the other hand, was not of statistical significance.

Associations between GHQ score and the social variables are shown in Table 9.4. It appears that non-employed respondents had a significantly higher morbidity rate than those who were employed. Although the psychiatric prevalence was relatively high in respondents of low social status, low educational level and a semi-urban area of residence, these differences failed to reach a significant level.

2 Multivariate analysis

The combined effect of physical illness and all the socio-demographic variables on the probability of psychiatric illness was examined by means of logistic modelling. Only main effects and two-way effects were included

Table 9.4 Psychiatric morbidity, according to selected social characteristics, in respondents with somatic pathology diagnosed by general practitioners (N = 313)

Social characteristic	No. of persons	High GHQ score		Estimated prevalence (%)	Statistical significance (Chi-square)
		No.	*%*		
Gainful employment:					
employed	122	30	24.6	13.7	
					P<0.005
non-employed	191	67	35.1	19.5	
Educational level:					
higher	43	9	20.9	11.6	
					NS
lower	270	88	32.6	18.1	
Social status:					
higher	33	8	24.2	13.4	
					NS
lower	280	89	31.8	17.6	
Area of residence:					
semi-urban	98	34	34.7	19.3	
					NS
rural	215	63	29.3	16.3	

in the analysis. The model found to fit the data best (deviance $[G^2]$ = 14.57; df = 29; P = 0.98) was:

$$Ln (P/ [1 - P] = GM + SEXi + AGEj$$

where:

P   is the proportion of respondents with psychiatric illness;
GM   is a constant (Grand Mean);
SEXi is the effect of sex when i takes the value of 1 for males and 2 for females;
AGEj is the effect of age when j takes the value of 1 for persons under 45 years of age and 2 for persons aged 45 years or over.

Details of the model are given in Table 9.5. The model indicates that sex and age each have an independent effect on the prevalence of psychiatric disorders. There were no two-way effects. The model shows a significant excess of morbidity in females and in the older age range. The probabilities of psychiatric illness for each of the four age and sex groups, derived from this model, are presented in Table 9.6.

Table 9.5 Significant joint effects of socio-demographic variables on the frequency of psychiatric morbidity of respondents with diagnosed somatic pathology (N = 313)

	Estimate	(SE)	Difference in deviance	Statistical significance
GM	−1.671	0.3177	−	−
Sex (2)	0.6373	0.2542	6.51	d.f. = 1; P < 0.01
Age (2)	0.6582	0.3034	5.03	d.f. = 1; P < 0.025

Sex 1, Age 1, were all constrained to be zero by the model

DISCUSSION

We have estimated that 17.2 per cent (11.9 per cent of males and 20.6 per cent of females, over the age of 17 years) among physically ill persons who consulted a general practice clinic also manifested psychiatric disturbance, as measured by the GHQ-60. Although these estimates are markedly higher than those previously made by us for the general population of Cantabria (Vázquez-Barquero *et al*. 1987), they are somewhat lower than has been found in studies in the general practice setting conducted in other countries (Goldberg and Huxley 1980). A possible explanation for the lower figures in Cantabria may be that the present study was based on physically ill community residents who retrospectively reported contact with general practitioners in the two weeks preceding interview. In these circumstances one might expect to detect fewer cases of psychiatric morbidity than when assessing patients at the stressful time at which they are seeking medical help. We have also to take into account that in this study the psychiatric assessment was based on a self-report questionnaire and this may increase the possibility of the reported rates being influenced by under-reporting.

Our findings tend to confirm that, as has been reported from a number of other surveys (Schwab *et al*. 1979; Vázquez-Barquero *et al*. 1981; 1987; 1990), the prevalence of psychiatric illness, among physically ill persons who consult a general practitioner, is considerably higher in women than in men, the male–female ratio in this instance being 1.0 : 1.7. This female predominance has been interpreted in two ways: first, as a reflection of differences in morbidity and, second, as due to sex-specific patterns of illness behaviour. There is evidence to suggest that females are more likely to consult, especially with vague complaints or when looking for reassurance, and are also more predisposed than men to report symptoms (Goldberg and Huxley 1980; Vázquez-Barquero *et al*. 1990).

In most surveys, age appears to exert a significant effect on the frequency of physical illness and also on the likelihood of consulting a general practitioner. The direction of this effect has been towards an increase of

Table 9.6 Estimated probability of psychiatric morbidity, according to demographic profile

Demographic profile	Probability of psychiatric morbidity (%)
Male, younger age-group	15.8
Male, older age-group	26.6
Female, younger age-group	26.2
Female, older age-group	40.7

physical illness and consulting frequency with increasing age. Our analysis is in agreement with the findings of earlier studies in this respect.

Certain 'negative' social characteristics, such as being out of work, or having a low social status and educational level, have been found to strengthen the association between physical and psychiatric morbidity, both in community surveys and in various medical settings. Our present findings, however, do not provide confirmation for this hypothesis. Furthermore, in our survey social factors did not exert a significant effect on the logistic model, once the effects of age and sex had been allowed for.

Finally, one of the main benefits of the logistic modelling is that it permits quantification of the probability of a psychiatric illness in the groups defined by the model. It appears from Table 9.6 that:

1 both in males and females the increase in probability of psychiatric illness from the lower to the higher risk groups was about 1.5;
2 in the groups defined by age the probability of psychiatric morbidity was higher in women than in men; and
3 in the groups defined by sex the probability of psychiatric morbidity was increased significantly in the older age-group.

To summarize: we have presented data illustrating, first, that a high proportion of persons who establish contact with primary-care doctors have both physical and psychiatric disorders; second, that among the physically ill the risk of psychiatric disorder is higher in women and in the older age-groups; and lastly that socio-demographic characteristics such as marital status, social class, education level, area of residence or employment status do not appear to influence the interaction between the two types of ill health. These findings, which have important implications for health services, emphasize the need to develop strategies aimed at improving the process by which mental disorders are recognized and treated in general practice settings, as well as the need to continue investigation of the factors determining the coexistence of physical and mental illness in many patients.

ACKNOWLEDGEMENTS

This study was supported by grants (Exp. No. 88/2147, 89/0361) from the Spanish Institute of Health (FIS). Thanks are due to Dr P. Williams and Dr G. Wilkinson, formerly of the Institute of Psychiatry, London, for their helpful suggestions on the draft manuscript.

REFERENCES

Andrews, G., Tennant, C., Hewson, D., and Schonell, M. (1978) 'The relation of social factors to physical and psychiatric illness', *American Journal of Epidemiology* 108:25–37.

Baker, R.J. and Nelder, J.A. (1987) *The GLIM System Release 3.77 NAG*, London: Royal Statistical Society.

Ballinger, C.B. (1976) 'Psychiatric morbidity and the menopause: clinical features', *British Medical Journal* i: 1183–5.

Bentsen, B.G. (1970) *Illness and General Practice: a Survey of Medical Care in an Island Population in south-east Norway*, Oslo, Bergen, Trømso: Universitets-Forlaget (Scandinavian University Books).

Bremer, J. (1951) 'A social psychiatric investigation of a small community of northern Norway', *Acta Psychiatrica Scandinavica*, Supplement 62.

Brown, G.W. and Harris, T. (1978) *Social Origins of Depression: a Study of Psychiatric Disorders in Women*, London: Tavistock.

Catalano, D.W. and Dooley, D.C. (1977) 'Economic predictions of depressed mood and stressful life events in a metropolitan community', *Journal of Health and Social Behaviour* 18:292–307.

Eastwood, M.R. (1975) *The Relation between Physical and Mental Illness*, Toronto: University of Toronto Press.

Goldberg, D.P. and Huxley, P. (1980) *Mental Illness in the Community: the Pathway to Psychiatric Care*, London: Tavistock.

Goldberg, D. and Williams, P. (1988) *A User's Guide to the General Health Questionnaire*, Windsor, UK: NFER-Nelson.

Kasl, S.W., Gore, S., and Cobb, S. (1975) 'The experience of losing a job: reported changes in health, symptoms and illness behaviour', *Psychological Medicine* 37:106–22.

Koranyi, E.K. (1972) 'Physical health and illness in psychiatric out-patient department populations', *Journal of the Canadian Psychiatric Association* 17:109–21.

Levin, M.L. (1953) 'The occurrence of lung cancer in man', *Acta Unio Internationale Contra Cancrum* 19:531–41.

Maguire, G.P. and Granville-Grossman, K.L. (1968) 'Physical illness in psychiatric patients', *British Journal of Psychiatry* 114:1365–9.

Schwab, J.J., Bell, R.A., Warheit, G.J., and Schwab, R.B. (1979) *Social Order and Mental Health: the Florida Health Survey*, New York: Brunner Mazel.

Shepherd, M., Cooper, B., Brown, A.C., and Kalton, G. (1966) *Psychiatric Illness in General Practice*, London: Oxford University Press.

Vázquez-Barquero, J.L., Muñoz, P.E., and Madoz Jauregui, V. (1981) 'The interaction between physical illness and neurotic morbidity in the community', *British Journal of Psychiatry* 139:328–35.

Vázquez-Barquero, J.L., Padierna Acero, J.A., Ochoteco, A., and Diez Manrique, J.F. (1985) 'Mental illness and ischaemic heart disease: analysis of psychiatric morbidity', *General Hospital Psychiatry* 7:15–20.

Vázquez-Barquero, J.L., Diez Manrique, J.F., Peña, C., Quintanal, R.G., and Labrador Lopez, M. (1986) 'Two-stage design in a community survey', *British Journal of Psychiatry* 149:88–97.

Vázquez-Barquero, J.L., Diez Manrique, J.F., Peña, C., Aldama, J., Samaniego, C., Menendez, A.J., and Miropeix, C. (1987) 'A community mental health survey in Cantabria: a general description of morbidity', *Psychological Medicine* 17:227–41.

Vázquez-Barquero, J.L., Peña, C., Diez Manrique, J.F., Arenal, A., Quintanal, R.G., and Samaniego, C. (1988) 'The influence of socio-cultural factors on the interaction between physical and mental disturbances in a rural community', *Social Psychiatry and Psychiatric Epidemiology* 23:195–201.

Vázquez-Barquero, J.L., Wilkinson, G., Williams, P., Diez Manrique, J.F., and Peña, C. (1990) 'Mental health and medical consultation in primary care settings', *Psychological Medicine* 20:681–94.

Chapter 10

Mental disorders in primary care in a health district of Bahia, Brazil

N. M. de Almeida-Filho, V. S. Santana, E. C. Moreira, M. G. Modesto and M. B. Oliveira

Many epidemiological studies of mental disorders in primary-care settings have been conducted in developed countries (Shepherd *et al*. 1966; Hankin and Oktay 1979; Bebbington *et al*. 1981; Barrett *et al*. 1988) and in some Third World countries (Harding *et al*. 1980). In Brazil, up to 1989, only three investigations of this kind have been reported. Santana (1977) studied retrospectively the frequency of psychiatric problems in a sample of 208 persons registered for care in a community health centre in Salvador, Bahia. The results indicated that 15 per cent of the patients presented psychiatric complaints at their first visit to the clinic. An additional 6 per cent received psychotropic drug prescriptions without any psychiatric diagnosis being recorded. Although recognizing that the study dealt with a poor quality of case recording, the author did not make any attempt to evaluate the influence of the recording system on the data collected. Busnello *et al*. (1983) investigated the occurrence of psychiatric problems in a sample of 242 patients of a community health centre in Porto Alegre, Rio Grande do Sul. In this study, a short standardized questionnaire (the Self-Report Questionnaire – SRQ) was completed by each patient. The authors estimated an overall frequency of emotional problems of around 55 per cent. However, they did not provide detailed information on their methodology or on the data analysis.

Finally, Mari (1987) studied the frequency of psychiatric disturbances in two health centres and one out-patient clinic of a general hospital on the periphery of São Paulo, with a selected sample of 875 patients. This study was based on an application of the SRQ together with the General Health Questionnaire (GHQ) as screening instruments, validated by comparison with a diagnostic assessment made using the Clinical Interview Schedule (CIS). The frequency of minor psychiatric morbidity was found to be very high – around 50 per cent in all three services – while one-quarter of those attending the clinics presented relatively severe psychiatric disturbances. Women had proportionately more minor mental disturbance than men, and the frequency was also raised in the low-income groups of the population.

Two of these three studies had problems of sample size, which did not allow them to go beyond presenting crude total morbidity estimates. In addition, because they were based on individual treatment agencies, none of them covered the entire population demanding primary care in the respective catchment areas. For this reason, their findings may have been affected by selection biases. Even so, it is of interest to note the large differences in frequency estimates between the first of the studies, which was based on a simple case registry, and the other two, which made use of the direct application of standardized questionnaires.

The present study is aimed at drawing a profile of psychiatric morbidity for the adult clientele of primary health services in one health district of Salvador, Bahia. In addition, it is intended to evaluate the quality of data recording of the health registry, with regard to information on mental and emotional disorders.

SURVEY METHOD

1 The research setting

The health district of Itapagipe is located on the west side of Salvador (population, 1.9 million), capital city of the state of Bahia, north-east Brazil. Covering an area of approximately 146 sq km and a population of 145,000 people (1986 projection), the health district includes 13 *bairros* (neighbourhoods), mostly low-income and with poor housing and sanitary conditions. There are seven primary health-care institutions in the district: one municipal medical/dental centre, two small out-patient clinics and two community health centres administered by the state government, one small health centre of the LBA (a federal welfare institution) and, finally, the out-patient service of the Santo Antonio Hospital, a medium-sized general hospital used as a teaching setting for medical students.

2 Sampling procedure

In 1986, there were 18,990 new registrations for primary health care at the health institutions of the district. The LBA centre was not included in this census because at that time it had only a paediatric clinic open. The municipal medical/dental centre also had to be excluded because it was closed for restoration. Patients receiving 'secondary level' care in specialist clinics were also not counted. Of the services which were included in the census, the Santo Antonio out-patient service recorded 14,609 patient registrations, or 77 per cent of the total.

A proportional sampling technique was employed, with random starting assignment for each service, and selected one in thirty patients of the Santo

Table 10.1 Demographic characteristics of the survey sample

Characteristic	No. of persons	Adjusted (%)[1]
Age-group:		
under 25	331	31.3
26–35	197	19.4
36–45	119	15.0
46–55	103	11.5
56+	148	19.4
unknown	63	3.4
Gender:		
female	590	61.8
male	295	34.0
unknown	76	4.2
Total	961	100.0

[1]Adjustment for sampling weights in the different health-care facilities

Antonio clinic and one in ten of the pooled registered patients from all the other clinics. The final sample was made up of 961 individuals. Table 10.1 shows that the majority of these are female (62 per cent) and under 35 years old (51 per cent). Both groups are over-represented by comparison with the general population of the district (IBGE 1985).

3 Data gathering

Initially, a pilot study was conducted in order to explore the prospects for institutional co-operation, the state of the medical files and the feasibility of data gathering. The collection of data was undertaken by three third-year medical students (E.C.M., M.G.M. and M.B.O.), who were intensively trained and eventually became active participants in planning and carrying out the research project as a whole. Sampled case-records were subjected to a detailed examination, making use of standard evaluation procedures. Information on the study topics was transferred to a special form, whose eight sections covered: (1) identification; (2) personal data; (3) types of care delivered; (4) findings on clinical examination; (5) laboratory tests; (6) other diagnostic information; (7) prescriptions, and (8) assessment of the data quality. The data-gatherers were instructed to consider every item of information found in the patients' records, and to search for misplaced information; for example, a missing diagnosis noted on a prescription form, or reasons for consultation entered on the diagnosis sheet. They were also trained to decipher illegible entries, such as are universally attributed to medical records. Missing or illegible information was noted as such and contributed to the assessment of data quality. The data gathering was closely supervised, and each case carefully reviewed by the research group, to detect possible errors or ambiguities on the recording forms.

4 Data analysis

The relative frequencies of psychiatric morbidity were estimated in three ways: (1) psychiatric symptoms or emotional or behavioural disturbance noted as the main reason for consultation; (2) psychiatric diagnosis recorded by the treating physician, and (3) prescription of psychotropic medication. In the first approach, a comprehensive list of symptoms and complaints was drawn up from a content analysis of the data and, following discussion by the research team, was used as the basis for a classification suitable for the research objectives. The second approach was fairly straightforward, since most diagnoses had been recorded according to the International Classification of Diseases, Ninth Revision, the classification system officially adopted in Brazil, and the few exceptions were carefully reviewed and classified by the research team. For the third approach, a list of brand-name psychopharmacological substances marketed in Brazil was available as a basis for classifying the drugs prescribed.

At this stage, clinical experts from the faculty of the university medical school were consulted about many of the cases, in order to minimize any misclassification of complaints, diagnoses or medication. The data were analysed on a microcomputer IBM-AT compatible with SPSS-PC+ software.

In this report, indicators of psychiatric morbidity are presented by sex and age, with frequency estimates adjusted for the differential weightings of the proportional sub-sample. Mantel-Haenszel estimators of odds ratios (mOR) are employed for the comparisons between these adjusted estimates, and 95 per cent confidence intervals calculated by the test-based method (Kleinbaum, Kupper and Morgenstern 1982). These special summary estimators are particularly suitable, because some zero frequencies had to be expected in stratum-specific tables, as a result of simultaneous adjustment for the sampling-design effect and for confounding variables.

SURVEY FINDINGS

Table 10.2 reveals that some 5 per cent of the sample had emotional or behavioural disturbance recorded as the main reason for consultation. In a further 5 per cent, the reason for consultation was unrecorded. There were virtually no differences in relative frequency according to gender, yielding a non-significant odds ratio of 1.09 (0.43, 2.14). Clearer differences emerged with respect to age (collapsed into three groups for this analysis), there being a marked rise in frequency of psychiatric complaints with rising age, from 5 per cent for the age-groups under 45 years to 8 per cent for the

Table 10.2 Type of medical complaint given as main reason for consultation, by age and gender

Characteristic	No. of persons	Neuro-psychiatric[1] (%)	Other conditions[1] (%)	Not recorded[1] (%)
Age-group:[2]				
under 25	331	4.6	88.4	7.0
26–45	316	4.8	92.0	3.2
46+	251	8.0	88.8	3.2
unknown	63			
Gender:[3]				
female	590	5.0	89.7	5.3
male	295	5.4	90.1	4.4
unknown	76			
Total	961	5.4	89.8	4.8

[1] Proportions weighted for the sampling design effect
[2] Adjusted by gender
[3] Adjusted by age

groups above that age. The odds ratio of 1.41 (1.01, 2.83) for this trend is of borderline significance.

According to Table 10.3, 8.8 per cent of the sample had some form of neuropsychiatric diagnosis recorded, while an additional 0.8 per cent also received psychopharmacological prescriptions. However, just over one-quarter of the patients had neither a diagnosis nor details of treatment recorded in their case-notes. Here again, no gender differences were found, the odds ratios being insignificant both for diagnosis (1.26) and for drug prescription (1.09). The age patterns are similar for these two indicators, suggesting higher frequencies in the age-group 26–45 years. Gender-adjusted odds ratios between this and the younger age-group were 1.96 (0.89, 4.33) with respect to diagnosis and 1.92 (0.93, 3.98) with respect to psychotropic drug prescribing. Corresponding odds ratios for comparison between the 26–45-year and over-45-year age-groups were 2.48 (1.16, 5.30) for diagnosis and 1.88 (0.95, 3.73) for psychotropic drug-prescribing. Failure to record the necessary information was found most often for the younger age-group (35 per cent) and may thus have contributed to some under-estimation of case frequency in this age range. The same point does not, however, hold true for the oldest age-groups, for which incomplete case recording was less serious (17 per cent).

The frequency of neuropsychiatric diagnosis is presented in Table 10.4 according to gender and age-group. For men the lowest rates are found in the youngest and oldest groups, while there is a trend towards maximum rates in early and middle adult life. A similar trend is also discernible for

Table 10.3 Proportions of patients with (a) neuropsychiatric diagnoses and (b) psychopharmacological prescriptions recorded, by age and gender

Characteristic	No. of persons	Neuro-psychiatric diagnoses[1] (%)	Psychopharm. prescription only[1] (%)	No diagnosis or treatment recorded[1] (%)
Age-group:[2]				
under 25	331	6.0	1.3	35.0
26–45	316	13.1	0.6	24.0
46+	251	6.8	0.8	17.0
unknown	63			
Gender:[3]				
female	590	8.6	0.4	28.6
male	295	9.8	0.7	21.4
unknown	76			
Total	961	8.8	0.8	25.5

[1] Proportions adjusted for the sampling design effect
[2] Adjusted by gender
[3] Adjusted by age

women, but it is much less pronounced. The odds ratios for differences between the sexes are highest for the age-groups 36–45 and 46–55 years. None of the odds ratios shown in this table reaches statistical significance, though a significant excess among males was found when the age-groups from 26 to 55 years were collapsed into one.

Finally, Table 10.5 shows the distribution for recorded neuropsychiatric diagnoses by gender, broken down into major diagnostic categories. Neurotic and psychosomatic disorders constitute the largest groups (5 per cent in combination), followed by alcohol and drug abuse (2.5 per cent). Other severe psychiatric disorders (including two cases of schizophrenia and one of mental retardation) accounted for under 1 per cent of the sample. There is a strong, significant association between gender and frequency of substance-abuse disorders (mainly alcoholism, but also including three cases of narcotic addiction), with an odds ratio of 11.1 (3.00, 40.71) for males. Since most of the cases are men in the age-group 26–45 years, the prevalence of alcoholism could be responsible for the only clear-cut effect of gender found in this study, as shown in Table 10.4.

It can be seen from Table 10.5 that a small proportion (less than 1 per cent) of cases received a vague general diagnosis of mental disorder, with no further specification by the treating physician. One may also note that some 52 per cent of all diagnosed cases had no recorded prescription, while on the other hand nearly 1 in 10 of the patients with a psychopharmacological

Table 10.4 Weighted proportions of patients with neuropsychiatric diagnoses, by gender and age-group (N = 885)[1]

Age-group	Males (N = 295) (%)	Females (N = 590) (%)	Odds ratio (mOR)	(95% confidence interval)
Under 25	3.8	7.1	1.61	(0.56, 16.60)
26–35	16.8	9.7	1.88	(0.77, 4.60)
36–45	19.2	8.8	2.46	(0.76, 7.99)
46–55	17.9	6.8	3.00	(0.94, 9.61)
56+	2.5	5.7	2.36	(0.36, 15.63)

[1] Gender unknown in 76 cases

prescription had no recorded neuropsychiatric diagnosis. The overall quality of the medical records was very poor, suggesting that in this specific context at least, the primary-care providers simply were not trained to record adequately either their working diagnoses or the treatment they provided for psychiatrically disturbed patients.

DISCUSSION

Undoubtedly, these findings are subject to serious selection biases, due mainly to the unequal availability and access to health services in the Brazilian context. In addition, there are problems of the completeness and quality of health-service records which are bound to produce flaws in this type of investigation. In the present study, inaccuracy due to the indifferent quality of medical records was probably a more serious source of bias than any problems connected with the method of data collection. For these reasons, the frequencies of neuropsychiatric diagnosis, psychological complaints and prescribing of psychotropic drugs, as reported here, must be regarded as an under-estimate of the 'true' prevalence of psychiatric morbidity in this patient population.

Despite these limitations, the results indicate that, in the context of one urban area in north-east Brazil, psychiatric morbidity is being at least partially recognized and dealt with at the primary health-care level. In other words, general medical practitioners seem able to identify, and to some extent also to diagnose, to treat and when indicated to refer to specialists, psychiatric disturbance present in nearly 10 per cent of the patients who consult them in their everyday practice. Given the probability of under-estimation, the true case frequency is probably considerably higher than this, suggesting that primary health care has indeed become one of the most important resources for care of the mentally ill in urban areas in under-developed countries. Data from a population survey on the utilization of mental health services, conducted in another neighbourhood

Table 10.5 Weighted proportions of patients in the main neuropsychiatric Diagnostic categories, by gender (N = 841)[1]

Diagnostic category	Male (N = 282) (%)	Female (N = 559) (%)	Odds ratio (mOR)	(95% confidence interval)
Neurosis or psychosomatic disorder	3.1	6.0	1.92	(0.73, 5.04)
Alcoholism or drug abuse	6.0	0.5	11.11	(3.00, 40.71)
Other psychiatric disorders	–	0.5	–	–
Unspecified diagnoses	0.5	0.5	1.02	(0.00, ...)
All psychiatric disorders	9.6	7.8	1.27	(0.62, 2.60)

[1]Diagnosis not recorded in 120 cases

of Salvador (Santana *et al.* 1987), also indicate that general medical care is the type of service most in demand by persons who are in need of treatment and help for mental health problems.

Comparison of our findings with those of other investigations is limited because of methodological differences. The overall frequency of psychiatric morbidity found is only about half that reported by Santana (1977), who employed a similar methodology. The finding that there are no significant associations of psychiatric prevalence with gender, but an increased frequency among men in the middle age-groups, also fails to replicate the results of the other Brazilian studies (Santana 1977; Mari 1987), as well as of similar investigations conducted in other Third World countries (Harding *et al.* 1980). These discrepancies may arise from the diversity of socio-economic and cultural backgrounds involved, as well as from differences in the health-service structures in each country or region, and in the methods of data-gathering employed.

Paradoxically, given the serious methodological difficulties of conducting this type of study in developing countries, the principal achievement of the present project may lie in demonstrating that the use of case-record data for research purposes is not the exclusive prerogative of highly organized, sophisticated health-care systems. Careful, exhaustive and labour-intensive data collection, combined with simple but effective techniques of data analysis, make it possible to use routine medical records in psychiatric epidemiological studies in such developing countries, and at the same time to underline the need for an improved quality of case-recording. Studies of this type are especially important because of the still rudimentary status of mental health planning and care-provision in most Third World countries.

REFERENCES

Barrett, J.E., Barrett, J.A., Oxman, T., and Gerber, P. (1988) 'The prevalence of psychiatric disorders in a primary care practice', *Archives of General Psychiatry* 45:1100–6.

Bebbington, P., Hurry, J., Tennant, C., Sturt, E., and Wing, J.K. (1981) 'Epidemiology of mental disorders in Camberwell', *Psychological Medicine* 3:561–79.

Busnello, E., Bertolote, J., and Wildt, M. (1983) 'Psychiatric disorders in primary health care settings: incidence or prevalence?', WHO International Conference on Classification and Diagnosis of Mental Disorders: *Abstracts*, Copenhagen: WHO Regional Office for Europe.

Hankin, J. and Oktay, J. (1979) *Mental Disorders and Primary Medical Care. An Analytical Review of the Literature*, NIMH Series D, no. 5, DHEW Publication no. (ADM) 78–661, Washington, DC: US Government Printing Office.

Harding, T., de Arango, M.V., Baltazar, J., Climent, C.E., Ibrahim, H.A., Ladrido-Ignacio, L., Murthy, R.S., and Wig, N.N. (1980) 'Mental disorder in primary health care: a study of their frequency and diagnosis in four developing countries', *Psychological Medicine* 10:231–41.

IBGE (1985) *Anuario Estatistico Brasileiro*, Rio de Janeiro: Fundacão Instituto Brasileiro de Geografia e Estatistica.

Kleinbaum, D., Kupper, L., and Morgenstern, H. (1982) *Epidemiologic Research: Principles and Quantitative Methods*, Belmont, CA: Wardsworth.

Mari, J. (1987) 'Psychiatric morbidity in three primary medical care clinics in the city of São Paulo: issues on the mental health of the urban poor', *Social Psychiatry* 22:129–38.

Santana, V. (1977) 'Transtornos mentais em um centro de saúde de Salvador-Bahia', *Revista Baiana de Saude Pública* 4:160–7.

Santana, V., Almeida-Filho, N., Lima, F.B., and Nunes, M.D. (1987) 'Utilizacão de Serviços de Saude Mental em uma Área Urbana de Salvador, Bahia', *Revista Baiana de Saúde Pública* 13:194–211.

Shepherd, M., Cooper, B., Brown, A.C., and Kalton, G. (1966) *Psychiatric Illness in General Practice*, London: Oxford University Press.

Chapter 11

Use of services by homeless and disaffiliated individuals with severe mental disorders

A study in Melbourne

Helen Herrman, Patrick McGorry, Pamela Bennett, Katrina Varnavides and Bruce Singh

The numbers of obviously disturbed, homeless people in the cities of the western world, especially in the United States (Bassuk 1984), have increased in recent years. Concern about this has prompted several studies of mental disorder among homeless persons, and consideration of ways to provide appropriate services. Various sub-groups of the homeless population have been sampled in these studies, including frequenters of 'Skid Row', patients attending hospital emergency rooms, or occupants of single rooms. While the diagnostic criteria used and the skills of the interviewers have varied (Koegel *et al.* 1988; Morrissey and Levine 1987; Arce and Vergare 1986), it appears from American and British studies that somewhere between one-quarter and one-half of adult homeless persons are suffering severe and perhaps chronic mental disorder (Morrissey and Levine 1987; Koegel *et al.* 1988; Arce and Vergare 1986; Priest 1976; Bachrach 1984a). The number and proportion of the mentally ill appear to have increased significantly over the past twenty years, and the proportion of young chronically ill has apparently increased as the proportion of older substance abusers has decreased (Bachrach 1984a; Arce and Vergare 1984).

Previous reports of service use by single homeless people are concerned mainly with specialist mental health services in the United States. These reports suggest that between 20 per cent and 44 per cent of the people surveyed have a past history of psychiatric hospitalization; the higher rates have applied in those studies which include a past history of admission for drug or alcohol abuse (Gelberg *et al.* 1988). Gelberg and colleagues interviewed a randomly selected sample of over 500 homeless people in a Los Angeles beach community. A small proportion of respondents (15 per cent) had previous contact with out-patient psychiatric services only. Although a greater proportion (44 per cent) had a past history of hospitalization, very few with this history had made recent contact with out-patient or community mental health services.

The use of primary-care services by homeless, mentally ill people has received little attention, perhaps because in the United States the contribution of this service sector is relatively small. Elsewhere, as in Edinburgh (Powell 1988), there have been a number of attempts to provide acceptable and accessible primary health-care services for such people. In the British National Health Service overall, gaps remain in provision of general health (and social) services to the homeless despite elimination of hospital and medication charges, but Reuler (1988) believes that the emphasis on primary care facilitates problem-solving and provides a framework for 'mainstreaming the homeless into a single class system'. A recent study of single homeless people sleeping rough in London (Ramsden *et al.* 1989) found that most of those using a special mobile clinic either had no local general practitioner or did not consult about current problems. This special arrangement may, however, have provided a link to mainstream primary health care. In a survey of boarding-house occupants in Sydney, the primary-care physician was, by a long way, the main carer for many isolated mentally ill people (Harris *et al.* 1987). The extent to which homeless and disaffiliated people use these services, where they are available, remains unknown.

Debate continues about the most appropriate ways to provide primary and/or mental health care for single homeless people. Schemes which seek to isolate the single homeless as a group, and to provide for them by services separate from those for the rest of the population, have received criticism from the medical profession and from advocacy groups. The latter have expressed the view that access to normal health-care provision should be facilitated for the single homeless by efforts to increase their awareness and utilization of available services and by re-integration with the general population, rather than segregation through use of special facilities (Powell 1988).

In Australia, there has been limited study of mental disorder in homeless people. Doutney and colleagues (Doutney *et al.* 1985) diagnosed schizophrenia in 15 per cent of men living in a shelter in central Sydney. The national problem is not well documented otherwise, but members of the Victorian Council to Homeless Persons have expressed concern that staff in crisis accommodation centres, day centres and other services appear to be facing increasing difficulties in dealing with homeless and disaffiliated people with florid mental disorders. Lack of shelter and disaffiliation, or lack of social roots in a community, are often merged in the concept of homelessness (Fischer and Breakey 1986). Whereas people sleeping in crisis accommodation centres or shelters are clearly homeless, many other disaffiliated people are living in cheap, single-room accommodation. People in such marginal accommodation are probably more numerous in Melbourne than those living outdoors or in shelters, interchange with them to some extent, and appear to present a number of similar problems to service providers.

Although lack of shelter is an increasing problem in Melbourne, people without shelter are not encountered in the numbers known in recent times in the United States. A contributing factor may be that cheap single rooms are still more readily available in Melbourne, despite a shrinking supply, than in US cities.

AIMS AND METHOD

The aims of this survey were:

1 to estimate the prevalence of severe mental disorders in representative sub-groups of the homeless and disaffiliated populations, of persons aged 60 or under, of inner Melbourne, and
2 to describe the characteristics of people so affected, and their past and present use of services, with a view to guiding modifications and additions to service provision.

We set out to survey representative groups of homeless and disaffiliated people, as operationally defined below, with clinically experienced interviewers trained in the use of standardized methods of case definition.

1 Case definition and assessment

'Severe mental disorder' was defined as mental illness meeting the DSM-III-R criteria for schizophrenia, other psychotic disorders, major affective disorders, dysthymic disorder (as this indicates unremitting depressed mood for two years), and substance abuse or dependence (alcohol and other). We recorded indicators of organic mental disorder in addition, but did not make formal clinical assessments of organic mental disorder or mental retardation. We did not attempt to diagnose the severe personality disorders which are very disabling but difficult, and perhaps impossible, to diagnose in cross-section from the subject's report alone.

We used modules of the Structured Clinical Interview for DSM-III-R (SCID-R) (Spitzer et al. 1986) to construct the primary diagnostic tool. An exploratory screening section was followed by modules from the version for psychiatric patients, which allows for sub-categorization of psychotic disorders. The SCID-R is a flexible interview allowing cross-examination, and use of information from all available sources. We added the Mini-Mental State Examination (MMSE) to indicate whether or not a subject was cognitively impaired (Folstein et al. 1975), as well as questions on current accommodation, income and activities.

We recruited and trained six interviewers. They were all experienced professionals with backgrounds in psychiatric nursing, medicine, social work and psychology. We discussed and supervised the work in detail in weekly meetings through the three months of interviewing. One of the psychiatrists (PB) conducted thirty-eight independent repeat interviews within three weeks of the originals, to provide a measure of test–retest reliability. In addition, we obtained limited information about previous treatment contacts with state psychiatric services from the Victorian Psychiatric Case Register (Krupinski 1986).

2 Sampling procedures

The subjects were occupants of the Melbourne shelters for homeless people, and of the special accommodation houses and low-cost rooming houses in St Kilda, which is a needy inner city area of Melbourne with a high concentration of these types of accommodation. Only residents aged 15 to 60 years were interviewed. We regard the problems of elderly homeless people, especially those with organic mental disorder, as deserving separate study, with full clinical assessment of functional and organic mental disorder: this would be done best with instruments designed for use with the elderly, and would ideally include physical examinations. People with a command of English inadequate to complete the survey instruments were excluded.

The three main shelters for homeless men in Melbourne are located in inner areas of the city and have a total of 670 beds. One of these shelters houses a small number of women. We also approached a small (seven-bed) centre for women and a small youth crisis centre. The rooming houses (and private hotels) included were those with charges affordable for people on pensions; the great majority of rooming houses in St Kilda are in this price range. They were located from local government lists and the personal knowledge of social workers and community nurses. Special accommodation houses (SAHs) are state-registered premises established originally for the elderly disabled, but catering also to the physically and mentally handicapped in general. They provide full board and supervision. They operate on a commercial basis with no subsidies and mostly charge the amount of the invalid or older age pension as the price for accommodation.

We estimated the size of the study population and its distribution among the three types of accommodation, or three strata, after preliminary fieldwork in the area. We aimed to sample each of the three strata over as short a time as possible, to approximate to a point prevalence. In each of the shelters, we used the bed numbers on an overnight census list to select a one-in-two random sample, stratified by sex, of all occupants known or thought to be eligible on the basis of age. We did not attempt to replace those who refused to participate, had left, or could not be located after a number of return visits. A replacement was made when a subject was found to be over 60 years old or in the occasional case of an individual who had already been included in sampling at another site. In the early stages of the study, as a consequence of the unfamiliar and difficult conditions, the raters interviewed thirty-six men residing in the shelters who were not part of the random sample. We included the results of these interviews in the analyses after checking that the age and diagnostic profiles for this group did not differ significantly from those of the remainder of the group in the shelters.

The managers of all twenty-five special accommodation houses operating in the area were approached, and twenty-four agreed to participate. A one-in-two sample of all occupants less than 61 years of age was selected randomly from room or bed numbers in each house. The caretakers or owners of all eighty-three low-cost rooming houses and private hotels identified and operating in the area were approached, and forty-seven agreed to participate in the survey; there were no apparent differences in type or size of facility between those who participated and those who did not. In each participating house a one-in-three sample of all occupants known or thought to be eligible on the basis of age was selected randomly from room numbers. When necessary, several return visits were made to locate the residents.

Each respondent received $5 as recompense for time taken and inconvenience. Respondents gave informed verbal consent to the interview, and the information was used confidentially.

3 Construction of 'life-charts' for respondents

Information about major events was assembled from various sections of the interview, and in a few instances additional treatment information obtained from the case register (above). A lifeline was drawn for each respondent (Vaillant 1987) and accommodation, health and other events charted where information was available. Our main purpose in this was to chart the order in which onset of the first episode of severe mental disorder and of homelessness, as defined here, occurred in each individual's life history. We also expected to obtain an indication of patterns of use of this type of marginal accommodation.

FINDINGS OF THE SURVEY

1 Sample characteristics and response rate

The numbers of people sampled and interviewed are summarized in Table 11.1.

Of the individuals in the random sample (346 of 524) 66 per cent were located and interviewed. The proportions varied by type of accommodation: 64 per cent in the shelters, 93 per cent in the special accommodation houses and 57 per cent in the rooming houses and private hotels. Data from interviews with the 346 respondents and from the additional 36 men interviewed in the shelters are included in the analyses.

Table 11.1 Study population and sample by type of accommodation

Shelters	Special accommodation houses (SAHs)	Rooming houses & private hotels (RHs)
3 main shelters + 2 small shelters	Total number of houses in area = 25 with 563 occupants, including 212 aged 60 years and under	Total number of eligible establishments = 83 Estimated occupants 60 years and under = 1,000
	Participating houses = 24	Participating establishments = 47
Total census population = 667	Total census population = 525	Estimated total (census) population = 1,000
Estimated population 60 years and under = 439	Population 60 years and under = 198	Estimated population 60 years and under = 570
Sample size = 222	Sample size = 85	Sample size = 217
Interviewed = 143 (64%)	Interviewed = 79 (93%)	Interviewed = 124 (57%)
Non-random subjects interviewed = 36		
Total interviews = 179		

Total random sample = 524
Interviewed = 346 (66%)
Additional non-random sample = 36
Total interviewed = 382

Of the 382 subjects interviewed, 69 were female and 313 were male. Of the male subjects, 7 per cent were aged 15 to 24 years, 22 per cent were 25 to 34 years old, 29 per cent were 35 to 44, 23 per cent were 45 to 54, and 19 per cent were 55 to 60. Just under half (48 per cent) of the female subjects were between the ages of 35 and 54 years, and 28 per cent were below that age. Age and sex data were obtained on 140 of the 178 people sampled but not interviewed. The age and sex profile of this group (141 males, 34 females, 3 with sex unknown; 54 per cent between the ages 35 and 54, and 24 per cent below that age) was similar to that of the group interviewed.

Of the respondents (107 people) 28 per cent were born outside Australia, and 58 per cent of these in countries with national languages other than English. In comparison, the percentage of the general population born outside Australia is 40 per cent for the total population of inner Melbourne and 30 per cent for Melbourne. Two people were excluded from the study before interview because of an inadequate command of English. Over half (59 per cent) of those interviewed were receiving invalid pension or sickness benefits. Most of the remainder were receiving other pensions or benefits. Twenty-nine people (8 per cent) reported current paid employment, which was full-time for twenty-two (6 per cent).

2 Prevalence of psychiatric disorders

Results of reliability testing of the diagnostic instrument are reported elsewhere (Herrman *et al.* 1989). They show a good level of diagnostic agreement for the broad diagnostic groups, for which adequate base rates could be computed.

Findings on the prevalence of disorders are reported in greater detail elsewhere (Herrman *et al.* 1989). Alcohol dependence, dependence on other substances, schizophrenia and major depression were the most prevalent disorders. Eighteen per cent of the respondents received a diagnosis of a 'current' (past month) psychotic disorder, and 21 per cent of a 'lifetime' psychotic disorder. For the broad diagnostic categories of mood and substance-related disorders the rate of current diagnosis was less than half the lifetime rate. To the 'mood' disorder category we assigned the major affective disorders, including major depression and mania, and dysthymia (the latter occurring in only 4 per cent of the respondents). The category of 'psychotic disorders' includes all psychotic diagnoses apart from major affective disorder.

Of the people interviewed 47 per cent received a diagnosis of at least one severe mental disorder for the month before interview, and 72 per cent received a lifetime diagnosis. Nineteen per cent of those with 'current' disorder diagnosed (or 9 per cent of respondents) and 29 per cent of those with 'lifetime' disorder (or 21 per cent of respondents) received diagnoses in more than one broad diagnostic category. The overlap between substance abuse or dependence and the other disorders was especially notable.

The patterns of disorder varied among the three accommodation types. Substance-related disorders and co-morbidity were most prevalent in the shelters, with 37 per cent of the respondents diagnosed as having current (past month) substance-related disorder, alone or in combination. The pattern in the rooming houses was similar. The highest prevalence of psychotic disorder was found in the special accommodation houses.

3 Past psychiatric treatment

Summary indicators of past psychiatric treatment were derived from information in the SCID-R overview and other parts of the interview, and some additional information obtained from the Victorian Psychiatric Case Register. Overall rates for earlier hospitalization and psychiatric treatment among the respondents were 40 per cent and 56 per cent respectively. We defined treatment as hospitalization in a psychiatric or drug and alcohol treatment facility, and/or contact with a mental health or general medical professional for 'emotional problems'. Most of those with a lifetime diagnosis of psychotic disorder reported treatment (91 per cent) and hospitalization (83 per cent) at some time. Those with mood and substance-related disorders reported lower rates for previous psychiatric treatment or hospitalization (Table 11.2). Of the subjects who did not receive a lifetime diagnosis, 18 per cent reported past psychiatric hospital treatment. Overall rates for hospitalization and treatment were higher among the females interviewed: 57 per cent and 72 per cent, respectively; compared with 37 per cent of males 'ever hospitalized' and 52 per cent 'ever treated'.

4 Use of prescribed medication

Twenty-seven per cent of respondents reported current use of prescribed medication (Table 11.3a). Over half of these people (fifty-two persons, or 14 per cent of all respondents) were taking anti-psychotic medication, with or without antidepressants or benzodiazepines. Female respondents reported more frequent use of any medication (38 per cent) and of anti-psychotic medication (28 per cent). Seven per cent of men and 6 per cent of women reported benzodiazepine use (Table 11.3b).

Of the sixty-seven people who received a diagnosis of current psychotic disorder, 32 (48 per cent) reported taking anti-psychotic medication (calculated from Table 11.4). Twenty-six of the remaining thirty-five not taking anti-psychotic medication described previous hospitalization and another four, previous treatment for emotional problems. A further fourteen people without a SCID-R diagnosis of psychosis reported taking anti-psychotic medication currently (Table 11.4).

Seventeen of the twenty-five people (68 per cent) with a diagnosis of current psychotic disorder living in the special accommodation houses were confirmed to be taking medication. The proportions for people so diagnosed and living in the other accommodation sectors were lower: eight out of twenty-six (31 per cent) in the shelters; and seven out of sixteen (44 per cent) in the rooming houses and private hotels (see also Table 11.3c).

5 Current service use

In Australia, Commonwealth-funded universal health insurance facilitates access to primary health services, and to specialist health services by referral. Among the few specialist health services allowing direct access are state-funded community mental health services and psychiatric hospitals. Commonwealth payment for primary health services occurs on a

Table 11.2 Frequency of reported treatment for emotional problems and hospitalization for emotional problems by broad diagnostic category derived from SCID-R 'lifetime' diagnoses

Diagnostic category	No.of persons	History of treatment No. (%)	History of hospitalization No. (%)
Psychotic disorder	50	48 (96)	45 (90)
Mood disorder	31	16 (52)	8 (29)
Substance-related disorder	114	58 (52)	37 (33)
Mood and substance-related disorder	48	31 (65)	19 (40)
Mood and psychotic disorder	5	4 (80)	4 (80)
Psychotic and substance-related disorder	15	14 (93)	11 (73)
Mood, psychotic and substance-related disorder	12	9 (75)	8 (67)
No psychiatric disorder	101	30 (29)	18 (18)
	376	210 (56)	150 (40)
No psychiatric disorder and history of treatment unknown	6		
Total	382		

fee-for-service basis. Practitioners may accept the Commonwealth fee as complete payment by billing the government directly, or may charge the patient a higher scheduled fee. The patient then reclaims the government portion of the fee. There are additional to these arrangements a limited number of salaried, primary-care physicians working in community health centres, mainly in areas with high indices of social deprivation.

Residents in shelters may attend any primary-care physician, usually seeking one who agrees to direct bill charges, or they may attend a community health centre free of charge where available. In addition, each of the main shelters employs a nurse, and appoints a medical practitioner

Table 11.3 Current psychotropic medication by type of medication and (a) age
of respondent, (b) sex of respondent, and (c) type of accommodation
(N = 382)

	Total no.	All psychotropic medication (%)	Anti-psychotic (%)	Anti-[b] anxiety (%)	Anti-depressant (%)	Other (%)
				Medication type[a]		
(a) Age						
15–24	30	10.0	6.7	–	–	–
25–34	80	24.8	13.8	5.0	–	6.3
35–44	101	31.7	14.9	12.9	2.0	5.0
45–54	90	30.0	16.7	5.6	2.2	6.7
55–60	73	24.7	12.3	4.1	2.7	9.6
Total	374	26.7	13.9	6.7	1.6	6.4
Medication unknown	8					
(b) Sex						
Male	313	23.6	10.2	6.7	1.9	6.7
Female	69	37.7	27.5	5.8	1.5	4.3
(c) Type of accommodation						
Shelters	179	16.2	6.1	3.9	0.6	6.1
Special accom. houses	79	49.4	35.4	7.6	5.1	6.3
Rooming houses	124	25.8	11.3	9.7	1.6	6.5

[a] 6 respondents were taking a combination of two types of medication
[b] Benzodiazepines

to attend regularly, with remuneration from direct billing of patients seen.
In most special accommodation houses, and some large boarding houses
and private hotels of the types surveyed, primary-care physicians attend
regularly by arrangement with the accommodation managers. Again, the
physicians are paid by direct billing; this method of payment may be seen
as an encouragement to regular contact with residents. Many primary-care
physicians, however, see their interests and confidence in undertaking
mental health care as limited. They often have little contact with psychiatrists or other mental health workers. Other primary-care physicians
working outside these arrangements may be reluctant to see patients
whose pensioner or indigent status makes direct billing a requirement.
Their links with mental health-care professionals may be even more
limited. Professionals from community mental health clinics may see links
with primary-care physicians as important in their work, but often find
difficulty in making and maintaining working relationships.

Table 11.4 Frequency of current medication use by categories of DSM-III-R disorders (N = 382)

| Type of disorder | Total no. | Medication type[a] | | | | |
		All psychotropic medication (%)	Anti-psychotic (%)	Anti-[b] anxiety (%)	Anti-depressant (%)	Other (%)
Mood	25	32.0	16.0	0.8	0.4	0.4
Psychotic	52	61.5	53.8	–	–	3.8
Substance-related	67	19.4	–	6.0	–	7.5
Mood and substance-related	19	15.8	–	10.5	–	5.3
Mood and psychotic	2	–	–	–	–	–
Psychotic and substance-related	13	30.8	30.8	–	–	–
Mood, psychotic and substance-related	–	–	–	–	–	–
No psychiatric disorder	204	19.6	6.9	3.4	–	3.9

[a] 6 respondents were taking a combination of two types of medication
[b] Benzodiazepines

Nearly three-quarters of respondents in our survey reported current contact with primary or mental health services (Table 11.5) and the rates were higher in those with current disorder (Table 11.6). Only 7 per cent mentioned specifically contact with a primary-care physician, although this was more frequent (11 per cent) among those in rooming houses. Medication use was almost confined to those currently using services, and was reported by 42 per cent (90 of 213) of those who said they were in contact with a doctor (Table 11.5).

6 Accommodation profile

Eighty-two per cent of respondents who gave relevant information reported living for more than six months in one or more of the accommodation sectors surveyed; that is, 82 per cent had been homeless or disaffiliated for over six months. Forty-nine per cent had lived in this way for over five years (Table 11.7). Thirty people (twenty-eight men and two women), or 8 per

Table 11.5 Present service use in respondents by medication use

	Present service use		Of these, any medication use	
	No.	%	No.	%
Doctor in hospital out-patient or community clinic, including drug and alcohol	48	14	26	54
Primary-care physician	25	7	10	40
Physician, unspecified	140	39	54	39
Other professional	13	4	2	15
Unspecified professional	37	10	6	16
Sub-total	263	74	98	37
None	92	26	2	2
Total	355	100	100	26
Unknown	27			
Total	382			

Table 11.6 Category of psychiatric disorder (DSM-III-R) by current service use

Current diagnostic category (mutually exclusive)	Total no.	Current service use		Unknown no.
		No.	(%)	
Mood disorders	25	21	(88)	1
Psychotic disorders	52	42	(88)	4
Substance-related disorders	67	44	(71)	5
Mood and substance-related disorders	19	13	(72)	1
Mood and psychotic disorders	2	2	(100)	0
Substance-related and psychotic disorders	13	11	(92)	1
None	204	130	(69)	15
Total	382	263	(74)	27

Table 11.7 Distribution of respondents by current duration of homelessness

Time	Total no.	%
< 6 months	56	17
6–11 months	18	6
1–5 years	92	28
> 5 years	159	49
	325	
Unknown	57	
Total	382	

cent of those interviewed, said that they sometimes or often slept 'rough' – that is, without shelter of any kind. For men interviewed in the shelters, this percentage was higher (12 per cent). Forty-five per cent of respondents said that they had lived in the same place for at least one year, and another 23 per cent had moved only within the locality during the previous year. Thus, about two-thirds of those we saw were relatively stable geographically.

7 Chronology of disorder and homelessness

Information was not available for the 107 people without a diagnosed 'lifetime' disorder; and there was insufficient relevant information on another fifty-six people. The onset of homelessness was taken for this purpose as the first period of abode lasting at least six weeks in one of the accommodation sectors surveyed, or (for a small number) the first period of at least the same length in 'squats' or refuges or living without shelter, or the current episode for those homeless for less than six weeks. Age of onset of disorder was taken from the lifetime diagnostic interviews unless, as occurred in a small number, a prior treatment episode was ascertained from the case register. Age of onset of psychotic disorders using the SCID-R was considered exclusive of any disorder prodrome. In 85 per cent of these persons one or more episodes of mental disorder appeared to pre-date homelessness or disaffiliation as defined here, and in another 5 per cent 'homelessness' and disorder first occurred at about the same time (Table 11.8).

The life-charts allowed the discernment of four patterns of homelessness as defined here. In this instance 342 charts, relating to 279 men and 63 women, were deemed adequate for the purpose. Uninterrupted homelessness for at least six weeks, with no evidence of prior homelessness, was the most common pattern. This occurred in 145 men (52 per cent) and 38 women (60 per cent). For most of these people the duration of

Table 11.8 Apparent sequence in onset of first episode of severe mental disorder and homelessness, by sex

	Males		Females		Total	
	No.	(%)	No.	(%)	No.	(%)
Disorder preceded homelessness	151	(85)	34	(83)	185	(85)
Homelessness preceded disorder	18	(10)	6	(15)	24	(11)
Onset approximately coincident	9	(5)	1	(2)	10	(5)
	178	(100)	41	(100)	219	(100)
No lifetime disorder	84		23			
Sequence unknown	51		5			
	313		69			

homelessness was much greater than six weeks, and was usually measured in years (see also Table 11.7). The second pattern consisted of periods of homelessness interrupted by short times in other types of accommodation, such as a family home or other shared house. For these people at least 80 per cent of the time since entering marginal accommodation was spent homeless. This pattern applied to eighty-one men (29 per cent) and twenty women (32 per cent). A small proportion of respondents had spent short periods homeless over a variable period; this applied to sixteen men (6 per cent) and two women (3 per cent). The remainder, thirty-seven men (13 per cent) and three women (5 per cent), had been homeless for less than six weeks with no prior episodes of homelessness.

DISCUSSION

We used a standardized clinical diagnostic procedure, an approach unusual in studies of this type (Morrissey and Levine 1987; Koegel et al. 1988), to interview individuals selected as representative of homeless and disaffiliated people in inner Melbourne. The interview rate of 66 per cent is probably as good as can be achieved in this setting. We cannot be sure, however, what selection biases may have been introduced, even though the age distribution of the respondents was not obviously skewed.

Overall, the findings suggest a strikingly high prevalence of severe mental disorders in the target population compared to the general population – as reported, for example, from the American Epidemiologic Catchment Area study (Regier and Burke 1987). In addition, the major issues of physical illness and disability (Brickner *et al.* 1984; Rossi *et al* 1987; Gelberg and Linn 1988), mental retardation and late-life dementia in this section of the population are not addressed in the present study.

The high rates of mental disorder found in this project are consistent with the findings of other surveys of homeless people in Australia and elsewhere. The overall rates of past hospitalization and treatment for psychiatric and substance-related disorders were also close to those in Los Angeles, reported by Gelberg and colleagues (1988).

Individuals marginally accommodated in Melbourne appear to have problems of mental disorder on a scale similar to those of truly homeless people. It appears that disaffiliated people with severe mental disorders are less likely to live on the streets in Melbourne, where low-cost accommodation is more readily available, than in many US cities. Although those we interviewed all had some form of shelter, almost all had spent more than a few weeks living in these settings, and most some years. A high proportion were also relatively stably located in the area; although an important corollary is that, whereas the transient group is a minority on cross-sectional assessment, it is likely to be a numerically important component of the overall population of homeless people.

Vaillant (1987) has discussed the use of life-charts in epidemiologic work, adapting Adolf Meyer's clinical concept. He suggests the utility at certain times of interpreting broad patterns of events as ascertained in prospective studies, even when more precise measures are not available. We decided to apply this approach to the rich though retrospective information about life situations and events obtained from many of our respondents in the course of and additional to the lengthy diagnostic interviews. The process of becoming homeless (according to our definition) was charted retrospectively, although in very broad outline. We applied operational definitions for the onset of homelessness, while recognizing that this process is often without a clear onset, or may be a gradual 'drift-down' (Susser *et al.* 1988; Benda and Dattalo 1988).

From the life-charts we were able to discern patterns in the history of homelessness, and to make a judgement that in many of our respondents mental disorder preceded homelessness and disaffiliation. We judged the reverse to be the case in only a small number of instances. Previous work suggests that homelessness for any individual is usually determined by many factors (Rossi *et al.* 1987; Main 1988; Benda and Dattalo 1988; Koegel *et al.* 1988). The direction of causality for hypothesized risk factors may be unclear. For instance, drug abuse, single marital status and mental disorder are all plausible consequences as well as cause of homelessness. Date of onset of hypothesized risk factors has rarely been compared with that of homelessness (Susser *et al.* 1988). Our findings contribute to evidence that the occurrence of one or more severe mental disorders may be considered as one of the variety or series of risk factors for homelessness (Koegel *et al.* 1988; Herrman *et al.* 1989). The comparability of our results with the studies quoted above emphasizes the role of prevailing economic and social policies in 'setting the threshold' for homelessness in those with severe mental disorders.

The people we interviewed represent those in our community with the most severe types of disorders and gross social disadvantage. The most helpful response is likely to be flexible (Lamb 1988), so that a range of services is provided in a variety of hospital and community settings, and to maximize continuity of care (Bachrach 1984b; Goldfinger and Chafetz 1984; Fischer and Breakey 1986). The information obtained in this survey on current use of services suggests an area of further investigation and service development.

In contrast to the findings in Los Angeles (Gelberg *et al.* 1988), respondents in our survey reported high rates of current contact with primary and mental health services. We do not have detailed information on the quality and frequency of these contacts, although we do know that relatively few people were taking prescribed medication. Our health-care service setting differs from that in the United States, and is more closely comparable with that in the United Kingdom, in that primary medical services remain an important service element. The work from Edinburgh and Sydney, mentioned above, suggests that it is primary-care services which have most contact with people living in these settings; and these are people with multiple health, welfare and accommodation problems.

The problems of homeless people with severe mental disorder will not be alleviated by changes in any single service type or setting, nor by health services alone without attention to major social, welfare and housing issues. One logical response has been the establishment of specialized service programmes with potential to 'engage the disengaged' and provide a range of basic and specialized services (Levine 1984). Gelberg and colleagues (1988) propose the development of integrated health, housing and social services for homeless people, separate from traditional settings.

Another, perhaps complementary response arises from our observation, similar to those in Edinburgh and Sydney, that many of the people we surveyed do make contact with health services. Despite relatively stable location for a sizeable group, many people with severe disorders do not maintain that contact. The important question then becomes, what factors make these contacts helpful and lasting, both for the stably located groups and for those probably more difficult to engage, the transient and shelterless people? It is likely that doctors and other professionals in primary care have potentially a greater role in case management and treatment of homeless (and other) people with severe mental disorder than they generally have at the moment in Melbourne and in other places. In particular, these practitioners could become a focus for other services, with access to a range of preventive, rehabilitative, crisis and support services in a variety of hospital and community settings. Increasing financial incentives for primary-care physicians to undertake this work may be combined with more focused training in community mental health care at undergraduate and postgraduate levels, and with service changes.

Recently the Victorian Office of Psychiatric Services introduced 24-hour community assessment and treatment teams in some areas of metropolitan Melbourne. In some of the inner city areas we surveyed it is providing accommodation workers alongside community mental health and primary-care staff. Evaluation of these services will include long-term comparative studies of the various systems of care.

REFERENCES

Arce, A.A. and Vergare, M.J. (1984) 'Identifying and characterizing the mentally ill among the homeless', in H.R. Lamb (ed.) *The Homeless Mentally Ill: a Task Force Report of the American Psychiatric Association*, Washington, DC: American Psychiatric Association (pp. 75–89).

Bachrach, L.L. (1984a) 'Research on services for the homeless mentally ill', *Hospital and Community Psychiatry* 35:910–13.

Bachrach, L.L. (1984b) 'The homeless mentally ill and mental health services: an analytical review of the literature', in H.R. Lamb (ed.) *The Homeless Mentally Ill: a Task Force Report of the American Psychiatric Association*, Washington, DC: American Psychiatric Association (pp. 11–53).

Bassuk, E.L. (1984) 'The homelessness problem', *Scientific American* 251:28–38.

Benda, B.B. and Dattalo, P. (1988) 'Homelessness: consequence of a crisis or a long-term process?', *Hospital and Community Psychiatry* 39:884–6.

Brickner, P.W., Filardo, T., Iseman, M., Green, R., Conanan, B., and Elvy, A. (1984) 'Medical aspects of homelessness', in H.R. Lamb (ed.) *The Homeless Mentally Ill: a Task Force Report of the American Psychiatric Association*, Washington, DC: American Psychiatric Association (pp. 243–60).

Doutney, C.P., Buhrich, N., Virgona, A., Cohen, A., and Daniels, P. (1985) 'The prevalence of schizophrenia in a refuge for homeless men', *Australian and New Zealand Journal of Psychiatry* 19:233–8.

Fischer, P.J. and Breakey, W.R. (1986) 'Homelessness and mental health: an overview', *International Journal of Mental Health* 14:6–41.

Folstein, M.F., Folstein, S.E., and McHugh, P.R. (1975) '"Mini-mental-state": a practical method for grading the cognitive state of patients for the clinician', *Journal of Psychiatric Research* 12:189–98.

Gelberg, L. and Linn, L.S. (1988) 'Social and physical health of homeless adults previously treated for mental health problems', *Hospital and Community Psychiatry* 39:510–16.

Gelberg, L., Linn, L.S., and Leake, B.D. (1988) 'Mental health, alcohol and drug use, and criminal history among homeless adults', *American Journal of Psychiatry* 145:191–6

Goldfinger, S.M. and Chafetz, L. (1984) 'Developing a better service delivery system for the homeless mentally ill', in H.R. Lamb (ed.) *The Homeless Mentally Ill: a Task Force Report of the American Psychiatric Association*, Washington, DC: American Psychiatric Association (pp. 91–108).

Harris, R., Maley, M., and Szajanoha, S. (1987) 'Chronically mentally ill in boarding houses: a discussion of service utilization', *Community Medicine*

Project, 1987, University of Sydney. Quoted in I.W. Webster (1989) 'Finding homes for the mentally ill', *Australian Doctor Weekly* 3/3/89:16, 25.

Herrman, H., McGorry, P., Bennett, P., van Riel, R., McKenzie, D., and Singh, B. (1989) 'Prevalence of severe mental disorders in homeless and disaffiliated people in inner Melbourne', *American Journal of Psychiatry* 45:1085–92.

Koegel, P., Burnam, M.A., and Farr, R.K. (1988) 'The prevalence of specific psychiatric disorders among homeless individuals in the inner city of Los Angeles', *Archives of General Psychiatry* 45:1085–92.

Krupinski, J. (1986) 'Longitudinal analysis of psychiatric patient registers: the experience in Victoria, Australia', in G.H.M.M. ten Horn, W.H. Giel, J.H. Gulbinat, and J.H. Henderson (eds) *Psychiatric Care Register and Public Health*, Amsterdam: Elsevier Science Publishers (pp. 89–94).

Lamb, H.R. (1988) 'Deinstitutionalization at the crossroads', *Hospital and Community Psychiatry* 39:941–5.

Levine, I.S. (1984) 'Service programs for the homeless mentally ill', in H.R. Lamb (ed.) *The Homeless Mentally Ill: a Task Force Report of the American Psychiatric Association*, Washington, DC: American Psychiatric Association (pp. 173–200).

Main, T.J. (1988) 'What we know about the homeless', *Commentary* 85(5):26–31.

Morrissey, J.P. and Levine, I.S. (1987) 'Researchers discuss latest findings, examine needs of homeless mentally ill persons', *Hospital and Community Psychiatry* 38:811–12.

Powell, P.V. (1988) 'Qualitative assessment in the evaluation of the Edinburgh primary health care scheme for single homeless hostel dwellers', *Community Medicine* 10:185–96.

Priest, R.G. (1976) 'The homeless person and the psychiatric services: an Edinburgh survey', *British Journal of Psychiatry* 128:128–36.

Ramsden, S.S., Nyiri, P., Bridgewater, J., and El-Kabir, D.J. (1989) 'A mobile surgery for single homeless people in London', *British Medical Journal* 298:372–4.

Regier, D.A. and Burke, J.D. (1987) 'Psychiatric disorders in the community: the Epidemiologic Catchment Area Study', in *Psychiatry Update: American Psychiatric Association Annual Review*, vol. 6, R.E. Hales and A.J. Frances (eds), Washington, DC: American Psychiatric Press (pp. 610–24).

Reuler, J.B. (1988) 'Health care for the homeless in a national health program', *American Journal of Public Health* 79:1033–5.

Rossi, D.H., Wright, J.D., Fisher, G.A., and Willis, G. (1987) 'The urban homeless: estimating composition and size', *Science* 235:1336–41.

Spitzer, R.L., Williams, J.B.W., and Gibbon, M. (1986) *Structured Clinical Interview for DSM-III-R (SCID-R)*, New York State Psychiatric Institute, Biometrics Research, New York.

Susser, E., Lovell, A., and Conover, S. (1988) 'Unravelling the causes of homelessness – and of its association with mental illness', in B. Cooper and T. Helgason (eds) *Epidemiology and the Prevention of Mental Disorder*, London: Routledge (pp. 228–39).

Vaillant, G.E. (1987) 'Time: an important dimension of psychiatric epidemiology', in B. Cooper (ed.) *Psychiatric Epidemiology: Progress and Prospects*, London: Croom Helm (pp. 167–77).

Vergare, M.J. and Arce, A.A. (1986) 'Homeless adult individuals and their shelter network', in *The Mental Health Needs of Homeless Persons: New Directions for Mental Health Services Number 30*, San Francisco: Jossey-Bass (pp. 15–26).

Psychiatric and general medical services: issues of patient selection, referral and treatment

Chapter 12

The relationship of usual source of health care to the prevalence of psychiatric disorder and the utilization of ambulatory mental health services in the United States

Martha L. Bruce, Gary L. Tischler and Philip J. Leaf

The health-care system of the United States is pluralistic. Traditionally, Americans have received their primary medical care from solo practitioners on a fee-for-service basis. Recently, a common alternative has been to enrol in pre-paid health-care plans: multispecialty group practices which provide a specified set of health services at a fixed rate of payment. Although these two types of arrangement predominate, primary medical care can also be obtained in other settings, such as hospital-based or free-standing clinics and emergency rooms, or other episodic care centres.

Comparisons of practice patterns in different settings suggest that the pluralism of the American health-care system is associated with considerable variation in terms of access to ambulatory mental health care and the extent of services provided (Regier *et al*. 1982). In this chapter, we expand upon these findings by looking at a community sample of individuals categorized by their reported usual source of medical care. We begin by contrasting the socio-economic and diagnostic characteristics of individuals whose usual source of care is a private practitioner, a pre-paid health-care plan, a clinic or an episodic care centre. We then examine the relationship between usual source of medical care and the likelihood and frequency of use of ambulatory mental health specialty services. Concordance between the need for care and the use of services of this kind is also explored. We also provide information on people who report no usual source of health care, or who receive care only from small or unusual sources which are less likely to be included in organizational studies.

METHODS

1 Sources of data

The data presented here are derived from the first wave of interviews in the five-site Epidemiologic Catchment Area (ECA) Project. The project and its methodology have been described extensively (Regier *et al*. 1984; Eaton and Kessler 1985; Leaf and Myers 1991). Briefly, the ECA consists of surveys in five US communities for the purpose of estimating rates of psychiatric disorders and use of health and, in particular, mental health services. Although the ECA also surveyed residents of long-stay care institutions, this chapter considers only respondents living in independent households.

The five communities studied were made up as follows:

1 thirteen towns comprising the greater New Haven area in south-central Connecticut;
2 three mental health catchment areas in the eastern section of Baltimore, Maryland;
3 three diverse, non-contiguous areas within the greater St Louis, Missouri, community;
4 a five-county region in central North Carolina, including both rural counties and the primarily urban county of Durham;
5 two non-contiguous mental health catchment areas in the county of Los Angeles, California.

The first wave of interviews was conducted between 1980 and 1983. Sample sizes ranged from 3,004 to 5,034, and totalled 18,571. Response rates varied from 68 to 79 per cent, with refusals comprising the major reason for non-response.

2 Methods of measurement

As part of the ECA interviews, respondents were asked to name their usual source of health care. If a respondent reported more than one such usual source, he or she was asked to name the source more frequently used. We have aggregated the numerous types of facility named in the responses into five types:

Private practice: office-based, group or solo private practice with payment on a fee-for-service basis;
Health plan: health-care programmes whose enrolees pre-pay fees that cover the costs of a wide range of preventive and treatment services;

Out-patient clinics: ambulatory treatment facilities which may be either free-standing or hospital-based, and whose patients pay, usually, on a sliding or reduced fee-for-service schedule;

Emergency room: walk-in clinics, usually hospital-based but including also community clinics, that provide care on an emergency or episodic basis;

None: some respondents reported having no usual source of health care, while others, also included in this category, named only non-medical sources.

Other information recorded by the ECA surveys included basic socio-demographic data, use of mental health services, and an assessment of the individual's psychiatric status, based on the Diagnostic Interview Schedule (DIS) (Robins *et al.* 1981; 1985), an interview instrument designed to be used by lay interviewers to assess the presence, duration and severity of psychiatric symptoms, and whether these symptoms can be explained by physical illness, or alcohol or drug intake. Computer algorithms use DSM-III criteria (APA 1980) to establish the diagnosis, history and recency of a range of psychiatric disorders. In this chapter, the diagnosed disorders are grouped into two main categories: substance (alcohol or drug) abuse or dependency is compared with other disorders identified by the DIS/DSM-III system: major depression, bipolar disorder, dysthymia, panic disorder, phobias, obsessive-compulsive disorder, schizophrenia and schizophreniform disorder, anti-social personality disorder and anorexia nervosa.

Respondents were asked about their use of out-patient mental health specialty services during the six months prior to their interview. The range of such services inquired about included office-based psychiatry, services delivered by psychologists and social workers, and those provided in Community Mental Health Centres, Veteran Administration hospitals and drug-abuse clinics.

3 Statistical analysis

The ECA Project was not based on a national sample of the US population, but rather on separate samples from five fairly heterogeneous communities. Because the purpose of this analysis is to demonstrate general trends in the variation in use of mental health services according to the usual source of health care, the emphasis is placed on data aggregated across these five survey samples. Clearly, however, we should also expect to find differences in this respect between the communities. For the most part, we found considerable consistency in the relationship between reported usual source of health care and the use of mental health services across the five communities, but where strong regional differences were observed, these will be highlighted.

The data are weighted to adjust for deviations from simple random sampling inherent in the sampling designs (for example, household size; over-sampling of certain sub-groups) and for non-response. Aggregate data from the five sites are weighted to the demographic (sex, age and race) characteristics of the United States, according to the 1980 Census. Single-site data are weighted according to the demographic characteristics of the geographic area from which the data were drawn.

For analyses involving the entire ECA sample, the complex sampling designs and weighting strategies used in the five separate surveys are taken into account in estimating standard errors and conducting statistical tests, by using Taylor Series Linearization with the computer program 'SURREGR' (Shah and LaVange 1981). These procedures are more appropriate for use with such complex survey data than others which assume simple random sampling, and generally yield more conservative estimates of statistical significance (Freeman *et al.* 1985; Bruce *et al.* 1987). To ensure the stability of the statistical models, sub-group analyses (stratifying, for example, for psychiatric status) are used to estimate variance under the assumption of simple random sampling. When conducting statistical tests on the aggregated data from all five sites, the ECA site was entered as a control variable. The tests of significance also control for socio-demographic variation in those analyses in which the psychiatric status, or use of mental health services, represents the dependent variable (outcome measure).

RESULTS

1 Usual source of health care

Table 12.1 presents the distribution by usual source of health care for each of the five ECA survey samples. In each community, the most frequently reported source of care was private medical practice, ranging from a maximum of 69.9 per cent in New Haven to a minimum of 42.9 per cent in Los Angeles. Health-plan utilization was greatest in the New Haven and Los Angeles areas. The use of out-patient clinics was reported most frequently by respondents in St Louis and Durham, and of Emergency Rooms by those in Baltimore. Reports of having no usual source of health care ranged from 5.8 per cent in Baltimore to 25.4 per cent among Los Angeles residents.

Data aggregated across the five ECA samples and weighted to correspond to the US population distribution show that 59.5 per cent of persons report private practice physicians as their usual source of care, while 12.8 per cent report no usual source of care. The remainder report either a pre-paid health plan (6.3 per cent), an out-patient clinic (14.9 per cent) or an emergency room (6.5 per cent).

Table 12.1 Distribution according to usual sources of medical care in five ECA communities

Community	New Haven	Baltimore	St Louis	Durham County	Los Angeles
Sample size	5,032	3,339	2,944	3,892	3,072
Usual source of medical care (% of sample):					
private medical practice	69.9	51.8	55.5	55.9	42.9
pre-paid health-care plan	9.6	3.4	1.9	2.7	13.2
out-patient clinic	6.6	17.2	22.3	26.9	15.0
emergency room	6.8	21.8	7.2	5.6	3.5
none	7.1	5.8	13.1	8.9	25.4
Total	100.0	100.0	100.0	100.0	100.0

2 Socio-demographic characteristics

Using data weighted to the US population, we contrasted the distributions of socio-demographic characteristics among persons using each source of health care and that of the population as a whole, and found great variation (cf. Table 12.2). With respect to gender, males predominate in two groups – emergency-room users and persons with no usual source of health care – whereas females predominate among persons using private medical practice and out-patient clinics.

In general, the sharpest contrasts are found between private-practice patients, on the one hand, and the users of out-patient clinics and emergency rooms, on the other. Here there are marked differences in the distributions by age, race, marital status and socio-economic status. The patients of private medical practitioners tend to be older, white, married and financially secure, while those using out-patient clinics and emergency rooms tend to be younger, non-white, unmarried, of low socio-economic status and to be receiving disability and welfare payments.

Although they are demographically similar to the clinic and emergency-room users, health-plan enrolees are not as socio-economically disadvantaged. It should be pointed out, however, that there is much more across-site variability in the demography of health-plan enrolees than in the other groups. In the Baltimore ECA, for example, the members of pre-paid health-care plans are almost all non-white and mostly of low socio-economic status; in Los Angeles, on the other hand, the health-plan enrolees are an older population. This variability in the characteristics of health-plan enrolees is consistent with the tendency of such health-care plans in the United States to concentrate on specific target populations, such as employee groups or residents of certain types of neighbourhood.

Like health-plan enrolees, respondents who report no usual source of health care are disproportionately often male, young, non-white and unmarried. The group includes a larger proportion of individuals in the lowest socio-economic status quartile than is found among the private-practice or health-plan users. The proportion receiving social welfare or disability payments is, however, significantly smaller than is found in the out-patient clinic and emergency-room groups.

3 Psychiatric status

The psychiatric status of the respondents also varies according to the source of health care, even when socio-demographic differences are controlled for. For example, the one-year prevalence for any psychiatric disorder is 20.2 per cent. Health-plan enrolees (16.0 per cent) and private-practice

Table 12.2 Percentages of respondents with specific socio-demographic and economic characteristics, according to usual source of health care

Characteristic	Private practice	Health plan	Out-patient clinic	Emergency room	None
Female	57.2[acd]	51.1[cd]	55.0[cd]	36.4	36.5
Under age 45	48.9[abcd]	61.3[c]	59.9[cd]	71.9[d]	68.6
Non-white	12.5[abcd]	34.0[bcd]	37.4[cd]	41.2[d]	31.1
Married	62.6[abcd]	54.3[bc]	52.1[c]	45.3[d]	51.0
Low socio-econ. status	13.6[abcd]	6.7[bcd]	26.0[cd]	22.5[d]	17.9
On welfare payments	1.8[bc]	1.9[bc]	7.9[d]	7.7[d]	1.9
On disability payments	4.5[bcd]	3.8[bc]	9.3[d]	8.2[d]	3.1

[a] = $p < .05$ difference compared to health plan
[b] = $p < .05$ difference compared to out-patient service
[c] = $p < .05$ difference compared to emergency room
[d] = $p < .05$ difference compared to no usual source of care

Note: Statistical tests control for ECA site

users (18.1 per cent) have ratios that are lower than this and significantly lower than those found among emergency-room users (28.1 per cent), the out-patient-clinic group (24.9 per cent) or respondents with no usual source of care (22.1 per cent). The direction of the differences is consistent for each of the ECA sites, although their magnitude varies somewhat.

When psychiatric disorders are divided into substance-abuse disorders and all other types, differing distributions are found. The prevalence of substance-abuse disorders is highest among the users of emergency rooms (14.8 per cent) and those persons with no usual source of care (11.6 per cent), and lowest among those who use private medical practice (5.3 per cent). The rates for other forms of psychiatric disorder are highest among the users of out-patient clinics (19.0 per cent) and emergency rooms (18.6 per cent), and lowest among persons with no usual source of care (13.9 per cent) and those in pre-paid health plans (12.1 per cent). The fact that the highest overall psychiatric prevalence is found among the out-patient-clinic users reflects their high rate for disorders other than substance abuse, whereas the overall high rate among those with no usual source of care is rather a function of their disproportionately high prevalence of substance-abuse disorders. The emergency-room users exhibit high rates of both these main categories of mental abnormality.

Table 12.3 Proportion of respondents with current or recent (within one year) psychiatric disorder, according to usual source of health care

Type of disorder	All sources	Private practice	Health plan	Out-patient clinic	Emergency room	None
Any psychiatric disorder (DIS)	20.2	18.1[bc]	16.0[bcd]	24.9	28.1	22.1
Substance-abuse disorder	7.3	5.3[bcd]	5.6[bcd]	9.0	14.8	11.6
Other psychiatric disorder	15.1	14.3[b]	12.1[bc]	19.0[d]	18.6	13.9

[b] p < .05 difference compared to out-patient service
[c] p < .05 difference compared to emergency room
[d] p < .05 difference compared to no usual source of care

Note: Statistical tests control for ECA site and socio-economic variables

4 Use of mental health specialty services

Given the differences in demographic structure and morbidity between the health-care sectors, one would expect the use of ambulatory mental health specialty services to differ from one population to another. The top row of Table 12.4 sets out the six-month rates of use of these services by persons reporting each usual source of health care. Rates are highest for the health-plan enrolees (5.7 per cent) and users of out-patient clinics (4.9 per cent); lowest for private-practice users (3.0 per cent) and the group with no usual source of care (3.1 per cent). The high use of mental health specialty services by the pre-paid health-care group stands in sharp contrast to their relatively low prevalence of psychiatric illness.

By computing the one-year prevalence for all DIS/DSM-III psychiatric disorders against the frequency of mental health service usage, we get a rough indication of the ratio of 'need' to 'demand' for specialist care within each group. Among individuals with a psychiatric illness (that is, in 'need' of mental health services), the users of emergency rooms have the lowest utilization rate, only 7 per cent reporting contact with mental health services in the six months preceding interview. In contrast, 19.1 per cent of the pre-paid health-plan members with psychiatric disorders had received specialist treatment during this period.

Among the different ECA survey populations, use of specialist mental health services was reported most frequently by health-plan enrolees in New Haven, Baltimore and Los Angeles. Even of this group, however, less than one-fifth of those with a psychiatric disorder had received specialist treatment for it.

Among persons with no confirmed psychiatric disorder, there is less variation in the reported use of specialist mental health services. Contact with such services is especially rare among the private-practice patients (1.6 per cent) and persons reporting no usual source of care (1.1 per cent). Persons treated in emergency rooms (2.8 per cent) are as likely as those in pre-paid health plans (3.1 per cent) to make such contacts in the absence of any confirmed psychiatric condition. As can be seen from Table 12.4 (bottom row), the selective use ratio (patients with a diagnosis in treatment, divided by patients with no diagnosis in treatment) is approximately the same among health-plan enrolees (6.2:1) as among persons using office-based physicians (5.7:1) or out-patient clinics (5.5:1). In other words, health-plan enrolees are more likely to receive mental health care, irrespective of their psychiatric status. This suggests that pre-paid health plans are better able to secure treatment for those who need it, not so much by selective referral, but rather because their relatively liberal policy gives all enrolees easy access to mental health services. The effect of easy accessibility is particularly striking in relation to substance-abuse disorders, as can be seen from Table 12.5.

Table 12.4 Percentage of respondents in contact with mental health specialty services, according to usual source of health care and psychiatric status at interview

Psychiatric status	All sources	Private practice	Health plan	Out-patient service	Emergency room	None
All respondents	18,279	3.0[ab]	5.7[d]	4.9[d]	4.1	3.1
Psychiatric disorder (DIS)	3,774	9.1[ab]	19.1[bcd]	12.6[c]	7.1	10.1
No psychiatric disorder	14,397	1.6[bc]	3.1[d]	2.3[d]	2.8[d]	1.1
Selective use ratio*		5.7	6.2	5.5	2.5	9.0

[a] p ∨ .05 difference compared to health plan
[b] p ∨ .05 difference compared to out-patient service
[c] p ∨ .05 difference compared to emergency room
[d] p ∨ .05 difference compared to no usual source of care

* % using if any disorder / % using if no disorder

Note: Statistical tests control for ECA site and socio-economic variables

Table 12.5 Proportion of respondents using mental health specialty services, and frequency of visits, according to usual source of health care and psychiatric status at interview

	No.	Private practice	Health plan	Out-patient clinic	Emergency room	None
Proportion using mental health services (%)						
Substance-abuse disorder only	725	5.0[ax]	22.7[bcd]	10.3[c]	1.3[x]	5.3
Other psychiatric disorders	3,049	10.4[ab]	17.8	13.2	9.9	12.7
Mean no. of visits						
Substance-abuse disorder only	61	3.0	4.2	3.3	1.0	2.0
Other psychiatric disorders	312	2.9[b]	5.1	5.9[c]	2.1	2.1

[a] p < .05 difference compared to health plan
[b] p < .05 difference compared to out-patient service
[c] p < .05 difference compared to emergency room
[d] p < .05 difference compared to no usual source of care
[x] p < .05 difference between substance and nonsubstance abuse disorders

Note: Statistical tests control for ECA site and socio-economic variables

Among emergency-room users, we find *low* rates of specialist service use by persons with psychiatric disorders, but a relatively *high* use by individuals with no psychiatric diagnosis. This suggests that case identification is likely to be imprecise and referral non-selective: a finding consistent with the literature on the complexity of decision-making in the emergency room (Walker 1983). The picture is very different among those reporting no usual source of health care. Their overall use of mental health specialty services is low (3.1 per cent), but the probability of those who are referred having a DIS/DSM-III psychiatric disorder is high, as reflected by the selective use ratio (9.0:1). Indeed, over 70 per cent of persons in this group contacting mental health services have a psychiatric disorder, compared to only about 50 per cent among corresponding persons whose usual source of care is given as private practice physicians, pre-paid health plan or the emergency room.

Finally, for those persons with a psychiatric condition, the likelihood of receiving specialist treatment appears to depend both upon the usual source of health care and the type of psychiatric problem (Table 12.5). For example, persons whose usual source of care is a private medical practitioner are less likely to receive specialist treatment if they have a substance-abuse disorder than if they have another type of mental disorder, and the same is true of those using emergency rooms. Use of mental health services by substance abusers is also somewhat lower, relative to that by persons with other DIS/DSM-III psychiatric disorders, in the group reporting no usual source of health care. This relationship is not found, however, among pre-paid health-plan or out-patient-clinic users. On the other hand, there are no substantive differences between substance abusers and those with other forms of mental disorder in terms of the *quantity* of care consumed. For substance abusers, the mean number of mental health visits ranges from 1.0 for the emergency-room group to 4.2 for health-plan enrolees; for individuals with other forms of mental disorder, the mean number of visits ranges from 2.1 for the emergency-room group and those with no regular source of health care, to 5.9 for the out-patient-clinic users.

DISCUSSION

The need for treatment, as measured by indicators such as psychiatric diagnosis or mental distress, has consistently emerged as the primary factor determining whether or not a person receives care in the mental health specialty sector (Shapiro *et al*. 1984; Leaf *et al*. 1988). Recent studies, however, have emphasized the extent to which receipt of out-patient psychiatric care in the United States is also contingent on a variety of organizational factors. These include physician referral practices (Hankin and Oktay 1979; Schurman *et al*. 1985), the degree of willingness or ability of medical practitioners to treat mental health problems themselves (Regier *et al.* 1978), price and reimbursement schemes (Reed *et al.* 1972; Manning *et al.* 1984), and policies and procedures (Regier *et al.* 1982). A major topic of this volume is the extent to which primary health care serves as a filter to the mental health specialty sector. The findings of our study indicate that the nature of such filters depends, in part, upon the organizational setting in which primary care is provided.

Specifically, we found that the probability of contacting ambulatory mental health services varied significantly as a function of an individual's usual source of medical care. Moreover, the type of organization structure appeared to lie behind differences both in the socio-demographic composition and level of psychiatric morbidity in each type of facility's patient clientele. The greatest likelihood of receiving specialist services was found if the respondent was enrolled in a pre-paid health plan. Even here, however, the probability that a person with a psychiatric disorder was receiving specialty care was less than one in five. Additionally, our findings suggest that the greater use of ambulatory mental health services by the health-plan enrolees is a function less of rigorous case identification and selective referral than of the organizational policy governing access to such services.

The relatively high utilization rate stands in contrast to the relatively low prevalence of mental disorder among the health-plan users. Indeed, we were struck by the lack of concordance between psychiatric illness prevalence and the rate of service utilization. For example, utilization rates for emergency-room users – the most socio-economically and, in terms of psychiatric morbidity, clinically disadvantaged population – were the lowest among the groups studied. Again, while the prevalence of psychiatric illness was roughly the same among health-plan enrolees and users of private medical practice, a two-fold difference existed in the proportions receiving ambulatory mental health care. Once again, these findings highlight the role that the primary-care sector plays in mediating access to specialist mental health services.

Our findings concerning the low rates of service utilization by substance abusers are troublesome. Pre-paid group practices represent the only primary-care setting in which substance abusers are at least as likely to be in touch with psychiatric services as patients with other forms of mental disorder. In all other settings the obverse is the case, and the numbers of substance abusers in contact with specialist services never exceeds 10 per cent of all respondents with substance-abuse disorders. Among emergency-room users and those with no usual source of care, in particular, the combination of a high psychiatric prevalence with a low rate of service utilization underlines the difficulty in engaging this population in treatment. Unfortunately, our data do not provide insight into why pre-paid health plans achieve greater success in this regard.

In an era when increasing attention is being paid to the organization of health care in the United States, our documentation of significant differences in the demographic, socio-economic, systems dependence and clinical status of patient populations, according to their usual source of medical care, highlights the diversity of the system. The possibility of exploiting these data for policy purposes requires further exploration in the near future. Although we noted a lack of concordance between the prevalence of mental disorder in primary-care settings and the access to specialist treatment, we also found that certain organizational arrangements were associated with a greater availability of such care. These findings suggest that further research into health services is needed in order to isolate the critical variables in the organization and delivery of primary care that promote case-identification and facilitate access to needed services. Such studies should be designed not only to address the issue of accessibility, but also to evaluate the impact of differing treatment practices and organizational structures, policies and procedures on the outcome of care.

REFERENCES

American Psychiatric Association (1980) *Diagnostic and Statistical Manual*, third edn, DSM-III, Washington, DC: American Psychiatric Association.

Bruce, M.L., Freeman, D.H., and Leaf, P.J. (1987) 'Use of SAS procedures for estimating design-based logistic regression variances by balanced repeated replication', *SAS Users Group International Proceedings of the Twelfth Annual Conference*, Cary, NC: SAS (pp. 1066–70).

Eaton, W.W. and Kessler, L.G. (eds) (1985) *Epidemiologic Methods in Psychiatry: the NIMH Epidemiologic Catchment Area Program*, New York: Academic Press.

Freeman, D.H., Livingston, M.M., Leo, L., and Leaf, P.J. (1985) *A Comparison of Indirect Variance Estimation Procedures, American Statistical Association Survey Research Methods*, Washington, DC: American Statistical Association, pp. 313–16.

Hankin, J. and Oktay, J.S. (1979) *Mental Disorder and Primary Medical Care: an Analytical Review of the Literature*, NIMH Series D, no. 5. USDHEW (ADM) 78–661, Washington, DC: US Government Printing Office.

Leaf, P.J. and Bruce, M.L. (1987) 'Gender differences in the use of mental health-related services: a re-examination', *Journal of Health and Social Behaviour* 28:171–83.

Leaf, P.J., Bruce, M.L., Freeman, D.H., Weissman, M.M., Myers, J.K., and Tischler, G.L. (1988) 'Factors affecting the utilization of specialty and general medical mental health services', *Medical Care* 26:9–26.

Leaf, P.J., Myers, J.K., and McEvoy, L.T. (1991) 'Procedures used in the Epidemiologic Catchment Area studies', in L.N. Robins and D.A. Regier (eds) *Psychiatric Disorders in America*, New York: Free Press, pp. 11–32.

Manning, W.G., Wells, K.B., Duan, N., Newhouse, J.P., and Ware, J.E. (1984) 'Cost-sharing and the use of ambulatory mental health services', *American Psychologist* 39:1077–89.

Reed, L.S., Myers, E., and Scheidemandel, P. (1972) *Health Insurance and Psychiatric Care: Utilization and Cost*, Washington, DC: American Psychiatric Association.

Regier, D.A., Goldberg, I.D., Burns, B.J., Hankin, S., Hoeper, E.W., and Nycz, G.R. (1982) 'Specialist/generalist division of responsibility for patients with mental disorders', *Archives of General Psychiatry* 39:219–24.

Regier, D.A., Goldberg, I.D., and Taube, C.A. (1978) 'The de facto US mental health services system: a public health perspective', *Archives of General Psychiatry* 35:685–93.

Regier, D.A., Myers, J.K., Kramer, M., Robins, L.N., Blazer, D.G., Hough, R.L., Eaton, W.W., and Locke, B.Z. (1984) 'The NIMH Epidemiologic Catchment Area Program', *Archives of General Psychiatry* 41:934–41.

Robins, L.N., Helzer, J.E., Croughan, J. and Ratcliff, K.S. (1981) 'National Institute of Mental Health Diagnostic Interview Schedule: its history, characteristics and validity,' *Archives of General Psychiatry* 38:381–9.

Robins, L.N., Helzer, J.E., Orvaschel, H., Anthony, J.C., Blazer, D.G., Burnham, A., and Burke, J.D. (1985) 'The Diagnostic Interview Schedule', in W.W. Eaton and L.G. Kessler (eds) *Epidemiologic Field Methods in Psychiatry: the NIMH Epidemiologic Catchment Area Program*, New York: Academic Press, pp. 143–70.

Schurman, R.A., Kramer, P.D., and Mitchell, J.B. (1985) 'The hidden mental health network', *Archives of General Psychiatry* 42:89–94.

Shah, B.V. and LaVange, L.M. (1981) *Software for Inference on Linear Models from Survey Data*, Cary, NC: Research Triangle institute.

Shapiro, S., Skinner, E.A., Kessler, L.G., Korff, M. von, German, P.S., Tischler, G.L., Leaf, P.J., Bentham, L., and Regier, D. (1984) 'Utilization of health and mental health services', *Archives of General Psychiatry* 41:971–82.

Walker, J.I. (1983) *Psychiatric Emergencies: Intervention and Resolution*, Philadelphia: Lippincott.

Chapter 13

Care of mental health problems in Finland

Selection between primary medical and psychiatric specialist services

V. Lehtinen, M. Joukamaa, T. Jyrkinen, K. Lahtela, R. Raitasalo, J. Maatela and A. Aromaa

General medical services play an important role in the provision of mental health care. Most patients with emotional problems never reach the specialized psychiatric service but are treated by general practitioners. Many studies in different countries have shown that a large proportion of patients treated by primary health-care agencies suffer from significant psychological disorders. In addition, a number of studies have investigated the factors which determine the selection of the patients with psychological disorder to either primary care or specialized psychiatric service (Shapiro *et al*. 1984; Horgan 1985; Wells *et al*. 1986; Leaf *et al*. 1988). These studies, which are all from the United States, have shown that patients treated by primary health services for their psychological disorders tend to be more often women, older, less educated and with lower incomes than those persons who are treated by psychiatric specialist services.

In this chapter we present data bearing on these questions, derived from the Mini Finland Health Survey, an extensive epidemiological investigation of the Finnish adult population. Both the primary medical and psychiatric specialist services in Finland are characterized by good availability and reasonably equal distribution all over the country. The main part of these services are run by local authorities, and they are free of charge for the patients (Lehtinen 1988). In larger towns, in comparison to the countryside, there also exists a private sector, and in other ways the treatment alternatives are more abundant (Lehtinen *et al*. 1980).

MATERIAL AND METHODS

The Mini Finland research project is a two-phase health survey, intended to provide basic epidemiological information, in particular, on cardio-vascular, musculo-skeletal and mental disorders. In the psychiatric part of the survey the 36-item version of the General Health Questionnaire (Goldberg 1972) was used as the main screening method in the first phase,

Table 13.1 Sex and age distribution of the sample

Age	Males No. (%)	Females No. (%)	Total No. (%)
30–34	512 (15.4)	522 (13.4)	1,034 (14.3)
35–44	831 (25.0)	851 (21.8)	1,682 (23.3)
45–54	781 (23.5)	828 (21.3)	1,609 (22.3)
55–64	603 (18.2)	745 (19.1)	1,348 (18.7)
65+	595 (17.9)	949 (24.4)	1,544 (21.4)
Total	3,322 (100.0) (46.0)	3,895 (100.0) (54.0)	7,217 (100.0) (100.0)

and the short version of the Present State Examination (Wing 1980) was used as the principal method of case-identification in the second phase. In addition, information obtained from mental hospitals, and various national health and sickness registers were also analysed.

The stratified sample consisted of 8,000 persons aged 30 years or over. It was selected randomly from forty areas in Finland, which together represented the national population as a whole. Of the sample 90 per cent (7,217 persons) participated in the screening phase of the health examination. The sex and age distributions of these subjects are shown in Table 13.1.

Information on the use of mental health services was gathered from the registers and questionnaires, and directly at interview of the subjects. The term 'primary-care services' was used to cover mainly the public health centres, but also, in a smaller proportion of cases, private general practitioners. If a person was currently in contact with these services because of a mental or psychological disorder, he or she was classified as receiving 'primary mental health care'. The term 'specialist psychiatric service' was used to cover mental health centres, mental hospitals and psychiatrists and psychologists in private practice. In this chapter we report only current utilization of these services; namely, that the person was under treatment at the time of the investigation. If a person was currently in contact with both primary and specialist services for a psychological disorder, he was allocated to the second category; that is, specialist service care.

In analysing the data, we started with simple cross-tabulations in which utilization of either primary or specialist mental health service was analysed according to a range of independent variables. We then made use of a multiple logistic model to test the statistical significance of differences in age-adjusted, treated prevalence ratios. The multivariate logistic regression analysis used (YTULOG) calculates relative risk ratios based on the beta coefficient of the logistic model. These ratios express the size of the difference in treatment prevalences between the groups investigated.

Table 13.2 Frequency of utilization of primary or specialist mental health services, according to age and sex

| | No. | Proportion of persons reporting current care for mental health problems | | | Probability p(P/S) |
		Primary care (%)	Specialist services (%)	Total (%)	
Sex					.2420
Men	3,322	4.3	3.0	7.3	
Women	3,895	5.7**	3.8	9.5***	
Age					<.0001
30–34	1,034	1.5	3.7*	5.1	
35–44	1,682	2.1	3.4*	5.6	
45–54	1,609	4.7***	5.0***	9.8***	
55–64	1,348	7.8***	3.2	11.0***	
65+	1,544	8.7***	2.1	10.8***	
Total	7,217	5.0	3.5	8.5	

The asterisks refer to the statistical significance of the prevalence in comparison to the lowest prevalence category in question:
  *= p < 0.05
 **= p < 0.01
***= p < 0.001

RESEARCH FINDINGS

Treated prevalence ratios

Altogether 8.5 per cent of the sample were receiving care for psychological disorders (Table 13.2). The treatment prevalence in primary health care was 5.0 per cent, and that in specialist service 3.5 per cent. Women were in contact with primary-care services more often than men, but sex differences alone did not explain the selection of patients to these treatment settings. Age was very significantly associated with treatment prevalence in general, and also with the selection between the treatment categories. The older a person, the more likely he was to be treated by primary-care services for any psychological disorder. In the age-group of 65 years or over the utilization of primary care was four times that of psychiatric specialist services. In the youngest age-group, in contrast, specialist services were used more than twice as often as primary care.

Factors influencing demand for medical services

The factors influencing utilization of mental health services in general are analysed in a separate paper (Joukamaa *et al.* 1990). Here, we are chiefly concerned with those factors which may determine the selection of one or other type of treatment facility.

Like Leaf and his co-workers (1988), we have divided factors influencing the demand for medical services into three groups:

1 factors directly related to health and need for medical care:
   self-perceived general health,
   a diagnosed physical illness,
   GHQ-36 score,
   clinically assessed psychiatric 'caseness',
   psychiatric diagnosis,
   self-perceived need for psychiatric care,
   clinically assessed need for psychiatric care;
2 socio-demographic and other variables, which are known to vary with the level of demand:
   educational standard,
   social class,
   marital status,
   living alone,
   self-reported quality of interpersonal relationships,
   migration,
   outdoor hobbies,
   self-reported use of alcohol,
   unemployment during the last year,
   self-perceived work problems,
   self-perceived physical workload,
   self-perceived mental workload;
3 factors influencing the ease of access to medical care:
   income category,
   area of residence,
   degree of urbanization of the local community,
   mental health centre in the local community.

1 Factors related to health and need

Unadjusted, a number of health variables (which refer to the need for care) were significantly associated with the selection of treatment facility. Unexpectedly, the clinical assessments of psychiatric 'caseness' and need for psychiatric care did not show any significant association. On the other hand, both the patient's self-perceived need for psychiatric care and also

Table 13.3 Relationship of health factors with utilization of primary or specialist mental health services

| Health factors | No. | Proportion of persons reporting current care for mental health problems (age-adjusted) | | | Probability p(P/S) |
		Primary care (%)	Specialist services (%)	Total (%)	
Physical illness					.0204
No	4,537	3.2	3.0	6.2	
Yes	2,680	6.8***	5.5**	12.3***	
GHQ-36 score					.0425
0–4	5,073	1.7	1.7	3.4	
5–8	756	6.4***	4.0**	10.4***	
9–	1,388	12.2***	10.0**	22.2***	
Diagnostic category:					<.0001
Psychosis	167	25.9***	59.8***	85.6***	
Phobic or anxiety neurosis	452	16.8	10.1	26.9	
Depressive neurosis	336	16.4	14.8***	31.2	
Other neurosis	178	21.4	4.8	26.2	
Other disorder	138	45.0***	30.8***	75.8***	
Self-perceived need for psychiatric care					<.0001
No need	6,838	3.9	1.5	5.4	
Probably	266	29.5***	26.6***	56.0***	
Certainly	113	21.2***	65.3***	86.5***	
Total	7,217	5.0	3.5	8.5	

The asterisks refer to the statistical significance of the prevalence in comparison to the lowest prevalence in the column:
*   = p < 0.05
** = p < 0.01
*** = p < 0.001

the psychiatric diagnosis were clearly related to the selection of treatment facility. These two associations remained significant after adjustment by age (Table 13.3), and they were significant also in the multivariate logistic regression model.

In Table 13.3 the age-adjusted treatment prevalences for primary or specialized service are shown according to those 'need' factors with which the association was statistically significant following adjustment for age differences. The probability of current contact with specialist services was greater if the diagnosis was one of psychosis, or if the person himself was convinced of his need for mental health services. The probability of being in primary health care was especially high for the diagnostic category 'other neurosis' (that is, not anxiety, phobic or depressive neurosis).

2 Demographic and social factors

A number of demographic and social characteristics (such as level of education, marital status, migration and hobbies) were found to be associated with the selection of treatment facility. Less-educated persons, the unmarried and divorced, those who had changed their domicile (migrated), and those who had more outdoor hobbies were more likely to use specialized services than primary care for their psychological disorder. After age adjustment, however, only the marital status was significantly ($p < 0.05$) associated with the type of treatment agency. The age-adjusted treatment prevalences by marital status are shown in Table 13.4.

3 Factors related to access to medical care

Not surprisingly, persons living in communities with mental health centre were more likely to be under specialist care. This association, however, was not significant after adjustment for age. Income and degree of urbanization were the only statistically almost significant ($p<0.05$) variables in the logistic regression model, using age as the third independent variable. If the subject belonged to the lowest income category, or if he was living in the capital

Table 13.4 Relationship of marital status with utilization of primary or specialist mental health services

| Marital status[1] | No. | Proportion of persons reporting current care for mental health problems (age-adjusted) | | | Probability p(P/S) |
		Primary care (%)	Specialist services (%)	Total (%)	
					.0116
Single	769	6.9***	8.4***	15.3***	
Cohabiting	142	5.5	2.0	7.5	
Married	5,092	4.2	2.5	6.7	
Widowed	836	6.7***	5.0	11.6***	
Divorced	370	7.5**	8.1***	15.6***	
Total	7,209	5.0	3.5	8.5	

The asterisks refer to the statistical significance of the prevalence in comparison to the lowest prevalence in the column:
* = $p < 0.05$
** = $p < 0.01$
*** = $p < 0.001$
[1] Unknown in eight cases

Table 13.5 Relationship of income and area of residence to utilization of primary or specialist mental health services

Social characteristic	No.	Proportion of persons reporting current care for mental health problems (age-adjusted)			Probability p(P/S)
		Primary care (%)	Specialist services (%)	Total (%)	
Income category					.0317
V (highest)	1,444	3.4	2.1	5.5	
IV	1,495	3.4	2.6	6.0	
III	1,540	3.8	2.7	6.5	
II	1,371	6.2**	3.3**	9.5***	
I (lowest)	1,367	7.6***	11.6***	19.2***	
Degree of urbanization					.0671
VI (highest)	1,102	5.9**	4.3*	10.1***	
V	1,377	3.7	3.3	6.9	
IV	1,390	4.7	3.6	8.2	
III	1,436	4.3	3.4	7.7	
II	1,184	5.4	2.6	7.9	
I (lowest)	728	7.5***	3.7	11.3**	
Total	7,217	5.0	3.5	8.5	

The asterisks refer to the statistical significance of the prevalence in comparison to the lowest prevalence in the column:
* = $p < 0.05$
** = $p < 0.01$
*** = $p < 0.001$

region of Finland (the highest degree of urbanization), he was more likely to be in contact with specialist services (Table 13.5). The association with income was thus somewhat unexpected.

Towards a comprehensive model

In a final analysis, we examined a multivariate logistic regression model in which the most significant variables from the three categories described above were included: namely, psychiatric diagnosis, and self-perceived need for psychiatric care, age, marital status and income (Table 13.6). The analysis indicates the relative risk ratios in the different categories of the independent variables, adjusted for all the other variables in the model, for receiving mental health care from a primary health-care agency compared to the total utilization of mental health services.

In this final model two need-related factors and one demographic factor remained highly significant in explaining the selection of treatment category: namely, psychiatric diagnosis, self-perceived need for psychiatric

Table 13.6 Use of primary mental health services among those receiving some treatment indicated as adjusted relative risk ratios; results of logistic regression model

Risk factor	Adjusted relative risk ratio	Limits of confidence	Probability p(P/S)
Psychiatric diagnosis:			<.0001
Psychosis	1.0		
Phobic or anxiety neurosis	3.6	1.9 – 6.7	
Depressive neurosis	2.6	1.4 – 4.8	
Other neurosis	10.4	3.9 – 27.6	
Other disorder	3.3	1.7 – 6.3	
Self-perceived need for psychiatric care:			<.0001
No need	1.0		
Probably	0.3	0.2 – 0.6	
Certainly	0.1	0.1 – 0.3	
Age:			<.0001
30–44	1.0		
45–54	1.4	0.8 – 2.5	
55–64	4.6	2.4 – 8.6	
65+	4.6	2.3 – 9.4	
Marital status:			.2782
Single	1.0		
Cohabiting	1.0	0.6 – 1.8	
Married	1.8	0.4 – 8.8	
Widowed	1.9	0.8 – 4.2	
Divorced	0.7	0.3 – 1.6	
Income category:			.3462
I (lowest)	1.0		
II	1.7	1.0 – 3.1	
III	1.1	0.6 – 2.2	
IV	1.1	0.5 – 2.3	
V (highest)	1.7	0.8 – 3.7	

care and age; the influence of all other factors included in the analysis was insignificant.

DISCUSSION

The results of this analysis are in many respects easily understood or self-evident: the persons who are most likely to use primary care for their psychological disorder have the following characteristics. They are relatively old; they have a psychiatric diagnosis other than psychosis: and they do not perceive the need for psychiatric care as often as persons in specialist psychiatric care. The results concerning age and psychiatric diagnosis are in accordance with those of studies in other countries.

Our results do, however, differ somewhat from those reported by Leaf and his co-workers (1988). In contrast to our findings they found that physical dysfunction helped to explain the selection of treatment setting but that perceived mental health did not. The third significant variable in our study, that of age, was associated with the treatment selection also in the study by Leaf *et al.*, but somewhat differently. The probability of being treated in primary care increased with increasing age in our study, whereas in the American study, the probability of using specialist service was greater in the age-group 25–64 years than in either the younger or older age-groups. Comparison of the results is, however, hampered by the fact that in the Mini Finland survey the lower age limit was fixed at 30 years.

No index of accessibility of services was associated in the comprehensive model with the selection of treatment facility in our study population. This finding also differs from the New Haven study (Leaf *et al.* 1988), in which members of pre-paid health plans were more likely than others to receive specialist mental health care, while persons subject to instrumental barriers or family resistance were more likely to be treated in the general medical sector.

This difference in findings indicates that the selection of type of treatment service for mental health problems is largely determined by the kind of health-care structure and infrastructure in each country, and must be expected to differ accordingly as these differ. Here one can mention that Finland has a well-developed community mental health system with a well-developed network of community mental health centres covering the entire national population. Moreover, the services of mental health centres, unlike those in the USA, are free of charge to the patients.

One important factor in explaining the selection of patients with mental health problems is the attitudes of general practitioners towards such problems and their treatment. In Finland, the official health policy regards mental health problems as an essential part of the targets in the primary health care (Ministry of Social Affairs and Health 1987). On the other hand, there are problems in the attitudes of general physicians, and one can also say that their training in psychiatry is not sufficient for the task.

REFERENCES

Goldberg, D.P. (1972) *The Detection of Psychiatric Illness by Questionnaire*, Maudsley Monograph 21, London: Oxford University Press.

Health for All by the Year 2000: the Finnish National Strategy, Helsinki: Ministry of Social Affairs and Health, 1987.

Horgan, C.M. (1985) 'Specialty and general ambulatory mental health services:

comparison of utilization and expenditures', *Archives of General Psychiatry* 42:565–72.

Joukamaa, M., Lehtinen, V., Jyrkinen, T., Lahtela, K., Raitasalo, R., Maatela, J., and Aromaa, A. (1990) Treatment situation in different types of psychiatric disorders in Finland. Unpublished manuscript.

Leaf, P.J., Bruce, M.L., Tischler, G.L., Freeman, D.H., Weissman, M.M., and Myers, J.K. (1988) 'Factors affecting the utilization of specialty and general medical mental health services', *Medical Care* 26:9–26.

Lehtinen, V. (1988) 'The development of mental health services in Finland', *International Journal of Mental Health* 16:58–68.

Lehtinen, V., Salokangas, R.K.R., Holm, H., and Laakso, J. (1980) 'Treatment prevalence in psychiatric outpatient care in Finland: a comparative study of two areas', *Acta Psychiatrica Scandinavica* 62:221–35.

Shapiro, S., Skinner, E.A., Kessler, L.G., Korff, M. von, German, P.S., Tischler, G.L., Leaf, P.J., Bentham, L., Cottler, L., and Regier, D.A. (1984) 'Utilization of health and mental health services: three Epidemiologic Catchment Area sites', *Archives of General Psychiatry* 41:971–8.

Wells, K.B., Manning, W.G., Duan, N., Newhouse, J.P., and Ware, J.E. (1986) 'Sociodemographic factors and the use of outpatient mental health services', *Medical Care* 24:75–85.

Wing, J.K. (1980) 'The use of Present State Examination in general population surveys', in E. Strömgren, A. Dupont, and J.A. Nielsen (eds) 'Epidemiological research as basis for the organization of extramural psychiatry', *Acta Psychiatrica Scandinavica*, Suppl. 285:230–40.

Chapter 14

Psychiatric morbidity in general practice in Verona

The importance of parallel studies at the primary and specialist levels of health care

M. Tansella, C. Bellantuono and P. Williams

It is well known that the great majority of patients presenting with psychiatric symptoms are treated by general practitioners rather than by psychiatrists or psychologists (Shepherd *et al.* 1966; Wilkinson 1985). Goldberg and Huxley (1980) have proposed a model to describe psychiatric disorders and the pathway to psychiatric care, valid in settings where health services are organized in a way similar to the British National Health Service. It consists of five levels and four filters and, in order to move from one level to the next, it is necessary to pass through a filter. The model has been described many times and is now widely accepted as a useful framework for considering psychiatric disorder in the community (Level 1); in general practice – total morbidity (Level 2) and morbidity recognized by general practitioners (Level 3); in specialized psychiatric services – all cases (Level 4) and cases in in-patient care (Level 5).

Applying the Goldberg and Huxley model to countries other than the UK can give rise to problems if in practice the service structures and infrastructures are different. In Italy, the National Health Service was introduced in January 1979. Since that date health insurance has been compulsory for all citizens and is dealt with through one organization. All residents must register with a local general practitioner and are free to choose their doctor. Each doctor is in charge of no more than 1,500 patients. General practitioners are funded by the Local Health Unit with a fixed allowance per patient registered, regardless of the number of consultations and prescriptions and other provisions of care. In general, it is necessary for patients to see the practitioner before seeing the specialist or attending hospital or community departments. However, special rules exist for patients attending psychiatrists, paediatricians, gynaecologists, dentists and eye-specialists (only for optometric examinations), and they may refer themselves directly.

Since 1978 in Italy psychiatric care has been provided for specified geographical areas by comprehensive community-based psychiatric services which work closely with in-patient psychiatric units in general hospitals (with no more than fifteen beds) to ensure continuity of care. Admissions to mental hospitals are not possible and in these institutions only a declining number of old, long-stay patients continue to reside. Many psychiatrists and psychologists engage in part-time private practice, mainly for psychotherapy and treatment of neurotic patients. More information on the organization and provision of psychiatric care in Italy has been provided elsewhere (Tansella *et al.* 1987).

In spite of the differences between Britain and Italy in the structure of health services, the Goldberg and Huxley model has been defined as a 'useful descriptive framework for our country' (Marino *et al.* 1990).

The study of the full spectrum of psychiatric morbidity at all levels, in the same geographical area, can be regarded as providing relevant information for the evaluation of specialist services (Tansella and Williams 1989). In particular, if information about Level 1 and Filter 1 is less important from the point of view of the specialist services, evidence on psychiatric morbidity in the general practice setting (Levels 2 and 3 and Filters 2 and 3) may be very useful for interpreting data concerning the care provided by psychiatric services (Levels 4 and 5) and the changes which may occur over time in the provision of care in this setting.

The aim of this chapter is to summarize the results of research conducted in general practice in and around Verona in the past five years, and to report data on psychiatric morbidity collected at all five levels of Goldberg and Huxley's scheme, based upon the same geographical area (South-Verona, Italy) and within the same time frame (one week in 1987).

INSTRUMENTS

One of the most widely used psychiatric interviews in general practice is the Clinical Interview Schedule (CIS) (Goldberg *et al.* 1970). This instrument has been often used at the second stage of a two-stage screening procedure. The General Health Questionnaire (GHQ) (Goldberg 1972; 1978; Goldberg and Williams 1988) is the most commonly used first-stage instrument in general practice studies conducted in many cultural settings. Both instruments (CIS and GHQ-30) were translated into Italian, and the accuracy of the translation was checked by two independent Italian psychiatrists who were familiar with the English version. The performance of both the clinical interview and the questionnaire was tested in three studies which concurred in finding that the CIS was a useful and reliable instrument for case-identification and that the GHQ-30 is valid as a screening instrument in general practice (Lattanzi *et al.* 1988; Fontanesi *et al.* 1985; Bellantuono *et al.* 1987b). An instrument to standardize general practitioners' assessment of psychiatric morbidity, the General Practitioner Recording Schedule, GPRS (Bellantuono *et al.* 1988; 1989; Fiorio *et al.* 1989), was developed in our Unit and proved to be acceptable, economic and efficient for collecting patient information. It is structured in three parts, covering physical illness, psychiatric problems and social problems, and also permits the collection of information about drug prescribing and referral to specialist agencies.

TOTAL AND CONSPICUOUS PSYCHIATRIC MORBIDITY

Marino *et al.* (1990) collected data from patients attending thirty-two general practitioners in South Verona on one particular day (in May–June 1987). Out of the 505 patients who attended, 404 (80 per cent) completed the GHQ-30 and of these 211 (52 per cent) were high scorers (total score $\geq$ 5). Application of the predictive values from a pilot validation study (Bellantuono *et al.* 1987b) gave an estimate of 41 per cent for the prevalence of *total psychiatric morbidity* among consulters.

A parallel study conducted in ninety-two general practices in the Local Health Unit No. 25 of the Veneto region (comprising the city of Verona and a few small surrounding towns) estimated the extent of *conspicuous psychiatric morbidity* in the area; that is, the extent to which the general practitioners themselves identify psychiatric problems in the patients who present to them. Of the 2,559 patients who were seen by practitioners on one day, 32.2 per cent were rated by their doctors as presenting psychiatric problems.

Two other smaller studies (Bellantuono *et al.* 1987a; Fiorio *et al.* 1989) confirmed this result. The rates of 41 per cent and 32 per cent for general practice total and conspicuous psychiatric morbidity respectively correspond well with rates obtained using the same methodology in general practice settings conducted in other countries (Williams *et al.* 1986; Marks *et al.* 1979).

We also studied the permeability of the second filter (recognition by general practitioners) and found, in common with other studies (Goldberg and Blackwell 1970; Marks *et al.* 1979; Skuse and Williams 1984), that the practitioners identified about two-thirds of the psychiatric morbidity that presented to them, the remaining one-third thus constituting hidden psychiatric morbidity. Factors significantly increasing the relative risk of being identified as psychiatric cases were the presence of social problems, a history of previous psychiatric illness and, to a moderate extent, female sex (Marino *et al.* 1990).

PRESCRIPTION OF PSYCHOTROPIC DRUGS

After two pilot studies, each based on three practices in Verona (Fiorio *et al.* 1989) and in a rural area in northern Italy (Bellantuono *et al.* 1988), Bellantuono *et al.* (1989) studied psychotropic drug prescribing for patients who attended in ninety-two practices on one day. They found that 14 per cent of the patients surveyed received such a prescription, three-quarters of the substances involved being benzodiazepines. Psychotropics were more likely to be prescribed when there was conspicuous psychiatric morbidity and, in women only, when the practitioners identified a social problem; and less likely to be prescribed when the patient was physically ill. These findings confirm previous work conducted in other settings (Williams 1983; Corney and Williams 1987). Moreover, a follow-up study showed that 26 per cent of new recipients of psychotropic drug prescriptions (mainly benzodiazepines) were still consuming these drugs six months later (Fiorio et al. 1990).

REFERRAL TO SPECIALIST PSYCHIATRIC SERVICES

It is well known that information relating to Filter 3 (referral by practitioners to specialist psychiatric services) may be obtained from either the practitioners or the psychiatric services. We have used both approaches. Arreghini et al. (1991), in a study conducted in ninety-two general practices in Verona, reported that 22 per cent of the patients identified by the doctors as having psychiatric disorders were referred by them to specialist psychiatric care, a proportion much higher than that reported from other settings (for example, Shepherd et al. 1966). This proportion did not differ between doctors working in an area with a community-based comprehensive district service (South-Verona) and those working in an area with a hospital-based system of care (North-Verona). However, the proportion of patients referred to the private psychiatric services was significantly lower for those doctors practising in South-Verona than for those practising in North Verona (29 per cent and 51 per cent respectively). This confirms that, among the factors influencing GP-referral to specialist services, the characteristics of the available specialist services play a central role (Arreghini et al. 1991).

From the specialist side of the filter, two assessments have been made, using the South-Verona Psychiatric Case Register (PCR), which routinely collects information on referral source for all contacts made with the South-Verona Community Psychiatric Service (CPS), the main agency operating in the area (Tansella et al. 1985; 1991). First, Bellantuono et al. (1991) showed that the proportion of referrals from general practice to the South Verona service increased for first-time patients from 11.2 per cent in 1982 to 23.9 per cent in 1987. They also showed that the role of the general practitioners is relatively small when only new episodes of care are considered: 3.4 per cent of the referrals in 1982 and 6.4 per cent in 1987 (see Table 14.1). In South-Verona, although Filter 3 is becoming gradually more permeable, only a quarter of referrals are currently from general practitioners, and a substantial proportion of first-time patients either refer themselves or are referred by their relatives. As far as referral patterns according to diagnostic category is concerned, in the period 1982–87, 4.9 per cent of first-time patients referred by general practitioners to the specialist services

Table 14.1 Permeability of Filter 3 in South Verona (assessment made from the specialist side of the filter, using the Psychiatric Case Register): number and percentage of contacts referred to the South-Verona Community Psychiatric Service (CPS) by GPs in 1982–87

| | First-time contacts | | | New episodes | | |
| | All | Referred by GPs | | All | Referred by GPs | |
	No.	No.	%	No.	No.	%
1982	250	28	11.2	145	5	3.4
1983	272	34	12.5	155	8	5.2
1984	236	42	17.8	172	6	3.5
1985	249	34	13.6	174	9	5.2
1986	274	46	16.8	182	14	7.7
1987	255	61	23.9	204	13	6.4

Source: Bellantuono *et al.* (1991)

received a case-register diagnosis of psychosis, 66.9 per cent a diagnosis of neurosis or personality disorder, 4.5 per cent a diagnosis of alcohol or drug dependence and 23.7 per cent other diagnoses.

Second, as Table 14.2 shows, the percentage of first-time contacts referred to the South-Verona service by general practitioners was the same when periods of 3 months and one year before and after the completion of a general practice survey, involving 47 per cent of all practitioners in the area, were compared. In other words, the practitioners' behaviour, as far as referral to the local mental health service is concerned, was not affected by their participation in this study, in spite of the fact that it involved preparatory meetings and extensive discussions.

A common policy within the South-Verona community service is to refer back to the general practitioners those patients who, independently from diagnosis, in the psychiatrist's opinion may be more effectively treated

Table 14.2 Permeability of Filter 3 in South-Verona (assessment made from the specialist side of the filter, using the Psychiatric Case Register): number and percentage of first-time contacts referred to the South-Verona Community Psychiatric Service (CPS) by GPs before and after a general practice study conducted in the area

	First-time contacts					
	3 months			1 year		
	All	Referred by GPs		All	Referred by GPs	
	No.	No.	%	No.	No.	%
Before GP study	67	13	19.4	257	51	19.8
After GP study	62	12	19.3	244	48	19.7

in a general practice setting, as well as those who simply express such a preference and whose request is considered acceptable by both the psychiatrist and the general practitioner. However, all psychotic patients and many neurotic patients, even when mainly treated in general practice for their psychiatric symptoms, remain under specialist psychiatric care and are seen at intervals by the psychiatrists of the South-Verona service for a check on their condition, adjustment of psychotropic therapy, and so on, and therefore remain in the psychiatric case register.

THE SPECTRUM OF PSYCHIATRIC MORBIDITY IN SOUTH-VERONA

The prevalence of psychiatric morbidity at the different levels can be summarized as follows:

1 Information collected in South-Verona in 1987 from a community sample of 453 individuals, who completed the GHQ-30 and other questionnaires, gave an estimate for the one-week prevalence of psychiatric morbidity of 227/1,000 population (Siciliani et al. 1988) (Level 1).
2 Using an estimate of one-week consultation rate in general practice, it was possible to convert the patient-based rate of psychiatric morbidity found by Marino et al. (1990) (41 per cent of those consulting the general practitioner on one day) into a population-based, one-week prevalence rate of patients having a psychiatric disorder and consulting a general practitioner. This was 34/1,000 population weekly (Level 2).
3 Similarly, the patient-based rate of 27.9 per cent of consulters identified by practitioners as having a psychiatric problem (Marino et al. 1990) was transformed into a population-based, one-week prevalence rate of 23/1,000 population (Level 3).
4 The South-Verona case-register provided prevalence rates for patients contacting psychiatric services in one week and for those admitted to psychiatric hospitals and wards during the same period. These rates were 3.7/1,000 and 0.7/1,000, respectively (Levels 4 and 5).

These data from the five levels of Goldberg and Huxley's model (Table 14.3) all relate to the same geographical area (South-Verona) and to the same time frame (one week in 1987) (Tansella and Williams 1989). As far as we are aware, this is the first time that comparable data have been used to reveal the extent of morbidity at each of the levels and, by implication, the permeability of each of the filters. Our results demonstrate that the permeability of Filter 1 is 15 per cent, a finding consistent with the estimate of 27 per cent by Williams et al. (1986) for the permeability of the same filter over a two-week period, but much smaller than Goldberg and Huxley's (1980) estimate of 92 per cent over a time-frame of one year. It should be emphasized that, when considering a time-frame of one year,

Table 14.3 Estimated one-week prevalence rates of psychiatric morbidity in South-Verona

Goldberg–Huxley model	Psychiatric morbidity	Point prevalence
Level 1	Morbidity in the community	227/1,000
Level 2	Total primary care morbidity	34.2/1,000
Level 3	Conspicuous primary care morbidity	23.1/1,000
Level 4	Total morbidity in psychiatric services	3.7/1,000
Level 5	Morbidity in in-patient wards and hospitals	0.7/1,000

Source: Tansella and Williams (1989)

the first filter is less permeable than the figures suggest since, although many psychologically disordered patients consult their doctors during this period, the consultations may be for other reasons. On the other hand the chance of this 'non-specific' passage through Filter 1 is obviously smaller during a smaller time-frame (that is, one or two weeks). As Goldberg and Gask noted (1991), 'if the time frame is condensed from one year to one week the first filter (illness behaviour) becomes very much more important.'

The ratio of psychiatric morbidity present at Levels 3 and 4 (conspicuous morbidity in general practice to total morbidity in specialist services) is 16 per cent (3.7/23) – that is, higher than that found elsewhere (Shepherd *et al.* 1966); which may reflect the availability and the visibility of the community psychiatric services in South-Verona. However, comparison of the extent of psychiatric morbidity at Levels 1, 2, 3 and 4 confirms that in South-Verona also, in spite of the possibility that exists for patients to bypass the general practice services and refer themselves directly to psychiatric services, the bulk of psychiatric care is dealt with in general practice. It is clear that, under such circumstances, a relatively small increase in the permeability of Filter 3 (referral to psychiatric services) may well balance a major increase in the resources made available at the specialist level. This demonstrates the need to consider the influence of the extent of psychiatric morbidity at other levels within the model (in particular, at the general practice level) and the influence of the permeability of various filters on the development of community psychiatric services, as well as the influence of the work-style of community services on the expression of morbidity at other levels of care and on the permeability of filters. For example, an increase of resources made available in the community in places where community psychiatric services are complementary or additional to the in-patient services may result, in terms of Goldberg and Huxley's model, in an increase in the permeability of Filter 3 (more patients with minor psychiatric disorders, previously treated by general practitioners, are referred to specialist services) with no modifications to the permeability of Filter 4; that is, with no decrease in the number of psychiatric admissions to hospital. On the contrary, in places where community psychiatric services are designed to be alternative to, rather than a complement of, the in-patient psychiatric services (Tansella and Zimmermann-Tansella 1988), an increase of resources made available in the community may result in a decrease of the permeability of Filter 4 (more patients previously admitted to hospital are treated in community psychiatric services) with little or no change in the permeability of Filter 3 (the community facilities and resources are mainly dedicated to the most handicapped long-term patients as well as to acute psychiatric patients, while the general practitioners continue to assist the majority of patients with minor psychiatric disorders presenting to them). 'Dynamic' studies conducted in parallel, in the same area, at the general practice as well as at the specialist level would provide important information for the evaluation of specialist services and, if repeated over time, may be very useful in interpreting monitored changes in the provision of care in defined geographical areas.

ACKNOWLEDGEMENTS

The studies summarized in this review have been supported by the Consiglio Nazionale delle Ricerche (CNR, Rome), Progetto Finalizzato Medicina Preventiva e Riabilitativa 1982–87 and Gruppo Nazionale Scienze del Comportamento, Grants 1986–87, and by the Regione Veneto, Ricerca Sanitaria Finalizzata, Contract No. 212.01.88 to Professor M.Tansella.

REFERENCES

Arreghini, F., Agostini, C., and Wilkinson, G. (1990) 'General practitioner referral to specialist psychiatric services. A comparison of practices in North and in South-Verona', *Psychological Medicine* 21:485–94.
Bellantuono, C., Arreghini, E., Adami, M., Bodini, F., Gastaldo, M., and Micciolo, R. (1989) 'Psychotropic drug prescription in Italy: a survey in general practice', *Social Psychiatry and Psychiatric Epidemiology* 24:212–18.
Bellantuono, C., Fiorio, R., Williams, P., and Cortina, P. (1987a) 'Psychiatric morbidity in an Italian general practice', *Psychological Medicine* 17:243–7.
Bellantuono, C., Fiorio, R., Zanotelli, R., and Tansella, M. (1987b) 'Psychiatric screening in general practice in Italy: a validity study of the GHQ', *Social Psychiatry* 22:113–17.
Bellantuono, C., Fiorio, R., Williams, P., Arreghini, E., and Cason, G. (1988) 'Urban–rural differences in psychotropic drug prescribing in Northern Italy', *European Archives of Psychiatry and Neurological Sciences* 237:347–50.
Bellantuono, C., Williams, P., and Tansella, M. (1991) 'Psychiatric morbidity in

general practice', in *Community-based Psychiatry: Long-term Patterns of Care in South Verona* (ed. M.Tansella), *Psychological Medicine*, Monograph Supplement 19, Cambridge: Cambridge University Press, pp. 41–5.

Corney, R.H. and Williams, P. (1987) 'The effect of social dysfunction on the presentation and diagnosis of psychiatric disorder in general practice', *International Journal of Family Psychiatry* 7:137–48.

Fiorio, R., Bellantuono, C., Arreghini, E., Leoncini, M., and Micciolo, R. (1989) 'Psychotropic drug prescription in general practice in Italy: a two-week prevalence study', *International Clinical Psychopharmacology* 4:7–17.

Fiorio, R., Bellantuono, C., Leoncini, M., Montemezzi, G., Micciolo, R., and Williams, P. (1990) 'The long-term use of psychotropic drugs: a follow-up study in Italian general practice', *Human Psychopharmacology* 5:195–205.

Fontanesi, F., Gobetti, C., Zimmermann-Tansella, Ch., and Tansella, M. (1985) 'Validation of the Italian version of GHQ in a general practice setting', *Psychological Medicine* 15:411–15.

Goldberg, D.P. and Blackwell, B. (1970) 'Psychiatric illness in general practice. A detailed study using a new method of case identification', *British Medical Journal* 2:439–43.

Goldberg, D.P. (1972) *The Detection of Psychiatric Illness by Questionnaire*, London: Oxford University Press.

Goldberg, D.P. (1978) *Manual of the General Health Questionnaire*, Windsor: NFER.

Goldberg, D.P. and Gask, L. (1991) 'Primary care and psychiatric epidemiology: the psychiatrist's perspective' (this volume, pp. 44–56).

Goldberg, D.P. and Huxley, P. (1980) *Mental Illness in the Community: the Pathway to Psychiatric Care*, London: Tavistock.

Goldberg, D.P. and Williams, P. (1988) *A User's Guide to the General Health Questionnaire*, Windsor: NFER-Nelson.

Goldberg, D.P., Cooper, B., Eastwood, M.R., Kedward, H.B., and Shepherd, M. (1970) 'A standardised psychiatric interview suitable for use in community surveys', *British Journal of Preventive and Social Medicine* 24:18–23.

Lattanzi, M., Galvan, U., Rizzetto, A., Gavioli, I., and Zimmermann-Tansella, Ch. (1988) 'Estimating psychiatric morbidity in the community: standardization of the Italian versions of the GHQ and CIS', *Social Psychiatry and Psychiatric Epidemiology* 23:267–72.

Marino, S., Bellantuono, C., and Tansella, M. (1990) 'Psychiatric morbidity in general practice in Italy: a point-prevalence survey in a defined geographical area', *Social Psychiatry and Psychiatric Epidemiology* 25:67–72.

Marks, J.N., Goldberg, D.P., and Hillier, V.F. (1979) 'Determinants of the ability of general practitioners to detect psychiatric illness', *Psychological Medicine* 9:337–53.

Shepherd, M., Cooper, B., Brown, A.C., and Kalton, G. (1966) *Psychiatric Illness in General Practice*, London: Oxford University Press.

Siciliani, O., Donini, S., Turrina, C., and Zimmermann-Tansella, Ch. (1988) *A Community Survey on Mental Health in South-Verona*. Research Report, Cattedra di Psicopatologia Generale, Istituto di Psichiatria, Università di Verona, Verona.

Skuse, D. and Williams, P. (1984) 'Screening for psychiatric disorder in general practice', *Psychological Medicine* 14:365–77.

Tansella, M., Balestrieri, M., Meneghelli, G., and Micciolo, R. (1990) 'Trends in the provision of psychiatric care 1979–1981', in M. Tansella (ed.) *Community-based Psychiatry: Long-term Patterns of Care in South-Verona. Psychological Medicine*, Monograph Supplement 19, Cambridge: Cambridge University Press, pp. 5–16.

Tansella, M., De Salvia, D., and Williams, P. (1987) 'The Italian psychiatric reform: some quantitative evidence', *Social Psychiatry* 22:37–48.

Tansella, M., Faccincani, C., Mignolli, G., Balstrieri, M., and Zimmermann-Tansella, Ch. (1985) 'Il Registro Psichiatrico di Verona-Sud: Epidemiologia per la valutazione dei nuovi servizi territoriali', in M. Tansella (ed.) *L'Approccio Epidemiologico in Psichiatria*, Turin: Boringhieri, pp. 225–59.

Tansella, M. and Williams, P. (1989) 'The spectrum of psychiatric morbidity in a defined geographical area', *Psychological Medicine* 19:765–70.

Tansella, M. and Zimmermann-Tansella, Ch. (1988) 'From mental hospitals to alternative community services', in J.G. Howells (ed.) *Modern Perspectives in Clinical Psychiatry*, New York: Brunner/Mazel, pp. 130–48.

Wilkinson, G. (1985) *Mental Health Practices in Primary Care Settings: an Annotated Bibliography 1977–1985*, London: Tavistock.

Williams, P. (1983) 'Factors influencing the duration of treatment with psychotropic drugs in general practice: a survival analysis approach', *Psychological Medicine* 13:623–33.

Williams, P., Tarnopolsky, A., Hand, D., and Shepherd, M. (1986) *Minor Psychiatric Morbidity and General Practice Consultations: the West London Survey. Psychological Medicine*, Monograph Supplement 9, Cambridge: Cambridge University Press.

Chapter 15

Prescribing of psychotropic drugs by primary-care physicians and psychiatrists
A study in Iceland

Tómas Helgason

Despite decrease in the use of psychotropic drugs in many countries in recent years, there is nevertheless a growing concern among psychiatrists, public health authorities and the general public as to their prescription (Allgulander 1986; Greenblatt *et al.* 1983; Williams *et al.* 1989).

It is often assumed that psychiatrists are the ones responsible for the extensive use of psychotropic medication. However, a closer examination indicates that such an assumption is, in fact, incorrect. Psychiatrists mainly treat the most severely ill and only see a small minority of the many patients who consult physicians with the very common complaints of depression, anxiety and insomnia. Previous Scandinavian studies of prescribing have supported this view (Bergström and Westerholm 1972; Agenäs and Jacobsson 1980; Björndal 1983). In a more recent American survey of visits to physicians having an office-based practice, two-thirds of the psychotropic drug prescriptions were given by primary-care physicians and only 17 per cent by psychiatrists (Beardsley *et al.* 1988).

It is well known that the most commonly used treatment for mental disorder by the general practitioner is the prescription of a psychotropic drug (Williams *et al.* 1989). More than 80 per cent of patient contacts with general practitioners in Iceland on account of mental disorders resulted in the prescription of such a drug (Sigfússon 1981). This is considerably higher than in a Norwegian study (Ögar 1977). However, the studies were not quite comparable, since the Icelandic study included telephone contacts as well as face-to-face contacts with general practitioners. Following either form of contact the doctor can telephone a pharmacy and ask for a prescription to be posted for the patient. According to the results of studies from different countries (Jencks 1985; Aga *et al.* 1987), including Iceland, the primary-care physicians prescribe psychotropic drugs to approximately twice as many patients as are assigned a psychiatric diagnosis. In spite of this, a sizeable proportion of patients with mental disorders do not obtain any professional treatment (Lehtinen and Väisänen 1981; Shapiro *et al.* 1984; Helgason and Björnsson 1989). In 1984 the total sales of psychotropic drugs per 1,000 only three-quarters of the sales in Denmark (Nordiska läkemedelsnämnden 1988), yet there appear to be no major differences in the frequency of mental disorders in these countries.

Because of the difference in the patient clientele of primary-care physicians and psychiatrists, a difference in prescribing habits can be expected with regard to drugs prescribed; dosages prescribed; mode of prescription and combination with other drugs. Comparison of prescription habits of psychiatrists and other physicians can give further insight into the medical treatment of mental disorders and indicate how prescriptions for psychotropic drugs and their use could be reduced and kept within the limits necessary for effective usage.

METHOD AND MATERIAL

In order to elucidate these problems, all prescriptions for psychotropic drugs issued during one month to out-patients living in Reykjavik were collected for analysis from the National Health Insurance, which pays for prescribed drugs. The Icelandic data-protection authorities gave their permission for the study on the recommendation of the Director General of Health, provided that nobody except researchers and technicians working on the study under oath of confidentiality had access to the primary data. Further, nothing pertaining to individual patients or doctors was to be published. In accordance with the anatomical, therapeutic and chemical classification system (ATC) (Nordiska läkemedelsnämnden 1986), the drugs were classified as neuroleptics, anxiolytics, hypnotics/sedatives, antidepressants or stimulants. Each prescription was entered into a data base along with the identification number and age of the patient, as well as the identification number, age and specialty of the prescribing physician, grouped into psychiatry; primary care (general practice, family medicine); internal medicine; and all other specialties. Up to five psychotropic drugs were entered, along with the quantity prescribed in milligrams and the prescribed daily doses (PDD). It was noted if other drugs were also prescribed, and whether the prescription was issued personally to the patient or by telephone to the dispensary in the patient's name. Unfortunately, it is not possible to distinguish between first and repeated prescriptions. Repeats cannot be obtained on the same prescription.

The prescriptions were collected in March 1984, at which time the population in Reykjavik was approximately 88,000, 77 per cent being 15 years or older (Hagstofan 1985).

In the analysis of the data prescribed, daily doses are presented in proportion to the defined daily doses (DDD), which is a technical unit of measurement recommended by WHO (1979). It is defined as the assumed average daily dose of the drug for its main indication in adults

Table 15.1 Distribution of physicians, patients and prescriptions, and number of psychotropic drugs per prescription by specialty of the prescribing doctor

Specialty	Physicians	Patients	Prescriptions	Drugs per prescription
Psychiatry	7.8	11.5	13.6	1.6
Primary care	14.3	58.3	57.7	1.2
Internal medicine	14.3	11.5	11.2	1.2
Other	63.5	18.7	17.6	1.2
Total	99.9	100.0	100.1	1.3
Number	370	4,818*	6,371	7,990

* The sum of patients seen by different specialists is 5,159; i.e., 341 doctor–patient contacts are with more than one specialty

(16). Examples of DDD are Chlorpromazine 100 mg; Diazepam 10 mg; Amitryptiline 75 mg; and Triazolam 0.5 mg (though this last figure has recently been changed to 0.25 mg). It should be noted that the hypnotics and anxiolytics are practically all benzodiazepines although presented as separate drug groups. Statistical analysis were carried out with chi-square test and analysis of variance (ANOVA) in the SPSS/PC+ package (Norusis 1988).

RESULTS

During this one month, 6,371 prescription forms, comprising in all 7,990 prescriptions for psychotropic drugs, were issued to 4,818 persons by 370 doctors (see Table 15.1). Psychiatrists, who made up some 8 per cent of the doctors, issued 14 per cent of the prescriptions to 12 per cent of the patients. General practitioners made up only 14 per cent of the physicians, but issued 58 per cent of the prescriptions. About 9 per cent of the patients had consulted more than one physician, most often in different specialties. In this analysis internal medicine is grouped with other specialties as its practitioners do not function as primary-care physicians in Iceland. Table 15.1 already indicates differences in prescribing habits, as the psychiatrists' prescriptions include on average 1.6 psychotropic drugs, while those of other physicians include on average only 1.2. In the following analysis, fifty-five prescriptions for stimulants are left out.

The one-month prevalence of psychotropic drug use, estimated from the number of persons presenting such prescriptions, is 7 per cent for the population aged 15 years or more: 5.3 per cent for men and 8.3 per cent for women. This is only 60 per cent of the prevalence estimated by using

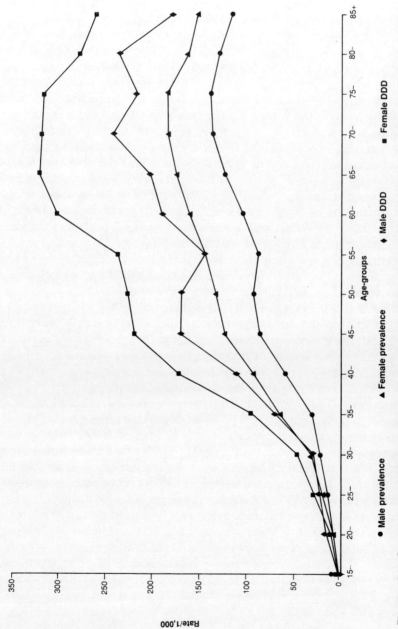

Figure 15.1 Comparison of the prevalence of psychotropic drug use, according to sex and age, with number of defined daily doses (DDD) per 1,000 inhabitants

the total number of DDDs prescribed and dispensed by the pharmacies. The prevalence increases with age up to 80 years (see Figure 15.1). But the number of DDDs prescribed per 1,000 inhabitants increases more steeply, especially for women, and reaches a plateau by the age of 65 years, slightly later for men.

Table 15.2 shows that the psychiatrists prescribed only 17 per cent of the psychotropic drugs while the primary-care physicians prescribed 55 per cent, and other kinds of specialists (namely, 78 per cent of the physicians) prescribed only 28 per cent of the drugs. The table shows the distribution of the amount of drugs, as measured by the number of prescriptions. The distribution of the amount of drugs measured by the number of DDDs prescribed gave similar results. The psychiatrists and the primary-care physicians prescribed the bulk of the neuroleptics and antidepressants, approximately 40 per cent of the prescriptions for these drugs being issued by each of these two groups of doctors. On the other hand, the primary-care physicians prescribed 58 per cent of the anxiolytics and hypnotics, which together accounted for more than 80 per cent of all psychotropic drugs. The distribution of drugs prescribed by each of the other three groups of doctors shows little variation between the four ATC categories, but that of the psychiatrists is quite different (Table 15.3).

Psychiatrists most often prescribed psychotropic drugs alone (Table 15.4), whereas the other physicians in about half the cases prescribed psychotropic drugs in combination with other drugs.

In Table 15.5 the mean PDD/DDD is shown according to drugs and specialty. These means have a large variance. The dosages vary between drug types and the prescribing doctor's specialty. Non-psychiatrists prescribe a relatively higher dosage of hypnotics than of other psychotropic drugs; whereas psychiatrists prescribe higher mean dosages than any other group of physicians, especially so in the case of antidepressants.

More than 40 per cent of the drugs were prescribed by telephone. The primary-care physicians prescribed 55 per cent of the drugs over the phone, whereas the psychiatrists prescribed only 15 per cent in that manner.

Not only were the psychiatrists probably seeing patients with more severe mental disorders, but their patients were also, on average, younger than the patients of all the other specialists. Almost 40 per cent of the psychiatrists' patients were under 45 years of age. The average age of the psychiatrists' patients was 50 years, compared to 58 years in the total group of patients.

Besides his specialty, the physician's age may also influence the prescribing habits. The mean number of DDD per prescription was 30.6. But the oldest physicians have issued more than their share of the prescriptions, with 35 DDD per prescription. From Table 15.6 it emerges that physicians under the age of 35 years and over the age of 75 prescribe the largest mean doses of all types of drugs.

These three factors – the type of drug, the physician's age and specialty –

Table 15.2 Distribution (%) of psychotropic drugs prescribed over one month by specialty of physicians

Specialty	ATC drug category				Total	No. of prescriptions
	Neuroleptics	Anxiolytics	Hypnotics, sedatives	Antidepressants		
Psychiatrists	38.4	13.4	10.3	38.8	16.7	1,323
Primary care	39.4	58.4	58.2	41.1	55.2	4,384
Internal medicine	7.7	11.8	11.6	7.4	11.0	873
Other	14.5	16.4	19.9	12.6	17.1	1,355
Total(%)	100.0	100.0	100.0	99.9	100.0	
Number of prescriptions	614	3,895	2,682	744		7,935

$\chi^2 = 592.79$; df = 9; p < 0.00001

Table 15.3 Distribution (%) of psychotropic drugs prescribed over one month by physicians of different specialties

| Specialty | ATC drug category | | | | Total | No. of prescriptions |
	Neuroleptics	Anxiolytics	Hypnotics, sedatives	Antidepressants		
Psychiatry	17.8	39.5	20.9	21.8	100.0	1,323
Primary care	5.5	51.9	35.6	7.0	100.0	4,384
Internal medicine	5.4	52.6	35.7	6.3	100.0	873
Other	6.6	47.2	39.3	6.9	100.0	1,355
Total(%)	7.7	49.1	33.8	9.4	100.0	
Number of prescriptions	614	3,895	2,682	744		7,935

$\chi^2 = 592.79$; df $= 9$; p < 0.00001

Table 15.4 Prescriptions with psychotropic drugs only or combined with other drugs by specialty of physicians

	Psychotropic drugs		
Specialty	Only (%)	Combined with other drugs (%)	No. of prescriptions
Psychiatry	78.3	21.7	866
Primary care	52.0	48.0	3,673
Internal medicine	44.1	55.9	712
Other	49.1	50.9	1,120
Total	54.2	45.8	6,371

$\chi^2 = 250.52$; df = 3; $p < 0.00001$

explain altogether only 14 per cent of the variance in the dosage measured by the proportion PDD/DDD (Table 15.7). The type of drug accounts for the greatest part of the variance. This is mainly because neuroleptics are prescribed in lower doses than the DDD by all physicians, though especially by non-psychiatrists. The interaction between drug, physician's age and specialty explains only a minor part of the variance, but nevertheless is sufficient to indicate that the age of the physician also has some effect on the mean prescribed dosage. As the focus of this study is on who prescribe psychotropic drugs, the patient variables, which would increase the explained variance, are not included here.

Table 15.5 Mean PDD/DDD (prescribed daily doses in proportion to defined daily doses) according to ATC drug category and specialty of prescribing physician

	ATC drug category			
Specialty	Neuroleptics	Tranquillizers	Hypnotics, sedatives	Antidepressants
Psychiatry	0.49	1.01	1.11	1.14
Primary care	0.28	0.73	0.86	0.74
Internal medicine	0.26	0.84	0.88	0.61
Other	0.37	0.76	0.88	0.70
Total	0.37	0.80	0.89	0.88

Table 15.6 Mean PDD/DDD (prescribed daily doses in proportion to defined
daily doses) according to ATC drug groups and age of
prescribing physician

Age	Neuroleptics	Anxiolytics	Hypnotics, sedatives	Antidepressants
− 34	0.45	0.86	0.91	1.09
35 − 44	0.28	0.72	0.85	0.84
45 − 54	0.41	0.82	0.83	0.84
55 − 64	0.36	0.82	0.88	0.68
65 − 74	0.27	0.73	0.93	0.91
75 +	0.39	0.89	1.05	1.25
All ages	0.37	0.80	0.89	0.88

DISCUSSION

The number of defined daily doses used per 1,000 population is a useful
measure for comparing the use of drugs in different districts or countries,
but cannot be used as an indirect measure to estimate the prevalence of
drug use. This is clearly borne out by Figure 15.1, which shows that the
one-month prevalence of psychotropic drug use is considerably lower, when
the number of drug users is counted, than that estimated from the number
of DDD dispensed according to the prescriptions. Although the average
prescribed daily dose is lower than the defined daily dose the too high
estimate of the prevalence derived from the number of DDD is explained
by the number of psychotropic drugs per prescription and by the fact that
a number of patients get repeated prescriptions during the month.

During this one month psychiatrists saw only 12 per cent of the patients
who were prescribed psychotropic drugs. They prescribed 17 per cent of
the drugs, whether measured by the number of prescriptions or by the sum
of DDDs prescribed. This is very similar to what has been reported from
the United States (Beardsley et al. 1988). Most of the drugs prescribed
(82 per cent) were anxiolytics and hypnotics, mainly benzodiazepines.
The psychiatrists prescribed only 12 per cent of these. In view of the risk
of long-term harmful effects associated with neuroleptics, it is worrying
that non-psychiatrists issued 60 per cent of the prescriptions for these
substances: probably often in place of anxiolytics or sedatives, as indicated
by the relatively low mean dose prescribed.

Since about half of the prescriptions issued from non-psychiatrists also
included other drugs, it can be assumed that the patients in question had
other disorders with or without mental disorders. Whether the psychotropic
drugs, which most often were benzodiazepines, were strictly indicated in

Table 15.7 Analysis of variance of prescribed daily doses as proportion of defined daily doses by ATC drug groups, specialty and age of physicians

Source of variation	Sum of squares	DF	Mean square	F	Significance level
Main effects:	247.26	9	27.47	117.26	.0001
A) Drug	174.63	3	58.21	248.46	.0001
B) Age of physician	5.71	4	1.43	6.10	.0001
C) Specialty	83.44	2	41.72	178.06	.001
2-way interactions:	33.16	26	1.28	5.44	.0001
A×B	14.34	12	1.20	5.10	.0001
A×C	6.47	6	1.08	4.60	.0001
B×C	11.78	8	1.47	6.29	.0001
3-way interactions:	11.84	24	.49	2.11	.001
A×B×C	11.84	24	.49	2.11	.001
Explained	292.26	59	4.95	21.14	.0001
Residual	1,844.80	7,874	.23		
Total	2,137.06	7,933	.27		

those instances, can be questioned. Supportive psychotherapy, explanation and reassurance (Catalan et al. 1984), in addition to any medication for physical illness, might have been sufficient.

Comparison with the prevalence of use of analgesics strongly suggests that the requirement of a prescription for dispensing psychotropic drugs is important in preventing their excessive use (Helgason 1989). Anxiety, depression and sleep disturbances are all common-place complaints, as are various aches and pains, which people treat freely by analgesics that can be purchased without prescription.

Looking at the mode of prescription for psychotropic drugs by the primary-care physicians and other non-psychiatrists, it may be possible to reduce the prescriptions for benzodiazepines considerably by curbing the practice of prescribing by telephone. Finally, the question may be raised as to whether antidepressants may be under-utilized relative to anxiolytics and in comparison to the prevalence of depressive disorders and other disorders for which they are effective (Shapiro et al. 1984; NIMH/NIH 1985).

On the whole, the mean daily doses prescribed by non-psychiatrists seem to be on the conservative side, sometimes to the extent that the adequacy of the medication may be questioned. This may be indicative of the non-psychiatrists' attitude to these drugs which they none the less continue to prescribe with too little attention to their effects and side-effects. Clearly, then, there is a need to inform non-psychiatrists better about these matters and about the rational prescribing of psychotropic drugs (Sellers 1988), as well as about alternative treatment methods.

REFERENCES

Aga, J., Fuglum, E., Nitter, L., and Bruusgaard, D. (1987) 'Forskrivning av benzodiazepiner til dagbrug' (Prescription of benzodiazepines for daytime use), *Tidsskrift for Norsk Lægeforening* 107:1568–71.

Agenäs, I. and Jacobsson, M. (1980) 'Psykiska störningar och psykofarmaka – et exempel' (Mental disturbances and psychopharmaca – an example), *Svensk Farmaceutisk Tidsskrift* 84:328–33.

Allgulander, C. (1986) 'History and current status of sedative-hypnotic drug use and abuse', *Acta Psychiatrica Scandinavica* 73:465–78.

Beardsley, R.S., Gardocki, G.J., Larson, D.B., and Hidalgo, J. (1988) 'Prescribing of psychotropic medication by primary care physicians and psychiatrists', *Archives of General Psychiatry* 45:1117–19.

Bergström, K. and Westerholm, B. (1972) 'Utköp av sedativa, hypnotika och ataraktika i Östersunds-området' (The purchase of sedative and hypnotic drugs and tranquillizers in the Östersund area), *Läkartidningen* 69:1366–70.

Björndal, A. (1983) 'Gagn eller ugagn? Forbruk av psykofarmaka i Norge' (Utilization of psychotropic drugs in Norway), Oslo, *Gruppe for helsetjenesteforskning* (Group for health services research), Report no. 4, Oslo.

Catalan, J., Gath, D., Edmonds, G., and Ennis, J. (1984) 'The effects of non-prescribing of anxiolytics in general practice', *British Journal of Psychiatry* 144:593–602.

Greenblatt, D.J., Shader, R.I., and Abernathy, D.R. (1983) 'Current status of benzodiazepines', *New England Journal of Medicine* 309:354–8.

Hagstofan (Statistical Bureau) (1985) 'Mannfjöldi 1. desember 1984 eftir heimili, kyni, aldri og hjúskaparstétt' (Population December 1 1984 by residence, sex, age and marital status'), *Hagtíðindi (Statistical Reports)* 70:24–7.

Helgason, T. (1989) 'Algengi notkunar róandi lyfja og verkjalyfja árið 1988' (Prevalence of the use of anxiolytics and analgetics in 1988), *Læknablaðið, Fréttabréf lækna* (Medical News) 7: 20–1.

Helgason, T. and Björnsson, J. (1989) 'Algengi minni háttar geðkvilla og ávísana á geðdeyfðarlyf og róandi lyf í Reykjavík 1984' (Prevalence of minor mental illness and prescriptions for antidepressants and anxiolytics in Reykjavik 1984), *Læknablaðið* 75:389–95.

Jencks, S.F. (1985) 'Recognition of mental distress and diagnosis of mental disorder in primary care' *Journal of the American Medical Association* 253:1903–7.

Lehtinen, V. and Väisänen, E. (1981) 'Epidemiology of psychiatric disorders in Finland. A five-year follow-up', *Social Psychiatry* 16:171–80.

NIMH/NIH (1985) 'Consensus Development Panel: NIMH/NIH consensus development statement: mood disorders: pharmacologic prevention of recurrences', *American Journal of Psychiatry* 142:469–76.

Nordiska läkemedelsnämnden (1986) 'Nordisk läkemedelsstatistik 1981–1983' (Nordic Statistics on Medicines 1981–1983), NLN Publication no. 14, Uppsala.

Nordiska läkemedelsnämnden (1988) 'Nordisk läkemedelsstatistik 1984–1986' (Nordic Statistics on Medicines 1984–1986), NLN Publication no. 21, Uppsala.

Norusis, M.J. (1988) 'SPSS/PC+ V2.0 Base Manual', SPSS Inc., Chicago, B 165–75, C 17–21.

Ögar, B. (1977) *Patienter i norsk almen praksis* (Patients in a Norwegian general practice), Universitetsforlaget, Oslo.

Sellers, E.M. (1988) 'Defining rational prescribing of psychoactive drugs', *British Journal of Addiction* 83:31–4.

Shapiro, S., Skinner, E.A., Kessler, L.G., Korff, M. von, German, P.S., Tischler, G.L., Leaf, P.J., Bentham, L., and Regier, D. (1984) 'Utilization of health and mental health services', *Archives of General Psychiatry* 41:971–8.

Sigfússon, S. (1981) 'Hlutur geðsjúkra í heilbrigðisþjónustu annarri en geðlæknisþjónustu' (Services for psychiatric patients outside psychiatry), *Læknablaðið* 67:50–64.

Williams, P., Wilkinson, G., and Rawnslay, K. (1989) 'Tranquillizer use: epidemiological and sociological aspects', in P. Williams and J. Gabe (eds), *The Scope of Epidemiological Psychiatry*, London: Routledge, pp. 328–42.

World Health Organization (1979) 'Studies in drug utilization', *WHO Regional Publications, European Series No. 8*, Copenhagen.

Part IV

Late-life mental disorders and primary health care

Chapter 16

Late-life mental disorders and primary health care

A review of research

Brian Cooper

The primary health-care setting represents the 'middle ground' of psychiatric epidemiology (Shepherd and Wilkinson 1988) and confers advantages for research in terms of case-definition, case-finding, population coverage and the representative nature of the picture it can provide of morbidity in the wider community. It also affords the possibility of a direct input of research findings into health-service planning and practice. Recognition of these advantages has led in recent decades to an impressive growth of psychiatric research in primary care. Hankin and Oktay (1979) reviewed 350 studies published up to the mid-1970s, while Wilkinson (1986) was able to list nearly 600 reported since that time. The trend received a new impetus from the Declaration of Alma-Ata (WHO 1978) and the mounting by the World Health Organization of its campaign, 'Health for All 2000' (WHO 1985), in which mental disorders are acknowledged as a public-health priority. It has since become extended both to developing Third World countries (WHO 1984a) and to the eastern-bloc socialist states (Tomov *et al.* 1990).

In western industrial countries, where general medical practice represents the main locus of primary health care, research has been pursued most vigorously on those populations which are covered by pre-paid health insurance schemes and, more especially, where medical practice is to some degree co-ordinated with community nursing and social work services. Such a network of professional agencies is of great value in the epidemiological study of mental illness, as well as for its effective management and – at least potentially – for its prevention. So far, however, attention has been concentrated on the 'minor' psychiatric morbidity of early and middle adult life (Shepherd *et al.* 1981; Goldberg and Huxley 1980), and few studies have been devoted to psychiatric disorders of the elderly. The purpose of this short review, therefore, is less to summarize an established body of scientific knowledge than to piece together the scattered and fragmentary information so far available, and to lay down some guidelines for future advance.

GENERAL PRACTICE AS AN EPIDEMIOLOGICAL FRAMEWORK

In some countries, lists of registered patients cover virtually the whole population, and so can be utilized as an epidemiological sampling frame. Many psychiatric illness surveys in the UK, in particular, have been based either on individual practice lists or on area Family Practitioner Committee (FPC) lists, and prevalence estimates computed by using these as the population denominator. A question arises as to how far such data are comparable with those obtained in area morbidity surveys, whose sampling has been based on residents' lists or electoral rolls. Dementia in the elderly can serve as a test case, because field-survey prevalence estimates for the severe and moderately severe grades of dementia show a good measure of agreement, and mean age-specific ratios have been computed by Jorm *et al.* (1987), using pooled data from twenty-two studies in different countries.

Table 16.1 indicates that recent British studies, based on general-practice lists, have yielded lower prevalence ratios than the pooled data from field surveys would lead one to expect. This has led to some speculation, either that earlier prevalence estimates for dementia were too high, or else that the prevalence of this group of disorders is currently declining in the UK and perhaps in some other countries also. Before drawing this conclusion, however, one must first exclude the possibility of an artefact due to differences between the studies in sampling or diagnostic methods. The choice of diagnostic tool may be an important factor. Thus in the surveys undertaken in Melton Mowbray (Clarke *et al.* 1986) and Nottingham (Morgan *et al.* 1987a; 1987b) the researchers relied on a simple rating scale, the information-orientation component of the Clifton Assessment Procedure for the Elderly (Pattie and Gilleard 1975) to detect cases of dementia. A more recent methodological study (Black *et al.* 1990) suggests that as many as 45 per cent of the cases would be missed by this technique, when applying the recommended cut-off score. Correcting for so high a proportion of 'false negatives' would bring the estimated prevalence among persons aged over 75 in Melton Mowbray up to 82 per cent, or four-fifths of the mean prevalence for that age-group computed by Jorm *et al.* (1987). The corresponding rates in Nottingham, following correction, would be 5.8 per cent for the age-group over 65 years and 10.2 per cent for that over 75 years, coinciding almost exactly with the mean rates. In both these surveys, therefore, the apparently low prevalence of dementia is probably due to reliance on a relatively insensitive screening instrument.

On the other hand, the two surveys in Cambridgeshire (O'Connor *et al.* 1988; Brayne 1989), both of which were based on general practice lists, also yielded lower than expected prevalence estimates for dementia, despite making use of more sophisticated methods of case-identification. In the rural survey (Brayne 1989), all women in the sample were examined with the aid of the CAMDEX schedule (Roth *et al.* 1986); in the urban study

Table 16.1 Prevalence of late-life dementia (severe or moderately severe) in general-practice-based surveys, compared with estimates from area field-survey data

Authors	Survey area	Survey period	Sample size	Method of case-identification	Prevalence of dementia Age-group 65 + (%)	Prevalence of dementia Age-group 75 + (%)
Gurland et al. (1983)	London	1972–76	489	CARE interview and rating scale	2.5	7.0
Maule et al. (1984)	Edinburgh	1979	487	Stand. Psychiat. Interview	2.9[1]	6.9
Clarke et al. (1986)	Melton Mowbray	1981	1,203	CAPE Info/Orient. scale	–	4.5[2]
Copeland et al. (1987)	Liverpool	1984	1,070	GMS/AGECAT interview	5.2	9.3
Morgan et al. (1987a)	Nottingham	1985	1,599	CAPE Info./Orient. scale	3.2	5.6
O'Connor et al. (1988)	Cambridge	1986–87	2,569	MMSE; CAMDEX interview	–	5.3[2]
Brayne (1989)	Cambridge	1985–87	410	CAMDEX and rating scales	–	2.8[3]
Jorm et al. (1987)	Estimates from pooled area field-survey data, applied to UK population				5.7	10.3

[1] Population aged 62–90 years
[2] Includes institutional cases
[3] Women aged 70–79 years

(O'Connor *et al.* 1988) a two-stage procedure was employed, based on the Mini-Mental State screening test (Folstein *et al.* 1975) and the CAMDEX interview. Although these approaches could be expected to miss very few cases of dementia in the survey samples (Black *et al.* 1990), the prevalence ratios given in Table 16.1 are clearly well below expectation. These findings must raise a question about the representativeness of the sampling frames on which the studies were based.

It thus remains a distinct possibility that reliance on general-practice lists may entail some risk of under-estimating the true prevalence of dementia in the elderly population, even if the research team makes its own diagnostic assessments independently of the practitioners and uses validated techniques to do so. This could affect cross-national comparisons such as that of the prevalence of organic mental disorders among old people in London and New York (Gurland *et al.* 1983), in which the London sample was drawn from general-practice lists and the New York sample from a professionally constructed probability sample of elderly residents. The reasons for under-estimation in practice-based samples are unclear and require more systematic study. In morbidity surveys based on metropolitan or urban areas, some residents will be missed because they are not registered with local doctors, as one recent study in a London borough has clearly demonstrated (Livingston *et al.* 1990). But this factor alone cannot account for the low prevalence estimates found, for example, in practice-based surveys of rural or semi-rural areas. Until this methodological problem has been resolved, it would be rash to conclude that the prevalence of late-life dementia is declining.

On present evidence one cannot decide how accurate practice-based sampling frames may be in investigating the frequency of functional mental illness and, in particular, of depressive states in the elderly. Estimates from field surveys have varied too widely to provide a firm basis of comparison against which to gauge the reliability of practice-based prevalence data. In this context, quite small differences in the time-span covered, the symptom check-lists employed for screening or the cut-off scores selected may result in disparities in the reporting rates so large as to preclude any meaningful comparison between individual studies, even within the same country.

If one can accept as a rough guide the estimates provided by the US Epidemiologic Catchment Areas programme, a point-prevalence of around 2.5 per cent is to be expected for the core group of major depressive disorder and dysthymia (Regier *et al.* 1988), with a wide penumbra of milder dysphoric states, affecting in all up to one-quarter of the elderly population (Blazer *et al.* 1987). Since this picture is fairly compatible with the findings of the recent practice-based British studies in Liverpool (Copeland *et al.* 1987) and Nottingham (Morgan *et al.* 1987a, 1987b), it appears that a practice-based approach does not necessarily miss any important focus of depressive illness in the elderly population. But this conclusion will remain a very tentative one until more precise comparisons become possible.

CASE-FINDING, SCREENING AND EARLY DETECTION

For early case-detection, 'opportunistic' screening, based on medical consultation, offers some advantages over the systematic screening of whole population groups. The potential for early detection of mental disorder in elderly patients at consultation has still to be explored. Although a number of geriatric screening programmes have been set up and tested in out-patient and general medical practice (Taylor and Ford 1987), these have paid hardly any attention to the mental health status. The omission is a striking one, given that mental impairment is known to be one of the leading causes of disability in old age. One must accept, however, that the inclusion of a psychiatric component would probably double the time required for screening, and might in some situations reduce its acceptability. To this extent, the reluctance of geriatricians to tackle the problem is understandable. The least satisfactory solution would be to pay lip-service to the psychiatric aspects of screening by including one or two items on mood or cognition, and to draw conclusions from the responses to them.

Screening tests are of two principal types: one makes use of standardized questionnaires or tests to elicit evidence of mental abnormality; the other relies upon the general practitioner and his co-workers to act as case-finding agents in the course of their daily routine. The former of these approaches is widely believed to be the more accurate and sensitive – and, indeed, for some conditions almost certainly is so. Alcohol abuse, for example, still goes largely undetected by general practitioners until social deterioration becomes evident. Systematic screening of consulting patients has shown that up to 10 per cent of males are drinking at unsafe levels, although in most cases no classical features of chronic alcoholism are present to alert the physician to the problem (Wallace and Haines 1985; King 1986). The same broad conclusion seems to apply to the detection of affective and neurotic disturbances among adult patients, for which standardized instruments such as the General Health Questionnaire (Goldberg 1972) have proved more sensitive than general practitioners' diagnostic assessments (Freeling *et al.* 1985; Goldberg and Bridges 1987). Hence the use of standardized techniques is widely assumed to be the method of choice for psychiatric screening.

Much less research has been carried out on psychogeriatric screening, and such evidence as we have is conflicting. German *et al.* (1987) carried out a study at a primary-care clinic in Baltimore, run by Johns Hopkins University. Comparing clinicians' assessments with scores on the General Health Questionnaire (GHQ), they concluded that the detection rate for psychiatric morbidity was lower for patients aged over 65 years than for those below that age. On the other hand, giving the doctors information about the patients' GHQ scores appeared to increase the likelihood of active treatment and intervention more for the elderly than for the younger adult patients.

The early detection of dementia poses a somewhat different problem from that of emotional disorder, calling for simple tests of cognitive function rather than the eliciting of symptoms. A number of short 'dementia scales', such as the Mental Status Questionnaire (Kahn *et al.* 1960) and the Mini Mental State Examination (Folstein *et al.* 1975), have been widely employed as screening instruments, both in field surveys and in general-practice studies, and have been shown to detect many undeclared cases. But these are for the most part relatively severe or advanced illnesses. Detection of early cognitive decline, or 'mild dementia', presents much greater difficulty and here the low specificity of dementia scales tends to result in an unmanageably high yield of false positives. It is doubtful whether any such scale, administered by interviewers without clinical experience or training, can fulfil this purpose.

HOW GOOD ARE GENERAL PRACTITIONERS AT RECOGNIZING MENTAL DISORDER IN ELDERLY PATIENTS?

A study by Williamson and others (1964) in Edinburgh has often been cited as showing that most cases of dementia go unrecognized by general practitioners; but this study was based on small numbers and its findings must be regarded with some caution (O'Connor *et al.* 1988). It seems in any case probable that there has been a distinct improvement of diagnostic standards over the past quarter-century, as indeed a number of more recent studies suggest. An American research group (Rubin *et al.* 1987), who conducted an interview survey of internists and family practitioners in an Illinois county, found a wide variation both in the physicians' familiarity with the causes of dementia and with the procedures for establishing a diagnosis. Younger doctors were generally better informed on this score, but nevertheless lacked confidence about making the diagnosis. Although the survey findings were considered to reflect favourably on the growth of medical awareness of dementia in the elderly, they implied that dissemination of information among practising physicians still leaves much to be desired.

In a recent British study (O'Connor *et al.* 1988), doctors in six Cambridge practices correctly identified 58 per cent of cases of cognitive impairment of all grades of severity (121/208), including 65 per cent of cases of severe or moderately severe dementia (73/112), among their registered patients aged over 75 years. A current study in Mannheim, Germany, has a sampling frame made up of all patients aged over 65 years who consult

Table 16.2 Accuracy of general practitioners in assessing cognitive status of elderly patients – selected samples: comparison of two research projects

Psychiatric int. assessment (standard diagnostic criteria)	General practitioners' ratings			
	In Cambridge, UK[1] (N = 444)		In Mannheim, FRG[2] (N = 206)	
	Definite or possible dementia	No evidence of dementia	Severe, moderate or mild dementia	No evidence of dementia
Severe, moderate or mild dementia	121	87	71	5
No evidence of dementia	51	185	28	102
Sensitivity	58.2%		93.4%	
Specificity	78.4%		78.5%	
Positive predictive value	70.3%		71.7%	
Negative predictive value	68.0%		95.3%	

1 O'Connor et al. (1988)
2 See Bickel in this volume

or are visited by each practitioner during a four-week period (Cooper and Bickel 1990). Each doctor is supplied with brief guidelines for rating the patient's cognitive status, and his ratings are subsequently compared with psychiatric interview assessments, based on a standard procedure, for a sub-sample of the consulting patients. A preliminary analysis of data from eleven practices shows that the doctors correctly classified 72 of 77 cases of dementia (93.5 per cent) and 104 of 133 patients with no cognitive impairment (78.2 per cent) (see Bickel, this volume). The accuracy of the doctors' ratings varied surprisingly little with the degree of severity of the patients' mental impairment. The higher sensitivity to cognitive disorder shown by the Mannheim physicians, as compared to that found in Cambridge, is probably due mainly to differences in design and method between the two research projects.

Both these latter investigations support the view that early detection of cognitive decline in the elderly is today feasible in general practice, using quite simple techniques, and that general practitioners are much more adept at recognizing dementia and cognitive impairment among their elderly patients than has commonly been supposed. The strategy applied in Mannheim, of providing the doctors with simple guidelines for rating the cognitive status, has some advantages over reliance on a routinely administered 'dementia scale', but calls for active participation and some degree of personal engagement on the doctor's part.

The prospects for early detection of depression among elderly patients in general practice are still unclear. Most surveys have indicated a failure to detect somewhere between one-third and half of clinically significant depressive states among adult patients in general (Freeling *et al.* 1985; Blacker and Clare 1987). One would not expect the proportion of 'false negatives' to decline with increasing age of the patients, and indeed a recent study in Canberra, Australia (Bowers *et al.* 1990) pointed to a very low level of recognition of depression among over-70-year-old patients. On the other hand, MacDonald (1986) has reported that doctors in three London practices tended to over-diagnose depression in the elderly, and that only one in eight cases of diagnostic disagreement between psychiatrist's and practitioner's assessments were due to cases being missed by the latter. He concluded that attempts to improve the recognition of depressive illness in the elderly may now be less urgent and less rewarding than corresponding efforts to improve its treatment and management in the primary-care setting. These are intriguing findings, which call for replication in other centres.

PHARMACOTHERAPY AND PRESCRIBING HABITS IN PRIMARY HEALTH CARE

The nexus of depression, physical ill-health and disability in old age (Cooper *et al.* 1982), the chronicity of many affective disorders in the elderly (Murphy 1983), the associated increase in mortality risk (Bickel 1987) and the relatively high rates of suicide due to self-poisoning (Nowers and Irish 1988), together constitute a formidable public-health challenge. Prospects for suicide prevention in this setting are uncertain, not least because, despite a high suicide risk among elderly patients (especially men), each practitioner will have had personal experience of only a few cases. Some reduction in fatal self-poisoning might nevertheless be achieved by means of general preventive measures: in particular, a more sparing and selective use of psychotropic drugs. Individual practitioners have tried to reduce the risk of suicide and drug dependency among their patients by cutting down on long-term repeat prescribing (Wilks 1975; Varnam 1981; Williams and Gabe 1989). In one British practice, both variety and frequency of psychoactive drug-prescribing were reduced until the net ingredient costs were down to one-third of the national average, without any increase in the rates of hospital admission or specialist referral; in fact, no ill effects on patients were observed (Wilks 1980).

That the prescribing of hypnotics and tranquillizers can be greatly reduced without detriment to patients has been demonstrated for younger age-groups by a randomized controlled trial in general practice (Catalan *et al.* 1984), in which adult patients consulting with new episodes of affective disorder were allocated randomly to two groups, one receiving psychotropic medication and the other brief counselling by the doctors. Similar degrees of improvement were found in both groups after seven months, on both clinical and social measures, and there was no associated increase in hospital admissions or referrals among the controls.

Evaluation of medical care is especially important for those old people who are in long-term residential care: a high-risk group of the population chiefly indebted to general practitioners for the treatment it receives. Existing patterns of medication in these establishments give some grounds for concern. In a recent British survey (Weedle *et al.* 1988), nearly one-quarter of geriatric-home residents were found to have been on hypnotics for a mean duration of 30 months. The proportion in each home varied between 4 and 60 per cent, with no obvious relation to the need for such medication. A more detailed study in Massachusetts, USA (Avorn *et al.* 1989) found that over half the residents of 'rest homes' were taking psychoactive drugs, including nearly 40 per cent on anti-psychotic medication. One-third of the residents showed evidence of serious cognitive impairment, and 6 per cent had severe tardive dyskinesia. The medication was administered by largely untrained care-givers with little understanding of its purpose or side-effects, and little control by physicians. There appears to be in many countries an urgent need for review of the use of psychotropic substances in geriatric homes and similar types of institution.

THE VALUE OF TEAMWORK IN PRIMARY HEALTH CARE OF THE ELDERLY

The growth of multidisciplinary teamwork in primary care affords opportunities for earlier case detection, improvement in patient management and increase in the support given to family care-givers. Practice-attached nurses, equipped with simple diagnostic guidelines, can correctly assess the mental health status of old persons they visit at home, and thus bring to light many undeclared cases of mental decline (Harwin 1973). Attachment schemes of this nature are an important step towards anticipatory care for the elderly (Robertson and Scott 1985), though they do not automatically ensure its development. The logical next step in research will be to compare and evaluate different teamwork strategies in primary care. Randomized controlled trials are notoriously difficult to mount in a community setting, even with the help of university-based research groups. So far, only a handful of such studies have been focused on the elderly, and each of these reveals unresolved problems of design and method.

Of the five projects included in Table 16.3, three were based directly on general practices, one on a defined area population and the fifth on patients discharged from acute-hospital care; hence they are not precisely comparable with one another. A general trend is, however, discernible towards a reduction in mortality over a defined time period, as well as a less distinct tendency towards reduction in the amount of time spent in hospital or geriatric-home care. These findings suggest that teamwork in primary health care can serve to improve the health status of elderly populations. The effect of such model programmes on mental health in the elderly is, however, unknown. Conversely, while a number of controlled trials have suggested that psychosocial intervention in general practice can be effective (Corney and Murray 1989), none of them was concerned specifically with problems of the elderly. Special studies of old people are undoubtedly necessary, since both the kinds of intervention required and the measures of outcome by which their efficacy can be judged, differ from those appropriate for younger patients.

HELPING THE FAMILY CARE-GIVERS

Community studies have shown repeatedly that the burden of caring for the disabled old people, especially those who are demented or confused, is borne chiefly by their families and above all by female relatives (Jones

Table 16.3 Randomized controlled trials of community intervention programmes for the elderly

Author & country	Sampling frame	Type & duration of intervention	Size of treatment group	Indicators of outcome		
				Crude death rate	Geriatric-home admissions	Hospital bed-days
Tulloch & Moore (1979) (England)	GP-registered patients, aged 70+	Screening & surveillance by GP team (2 yrs)	145	No diff.	No diff.	30% lower**
Vetter et al. (1984) (Wales)	GP-registered patients, aged 70+	Home visiting by practice-attached public health nurses (2 yrs)	471	28% lower*	No diff.	–
Hendriksen et al. (1984) (Denmark)	Copenhagen community residents, aged 75+	3-monthly home visits by research team; community services alerted (3 yrs)	285	14% lower*	20% lower (NS)	24% lower**
Rubinstein et al. (1984) (California, USA)	Discharged acute hospital patients, aged 65+	Assessment & rehabilitation by 'Geriatric evaluation clinic' (one yr)	63	51% lower**	42% lower*	25% lower (NS)
McEwan et al. (1990) (England)	GP-registered patients, aged 75+	Home visiting, screening and counselling by community nurses (variable: follow-up at 20 months)	151	33% lower	–	–

* $p < 0.05$
** $p < 0.01$

and Vetter 1984; Levin *et al.* 1989). Assistance with all kinds of task, ranging from household chores and shopping to intimate personal care and companionship, is as a rule undertaken by a spouse or a daughter, rather than by professional helpers (Jones and Vetter 1984; Luker and Perkins 1987). A high proportion of family care-givers manifest emotional distress, which is most pronounced when the supportive role has been long sustained. Distress may be due to the daily burden of routine, often strenuous or unpleasant tasks, the loss of a close personal relationship as a result of progressive mental deterioration, and the restrictions imposed upon the care-giver's own family life, occupation and social activities (Levin *et al.* 1989; Morris *et al.* 1988). Whereas admission of the old person to long-term residential care may result in lasting relief of relatives' distress, the use of day-care facilities appears to be less effective in this way (Henderson 1990).

Community support services are everywhere in short supply, and general practitioners have an important duty to act as 'gatekeepers' of these facilities. Though many are oppressed by a sense of having little to offer, they can actually do a great deal to improve the care-givers' morale by simple explanation and encouragement, by making regular home visits and by mobilizing social agency help (Philp and Young 1988). Mutual help and neighbourhood volunteer schemes are likely to be increasingly important resources for the primary-care team, if their efforts can be successfully channelled to those patients who are in the greatest need of support. Multidisciplinary workshops, in which general practitioners, medical specialists, community nurses and social workers participate together with self-help groups, can be effective in stimulating local initiatives (Davies 1988; Channing 1988).

No controlled studies have so far been reported of the efficacy of family support or self-help groups set up by primary-care workers. That the burden on families can be relieved is indicated by research carried out by hospital-based geriatricians. Kahan *et al.* (1985), for example, evaluated a scheme of this kind, using as a control group family care-givers who were placed on a waiting-list. Although the supportive programme, comprised of explanation, advice and group discussion of problems, was restricted to eight two-hour group meetings for the relatives, it had a beneficial short-term effect in reducing the sense of burden and alleviating depression. If such findings are confirmed, they will point the way to simple forms of supportive activity that can be provided by primary-care teams.

REFERRAL TO, AND LIAISON WITH, PSYCHIATRIC AGENCIES

Rates of referral to psychiatric out-patient services are usually found to decline in the higher age-groups, a trend unrelated to the age-specific prevalence of mental disorder. The explanation is often thought to lie in a tendency for general practitioners to under-diagnose mental disturbance, and the fact that many psychogeriatric conditions, in particular, are 'invisible' to them. More recent research findings, cited above, are inconsistent with this view (MacDonald 1986; Philp and Young 1988; Cooper and Bickel 1990). Probably other factors, including the system of specialist referral and consultation, are at least as important.

Since the 1960s a number of alternatives to hospital referral have been reported, in which psychiatrists undertake regular sessions in general practice and work closely with the primary-care team. The pace of change has been most striking in the UK. By 1984, one in five of consultant psychiatrists in England was in a scheme of this type (Strathdee and Williams 1984), while in Scotland the proportion was said to approach a half (Mitchell 1989). This silent growth of a new form of service suggests that it has been found valuable by practitioners and psychiatrists alike, and indeed a number of the latter have reported favourably on their experiences (Tyrer 1984; Tyrer et al. 1984; Mitchell 1985). Comparing the outcome of referrals to a team operating in general practice to those of conventional hospital referrals, McKechnie et al. (1981) found that the former were less likely to lead to hospital in-patient admission and that patients dealt with in this way spent on average 40 per cent less time in hospital than those in the latter group. A liaison service based on the practice encourages GPs and psychiatrists to work more closely together and to discuss individual cases, with or without transfer of patient care.

Three main modes of operation have been described (Strathdee and King 1989). First, there is the 'shifted out-patient' model, in which the psychiatrist sees patients in the practice, selected by the practitioner, and an agreed plan of treatment is undertaken by the latter. Second, the psychiatrist may both assess the case and treat the patient, keeping the family doctor informed of progress. Third, the psychiatrist may take on a largely consultative role, advising on the management of individual patients without the need for a formal referral. Mitchell (1989), in a short review of the 'state of the art', mentions two further possibilities: joint assessment of patients by GP and psychiatrist, and joint team consultations at which practice-attached nurses and social workers are also present. Each form of co-operation has its own advantages and limitations, and each can contribute to the mental health care of old people. None of them, however, is likely to prove a satisfactory substitute for the joint domiciliary visit, at which the family situation and housing conditions of the elderly patient can be observed and appraised.

TOWARDS AN INTEGRATED SERVICE MODEL

If it is to respond to patients' needs, a psychogeriatric service must offer facilities for in-patient, out-patient and day-patient care, and accept responsibility for a defined area population. Given current levels of demand in urban societies, a total population of about quarter of a million is probably a realistic basis for such special provision (Brook and Cooper 1975). While both national manpower statistics and regional levels of provision must be taken into account in planning the service, much will also depend on the way in which the different professional groups are deployed. In the UK, the growth of psychiatric liaison in primary care has undoubtedly been fostered by the existence of health centres and group practices in most parts of the country. It is feasible for psychiatrists running an area service to work quite closely with the local general practitioners if these are grouped in units of four or five, with attached nursing staff. It would be far more difficult to arrange such co-operation if up to 100 or more single-handed practitioners were involved, as would be the case in some European countries. For psychogeriatricians, who in any country are few in numbers, the logistic problems will be even more formidable.

In Table 16.4 the primary-care unit is assumed, for the sake of simplicity, to be a group practice with a patient population of around 12,500. The estimated numbers of old people with dementia and functional psychoses are computed from field-study data obtained in Mannheim (Cooper 1984) and updated in accordance with demographic trends. The prevalence ratios are similar to those reported from field surveys in a number of European countries. They suggest that a group general practice of this size would provide medical care for about 150 elderly persons with severe mental disorder, some 120 of them with dementing conditions. Only a fraction of these patients would be under psychiatric specialist care at any given time. If the practice doctors also provided medical cover for one or more local geriatric homes, the numbers involved would be considerably larger. It seems clear that a group practice carrying such a case load occupies a key position in the *de facto* psychogeriatric services, in terms both of specialist referral and of care for the great majority of affected persons who are not referred.

How many milder cases would present to the practice doctors each year is more difficult to estimate. Shepherd *et al.* (1981), who made a detailed survey in forty-six London practices, reported an annual consulting rate for psychiatric disorder of 135 per 1,000 among those aged over 65 years: a rate which corresponds to some 250 cases annually in the practice population featured in Table 16.4. This is probably an under-estimate, since field-study data would lead one to expect more than twice as many. But at the lower levels of morbidity, head-counting becomes a much less useful exercise, partly because case-definition is more problematic but also because the distribution of cases in the population fluctuates a good deal from year

Table 16.4 Expected numbers of mentally ill elderly in a standard area
population of 250,000, and in a group-practice patient population of
12,500 (severe and moderately severe cases only)

Psychiatric illness category	Standard area population of 250,000*		Health centre or group-practice population of 12,500
	In long-term care	In community	
1 Old long-stay psychiatric patients	75–80	–	–
2 Late-onset functional psychoses:			
with severe physical impairment	25–30	225	11
with no or only mild physical impairment	20	340	17
3 Dementia:			
with severe physical impairment	170	1,250	62
with no or only mild physical impairment	180	1,130	56
Total	470–480	2,945	146

* Mannheim estimates (Cooper 1984)

to year (Cooper *et al.* 1969; Jarman, this volume). More important is
the practice team's ability to recognize and respond to the psychosocial
factors which underlie many patients' symptoms; to intervene promptly
when the condition is reactive to family or other environmental stress,
and to detect as early as possible the emergence of chronic or progressive
mental illness.

CONCLUSION

The growth of collaboration with primary-care teams represents one of the
major advances of social psychiatry in the past twenty years: not least
because of its importance for epidemiological research. In this development, the issue of old-age mental disorders has been largely neglected,
but it is now attracting greater attention as the urgency of the problem
they present becomes increasingly apparent. A number of growing points
of research can now be distinguished. Prevalence and incidence studies
based on registered patient lists are not a substitute for field surveys,

but can supplement them and increase the opportunities for a research input to service planning and practice. Longitudinal research may be greatly facilitated and strengthened by the continuity of care provided in general practice. Case-control studies, whether focused on aetiology or on therapeutic evaluation, will have the brightest prospects for success if undertaken in a setting in which the comparison groups are drawn from the same background population and have been exposed to most of the same environmental risks: a condition fulfilled most readily in general practice.

An additional reason for pursuing this line of research vigorously is the rapid growth of old-age mental disorders in poor Third World countries. Earlier efforts to extend psychiatric diagnosis and treatment into the primary-care sector in these countries paid little attention to psychogeriatric illness, being understandably more concerned with the urgent problems of schizophrenia, mental retardation and epilepsy (Giel and Harding 1976; WHO 1984a). More recently, however, these attitudes and priorities have begun to change. Jablensky (1979) pointed out a decade ago that, while the frequency of mental illness among the old does not seem to vary much between cultures, its implications for the care services have so far differed between urban and rural societies. Social changes now occurring in many parts of the world may obliterate these differences in the next generation. Extended family groups and village communities will no longer be able to care for their mentally impaired old people as they have done in the past. Taken in conjunction with a rapid demographic transition – so that, for example, by the year 2000 two of every three inhabitants of the globe aged over 60 will be living in developing countries (WHO 1984b) – these changes mean that primary medical and social services will have to cope largely unaided with a rising flood of late-life mental illness, disability and dependency. A development of such magnitude must carry implications for future priorities in applied research.

Henderson (1990) has recently proposed as one outstanding priority in social psychiatry today 'studies of the contribution of general practice to the care of mental disorders of the elderly, and how to improve that contribution'. In thus correctly emphasizing the importance of treatment and management in primary health care, he may also have pointed to the most promising direction of advance for the new discipline of psychogeriatric epidemiology.

REFERENCES

Avorn, J., Dreyer, P., Connelly, K., and Soumerai, S.B. (1989) 'Use of psychoactive medication and the quality of care in rest homes', *New England Journal of Medicine* 320:227–32.

Bickel, H. (1987) 'Psychiatric illness and mortality among the elderly: findings of an epidemiological study', in B. Cooper (ed.) *Psychiatric Epidemiology: Progress and Prospects*, London: Croom Helm, pp. 192–211.

Black, S.E., Blessed, G., Edwardson, J.A., and Kay, D.W.K. (1990) 'Prevalence rates of dementia in an ageing population: are low rates due to the use of insensitive instruments?', *Age and Ageing* 19:84–90.

Blacker, C.V.R. and Clare, A.W. (1987) 'Depressive disorders in primary care', *British Journal of Psychiatry* 150:737–51.

Blazer, D., Hughes, D.C., and George, L.K. (1987) 'The epidemiology of depression in an elderly community population', *The Gerontologist* 27:281–7.

Bowers, J., Jorm, A. F., Henderson, S., and Harris, P. (1990) 'General practitioners' detection of depression and dementia in elderly patients', *Medical Journal of Australia* 153:192–6.

Brayne, C. (1989) 'Cognitive function and other indices of dementia in a rural elderly female population: preliminary findings', in B. Cooper and T. Helgason (eds) *Epidemiology and the Prevention of Mental Disorders*, London: Routledge, pp. 77–93.

Brook, C.P. and Cooper, B. (1979) 'Community mental health care: primary team and specialist services', in P. Williams and A. Clare (eds) *Psychosocial Disorders in General Practice*, London: Academic Press, pp. 183–200.

Catalan, J., Gath, D., Edmonds, G., and Ennis, J. (1984) 'The effects of non-prescribing of anxiolytics in general practice, I. Controlled evaluation of psychiatric and social outcome', *British Journal of Psychiatry* 144:593–682.

Channing, N. (1988) 'Caring for the carers', *Journal of the Royal College of General Practitioners* 38:140.

Clarke, M., Lowry, R., and Clarke, S. (1986) 'Cognitive impairment in the elderly – a community survey', *Age and Ageing* 15:278–84.

Cooper, B. (1984) 'Home and away: the disposition of mentally ill old people in an urban population', *Social Psychiatry* 19:187–96.

Cooper, B. and Bickel, H. (1990) 'Early detection of dementia in the primary care setting', in D. Goldberg and D. Tantam (eds) *The Public Health Impact of Mental Disorder*, Göttingen: Hogrefe-Huber, pp. 166–75.

Cooper, B., Fry, J., and Kalton, G. (1969) 'A longitudinal study of psychiatric morbidity in a general practice population', *British Journal of Preventive and Social Medicine* 23:210–17.

Cooper, B., Glettler, G., and Abt, H-G. (1982) 'Psychiatric disorder, physical impairments and disability among the elderly in an urban community', in G. Magnussen, J. Nielsen, and J. Buch (eds) *Epidemiology and Prevention of Mental Illness in Old Age*, Hellerup, Denmark: EGV, pp. 55–62.

Copeland, J.R.M., Dewey, M.E., Wood, N., Searle, R., Davidson, J.A., and McWilliam, C. (1987) 'Range of mental illness among the elderly in the community: prevalence in Liverpool using the GMS-AGECAT package', *British Journal of Psychiatry* 150:815–23.

Corney, R. and Murray, J. (1989) 'The evaluation of social interventions', in P. Williams, G. Wilkinson, and K. Rawnsley (eds) *The Scope of Epidemiological Psychiatry*, London: Routledge, pp. 343–54.

Davies, M. (1988) 'The role of general practitioners in supporting carers of the elderly in the community', *Journal of the Royal College of General Practitioners* 38:194–5.

Folstein, M.F., Folstein, S.E., and McHugh, P.R. (1975) 'Mini Mental State: a practical method for grading the cognitive state of patients for the clinician', *Journal of Psychiatric Research* 12:189–98.

Freeling, P., Rao, B.M., Paykel, E.S., Sireling, L.I., and Burton, R.H. (1985) 'Unrecognized depression in general practice', *British Medical Journal* 290: 1880–3.

German, P.S., Shapiro, S., Skinner, E.A., Korff, M. von, Klein, L.E., Turner, R.W., Teitelbaum, M.L., Burke, J., and Burns, B.J. (1987) 'Detection and management of mental health problems of older patients by primary care providers', *Journal of the American Medical Association* 257:489–93.

Giel, R. and Harding, T.W. (1976) 'Psychiatric priorities in developing countries', *British Journal of Psychiatry* 128:513–22.

Goldberg, D.P. (1972) *The Detection of Psychiatric Illness by Questionnaire*, London: Maudsley Monograph No. 21, London: Oxford University Press.

Goldberg, D. and Bridges, K. (1987) 'Screening for psychiatric illness in general practice: the general practitioner vs. the screening questionnaire', *Journal of the Royal College of General Practitioners* 37:15–18.

Goldberg, D.P. and Huxley, P. (1980) *Mental Illness in the Community: the Pathway to Psychiatric Care*, London: Tavistock.

Gurland, B., Copeland, J., Kuriansky, J., Kelleher, M.J., Sharpe, L., and Dean, L. (1983) *The Mind and Mood of Aging*, London: Croom Helm.

Hankin, J. and Oktay, J.S. (1979) *Mental Disorder and Primary Medical Care: an Analytical Review of the Literature*, NIMH Series D, No. 5 DHEW Publication No. (ADM) 78–661, Washington, DC: US Government Printing Office.

Harwin, B.G. (1973) 'Psychiatric morbidity among the physically impaired elderly in the community: a preliminary report', in J.K. Wing and H. Hafner (eds) *Roots of Evaluation*, London: Oxford University Press, pp. 269–78.

Henderson, A.S. (1990) 'The social psychiatry of later life', *British Journal of Psychiatry* 156:645–53.

Hendriksen, C., Lund, E., and Stromgard, E. (1984) 'Consequences of assessment and intervention among elderly people: a three-year randomized controlled trial', *British Medical Journal* 289:1522–4.

Jablensky, A. (1979) 'Priorities for cross-cultural mental health research in old age', in *Psychogeriatic Care in the Community: Public Health in Europe*, 10, Copenhagen: WHO Regional Office for Europe, pp. 103–10.

Jones, D.A. and Vetter, N.J. (1984) 'A survey of those who care for the elderly at home: their problems and needs', *Social Science and Medicine* 19:511–14.

Jorm, A.F., Korten, A., and Henderson, A.S. (1987) 'The prevalence of dementia: a quantitative integration of the literature', *Acta Psychiatrica Scandinavica* 76:465–79.

Kahan, J., Kemp, B., Staples, F.R., and Brummel-Smith, K. (1985) 'Decreasing the burden in families caring for a relative with a dementing illness', *Journal of the American Geriatric Society* 33:664–70.

Kahn, R.L., Goldfarb, A.I., Pollack, M., and Peck, A. (1960) 'Brief objective measures for the determination of mental status in the aged', *American Journal of Psychiatry* 117:326–8.

King, M. (1986) 'At-risk drinking among general practice attenders: prevalence, characteristics and alcohol-related problems', *British Journal of Psychiatry* 148:533–50.

Levin, E., Sinclair, J., and Gorbach, P. (1989) *Families, Services and Confusion in Old Age*, Aldershot: Avebury.

Livingston, G., Hawkins, A., Graham, N. Blizzard, B., and Mann, A. (1990) 'The Gospel Oak study prevalence rates of dementia, depression and activity limitation among elderly community residents in inner London', *Psychological Medicine* 20:137–46.

Luker, K.A. and Perkins, E.S. (1987) 'The elderly at home: service needs and provision', *Journal of the Royal College of General Practitioners* 37:248–50.

MacDonald, A.J.D. (1986) 'Do general practitioners "miss" depression in elderly patients?', *British Medical Journal* 292:1365–8.

McEwan, R.T., Davison, N., Forster, D.P., Pearson, P., and Stirling, E. (1990) 'Screening elderly people in primary care: a randomized controlled trial', *British Journal of General Practitioners* 40:94–7.

McKechnie, A.A., Philip, A.E., and Ramage, J.G. (1981) 'Psychiatric services in primary care: specialized or not?', *Journal of the Royal College of General Practitioners* 31:611–14.

Maule, M., Milne, J.S., and Williamson, J. (1984) 'Mental illness and physical health in older people', *Age and Ageing* 13:349–56.

Mitchell, A.R.K. (1985) 'Psychiatrists in primary health care settings', *British Journal of Psychiatry* 147:371–9.

Mitchell, A.R.K. (1989) 'Participating in primary care: differing styles of psychiatric liaison', *Psychiatric Bulletin of the Royal College of Psychiatrists* 13:135–7.

Morgan, K., Dallosso, H.M., Arie, T., Byrne, E.J., Jones, R., and Waite, J. (1987a) 'Mental health and psychological well-being among the old and the very old living at home', *British Journal of Psychiatry* 150:801–7.

Morgan, K., Dallosso, H., Ebrahim, S., Arie, T., and Fenton, P. (1987b) 'Mental health and contact with primary care services in old age', *International Journal of Geriatric Psychiatry* 2:223–6.

Morris, R.G., Morris, L.W., and Britton, P.G. (1988) 'Factors affecting the emotional wellbeing of the caregivers of dementia sufferers', *British Journal of Psychiatry* 153:147–56.

Murphy, E. (1983) 'The prognosis of depression in old age', *British Journal of Psychiatry* 142:111–19.

Nowers, M. and Irish, M. (1988) 'Trends in the reported rates of suicide by self-poisoning in the elderly', *Journal of the Royal College of General Practitioners* 38:67–9.

O'Connor, D.W., Pollitt, P.A., Hyde, J.B., Brooke, C.P.B., Reiss, B.B., and Roth, M. (1988) 'Do general practitioners miss dementia in elderly patients?', *British Medical Journal* 297:1107–10.

Pattie, A.H. and Gilleard, C.J. (1975) 'A brief psychogeriatric assessment scale – validation against psychiatric diagnosis and discharge from hospital', *British Journal of Psychiatry* 12:489–93.

Philp, I. and Young, J. (1988) 'Audit of support given to lay carers of the demented by a primary care team', *Journal of the Royal College of General Practitioners* 38:153–5.

Regier, D., Boyd, J.H., Burke, J.D., Rae, D.S., Myers, J.K., Kramer, M., Robins, L.N., George, L.K., Karno, M., and Locke, B. L. (1988) 'One-month prevalence of mental disorders in the United States', *Archives of General Psychiatry* 45:977–86.

Robertson, H. and Scott, D.J. (1985) 'Community psychiatric nursing: a survey of patients and problems', *Journal of the Royal College of General Practitioners* 35:130–2.

Roth, M., Tym, E., Mountjoy, C.Q., Huppert, F.A., Hendrie, H., Verma, S., and Goddard, R. (1986) 'CAMDEX: a standardized instrument for the diagnosis of mental disorder in the elderly, with special reference to the early detection of dementia', *British Journal of Psychiatry* 149:698–709.

Rubin, S.M., Glasser, S.L., and Werckle, M.A. (1987) 'The examination of physicians' awareness of dementing disorders', *Journal of the American Geriatric Society* 35:1051–8.

Rubinstein, L.Z., Josephson, K.R., Wieland, G.D., English, P.A., Sayre, J.A., and Kane, R.L. (1984) 'Effectiveness of a geriatric evaluation unit: a randomized controlled trial', *New England Journal of Medicine* 310:1664–70.

Shepherd, M., Cooper, B., Brown, A.C., and Kalton, G. (1981) *Psychiatric Illness in General Practice*, second edn, Oxford: Oxford University Press.

Shepherd, M. and Wilkinson, G. (1988) 'Primary care as the middle ground for psychiatric epidemiology', Editorial, *Psychological Medicine* 18:263–7.

Strathdee, G. and King, M. (1989) 'The interface between primary and secondary psychiatric care', in P. Williams, G. Wilkinson, and K. Rawnsley (eds) *The Scope of Epidemiological Psychiatry*, London: Routledge, pp. 420–33.

Strathdee, G. and Williams, P. (1984) 'A survey of psychiatrists in primary care: the silent growth of a new service', *Journal of the Royal College of General Practitioners* 34:615–18.

Taylor, R. and Ford, G. (1987) 'Functional geriatric screening: a critical review of current developments', in R.C. Tylor and E.G. Buckley (eds) *Preventive Care of the Elderly: a Review of Current Developments*, Occasional Paper No. 35, London: Royal College of General Practitioners.

Tomov, T., Temkov, I., Ivanov-Savor, Z., and Todorov, C. (1990) 'Frequency and recognition of mental health problems in general medical practice: a report from Bulgaria', Medical Academy, Sofia (unpublished manuscript).

Tulloch, A.J. and Moore, V. (1979) 'A randomized controlled trial of geriatric screening and surveillance in general practice', *Journal of the Royal College of General Practitioners* 29:733–42.

Tyrer, P. (1984) 'Psychiatric clinics in general practice: an extension of community care', *British Journal of Psychiatry* 145:9–14.

Tyrer, P., Seivewright, N., and Wollerton, S. (1984) 'General practice psychiatric clinics: impact on psychiatric services', *British Journal of Psychiatry* 145:15–19.

Varnam, M.A. (1981) 'Psychotropic prescribing: what am I doing?', *Journal of the Royal College of General Practitioners* 31:480–3.

Vetter, N.J., Jones, D.A., and Victor, C R. (1984) 'Effect of health visitors working with elderly patients in general practice: a randomized controlled trial', *British Medical Journal* 288:369–72.

Wallace, P. and Haines, A. (1985) 'Use of a questionnaire in general practice to increase the recognition of patients with excessive alcohol consumption', *British Medical Journal* 290:1949–52.

Weedle, ᴬB., Poston, J.W., and Parish, P.A. (1988) 'Use of hypnotic medicines by elderly people in residential homes', *Journal of the Royal College of General Practitioners* 38:156–8.

Wilkinson, G. (1986) *Mental Health Practices in Primary Care Settings: an Annotated Bibliography 1977–1985*, London: Tavistock.

Wilks, J.M. (1975) 'The use of psychotropic drugs in general practice', *Journal of the Royal College of General Practitioners* 25:731–44.

Wilks, J.M. (1980) 'Psychotropic drug prescribing: a self-audit', *Journal of the Royal College of General Practitioners* 30:390–5.

Williams, P. and Gabe, J. (1989) 'Tranquillizer use: epidemiological and sociological aspects', in P. Williams, G. Wilkinson, and K. Rawnsley (eds) *The Scope of Epidemiological Psychiatry*, London: Routledge, pp. 328–42.

Williamson, J., Stokoe, I.H., Gray, S., Fisher, M., Smith, A., McGhee, A., and Stephenson, E. (1964) 'Old people at home: their unreported needs', *Lancet* 1:1117–20.

World Health Organization (1978) *Psychogeriatric Care in the Community. Public Health in Europe, 10*, Copenhagen: WHO Regional Office for Europe.

World Health Organization (1984a) *Mental Health Care in Developing Countries: a Critical Appraisal of Research Findings*, Technical Report Series 698, Geneva: WHO.

World Health Organization (1984b) *The Uses of Epidemiology in the Study of the Elderly*, Technical Report Series 706, Geneva: WHO.

World Health Organization (1985) *Targets for Health for All*, Copenhagen: WHO Regional Office for Europe.

Chapter 17

Prevalence and one-year course of dementia in an English city

An application of CAMDEX

Daniel W. O'Connor and Penelope A. Pollitt

The prevalence of dementia has been measured by so many investigators over the last fifty years that further studies might seem superfluous. Indeed, from a purely practical point of view, it may not matter very much whether 5 or 6 or 7 per cent of elderly people suffer from dementia if the psychiatric services can barely cope with the small proportion of sufferers known to them already, but epidemiological research consists of more than mapping practical needs and a great deal remains to be discovered of the borderland between normal ageing and mild dementia, the evolution of dementia in community populations and the validity of the assessment procedures used to diagnose it.

Research psychiatrists in the 1950s and 1960s produced remarkably consistent prevalence rates for moderate and severe dementia by interviewing subjects in a flexible, semi-structured fashion and basing their diagnoses on textbook descriptions. This approach works satisfactorily in the hands of skilled, experienced clinicians who work and train together as a team, but difficulties arise in comparing the diagnostic threshold employed in one study with the threshold employed in others and in measuring the prevalence of mild dementia which, quite understandably, barely figures in textbook accounts.

Most of the studies carried out in recent years have used structured assessment procedures which, in many cases, comprised just a few, brief cognitive test items, either alone or in combination with questions about social, medical and psychiatric difficulties. Such procedures are efficient, economical and highly reliable, but the validity of the resulting diagnoses remains in doubt. Most severely demented individuals can be identified using the simplest tests, but what of the mildly demented individuals who score above the selected cut-point and are missed in error, or of the cognitively intact, poorly educated or deaf or depressed individuals who score below it and are diagnosed as demented as a result?

The task in future prevalence studies will be to combine efficiency, reliability and validity in equal measures, but this requires that a proportion of respondents be assessed in detail and that cases be followed over a period of years, to post-mortem if possible, to confirm the diagnoses made initially. The two-stage study described here is far from perfect, but it incorporates a number of features which make our findings of special interest. These features can be summarized as follows. The study population included the residents of nursing homes and hospitals; the screening test, the Mini-Mental State Examination (Folstein et al. 1985), is more than usually taxing and should therefore detect the majority of mildly demented individuals; low scorers were assessed using the a new, standardized diagnostic interview, the Cambridge Examination for Mental Disorders of the Elderly (Roth et al. 1986), which replicates a full clinical assessment and, finally, demented subjects have been followed over a period of one year (findings at two years will be available shortly).

RESEARCH METHODS

The names of all patients aged 75 years and over on 1 April 1986 were taken from the registers of five Cambridge general practices, together with a one-in-three sample of names from a sixth practice to make up the numbers required for the experimental part of the project. Patients were screened over a 12-month period by trained lay interviewers who administered the community version of the Mini-Mental State Examination (MMSE) (Folstein et al. 1985) which required only two minor modifications to make it suitable for use in a British setting (O'Connor et al. 1989a). Inter-observer reliability was measured during the course of the survey and found to be very high, with a mean kappa value of 0.97 for the MMSE as a whole (O'Connor et al. 1989a). Missing test items were scored as zero but, fortunately, only 40 subjects (2 per cent) refused items worth more than five out of a maximum of 30 points and only 36 (2 per cent) missed items worth more than five points because of physical or sensory disability (O'Connor et al. 1989a).

Subjects who scored 23 points or less on the MMSE were selected for CAMDEX interviews on the basis of a report by Folstein et al. (1985) that no demented people scored above this cut-point but additional steps were taken to help ensure that the number of missing cases was kept to a minimum. A one-in-three sample of respondents who scored 24 or 25 points on the MMSE was also assessed in detail; general practice records were searched to identify patients who were known to be demented by the geriatric or psychogeriatric services but who were missed by the survey; and all the larger public and private institutions in and around Cambridge were checked to ensure that no long-term residents had been overlooked.

CAMDEX takes 90 minutes to complete on average, and comprises a mental state examination, a past medical and psychiatric history, detailed cognitive testing, a brief physical examination and an interview with an informant, usually the next-of-kin, which enquires into changes in memory, intellectual function, behaviour, mood, competence in everyday tasks and physical health. CAMDEX is entirely structured, and diagnoses of dementia were made using operational criteria virtually identical to those in DSM-III (APA 1980). The descriptive criteria used to grade dementia as minimal, mild, moderate or severe have been summarized elsewhere but, briefly, mild dementia is defined as a loss of intellect sufficient to compromise daily function but not sufficient to render independent existence impossible (O'Connor *et al.* 1989b). Initial CAMDEX interviews were conducted by psychiatrists, all of whom had practical experience in caring for elderly patients. Inter-observer reliability values were acceptably high in a small series of twenty-three joint interviews. Mean phi values were 0.885 for the mental state examination, 0.984 for the medical and psychiatric history, 0.873 for the cognitive test section and 0.735 for the observational ratings (unpublished data).

Demented subjects were reviewed using CAMDEX as closely as possible to 12 months later, and a one-in-ten sample of normal subjects were reviewed using the MMSE. Normals (or presumed normals) included those who scored 26 points or more on the initial MMSE; those who scored 24 or 25 points but were not part of the one-in-three sample selected for CAMDEX interviews, and, finally, those who scored 25 points or less and were selected for CAMDEX interviews but judged to be cognitively intact. Subjects given CAMDEX interviews and found to have major depressive disorders were reviewed separately. Approximately half the follow-up CAMDEX assessments were conducted by a nurse, and diagnoses were assigned by the senior author in consultation with her. Both of us were aware of the initial diagnoses, but the CAMDEX schedule's highly structured nature reduced the likelihood that follow-up diagnoses were biased in consequence.

RESEARCH FINDINGS

Screening and diagnostic survey

We aimed to administer CAMDEX interviews within four weeks of the screening interview but the interval between the two was actually 3.1 months on average. The majority of assessments (78 per cent) were completed within four months but a small number were delayed for up to six months, usually because of admissions to hospital, and one was delayed for a year. Response rates in the screening and diagnostic phases of the study were 90 per cent (2,311/2,569) and 82 per cent (481/586) respectively. However, informant interviews were completed for only 89 per cent (430/481) of the subjects assessed using CAMDEX. We were reluctant at first to contact informants by telephone and made no approach in the case of subjects whom the psychiatrists were entirely confident were not

Table 17.1 Demographic characteristics of study population (N = 2,311)
compared with the whole of the same age-group (N = 7,309) in
the Cambridge urban area census (Office of Population
Censuses and Surveys 1981)

Age-group	Study population		Cambridge population (1981 Census)
	No.	(%)	(%)
75–79	1,037	45	49
80–84	786	34	30
85–89	356	15	21
90 +	132	6	
Sex:			
Male	811	35	33
Female	1,500	65	67
Type of residence:			
Private household	2,175	94	91
Institution	136	6	9

demented and whose next-of-kin lived too far away to be visited. As it happened, our concern that telephone contacts would cause unnecessary worry was unfounded and informant interviews were obtained in virtually every case from the third general practice onwards. This explains our failure to obtain informant interviews for 17 per cent (40/230) of subjects eventually judged to be normal but only 4 per cent (10/251) of those judged to be demented.

The 2,311 respondents who completed the screening interview were highly representative of the whole of this age-group in Cambridge (Table 17.1). Patients who refused the interview were similar to those who agreed to take part with respect to age, sex and type of accommodation, but subjects who declined the diagnostic interview were significantly younger and less likely to live in institutions than those who co-operated (O'Connor et al. 1989b).

The prevalence of mild, moderate and severe dementia combined was 10.5 per cent and rates increased steadily with age, from 4.1 per cent in subjects aged 75–79 years to 32.6 per cent in subjects aged 90 years and over (Table 17.2). Note that respondents who scored 24 or 25 points on the MMSE have been weighted to adjust for sampling, and that Table 17.2 includes thirteen subjects who were missed in the survey but were judged to be indisputably demented on the basis of detailed reports written by geriatricians or psychiatrists. Note also that forty-four minimally demented cases have been excluded because they failed to meet criteria for dementia proper. Minimal dementia, which CAMDEX defines as 'a limited and variable impairment of recall, minor and variable errors in orientation, a

Table 17.2 The prevalence of mild, moderate and severe dementia by age-group

Degree of dementia	75–79 (N = 1,037)	80–84 (N = 786)	Age-group 85–89 (N = 356)	90+ (N = 132)	All ages (N = 2,311)
Mild	23 (2.2%)	45 (5.7%)	33 (9.3%)	18 (13.6%)	119 (5.2%)
Moderate	16 (1.5%)	33 (4.2%)	28 (7.9%)	15 (11.4%)	92 (4.0%)
Severe	3 (0.3%)	11 (1.4%)	7 (2.0%)	10 (7.6%)	31 (1.3%)
All cases	42 (4.1%)	89 (11.3%)	68 (19.1%)	43 (32.6%)	242 (10.5%)

blunted capacity to follow arguments and solve problems, and occasional errors in everyday tasks', is an experimental concept and the difficulties involved in applying these guidelines will become apparent shortly.

One year follow-up

Initial and follow-up CAMDEX assessments were separated by a mean of 13.4 months. The majority of follow-ups (85 per cent) were completed between 9 and 15 months, with a maximum interval of 18 months in seven cases because of illness or change of address. The initial and follow-up MMSE tests administered to normal subjects were separated by 14.5 months on average. The majority (88 per cent) were re-tested between 11 and 16 months, with a maximum interval of 17 months in eight cases. Crude one-year mortality rates increased according to dementia severity, rising from 6 per cent (29/478) for normal subjects to 25 per cent (11/44) for minimal, 22 per cent (21/94) for mild, 33 per cent (28/85) for moderate and 52 per cent (15/29) for severe cases. Only 4 per cent (11/252) of surviving demented subjects (minimal cases included) refused to be seen again, or could not be contacted despite repeated visits, compared with 18 per cent of normal subjects (O'Connor *et al.* 1990a).

Only six out of twenty-nine surviving minimal cases had deteriorated over the course of the year, and thirteen were judged to be cognitively intact, largely because they recalled the questions and tests put to them the year before, but diagnoses of mild, moderate and severe dementia stood the test of time much better (Table 17.3). The down-grading of three moderate cases to mild, and of one severe case to moderate dementia reflected shifts in interviewers' judgements rather than clinical improvement, but two mild cases were changed to minimal dementia and another two were judged to be

Table 17.3 Comparison of initial and follow-up dementia severity ratings

Initial rating			Follow-up rating			
	Normal	Minimal	Mild	Moderate	Severe	Total
Minimal	13	10	5	1	–	29
Mild	2	2	38	23	2	67
Moderate	–	–	3	37	16	56
Severe	–	–	–	1	13	14

normal. The first two cases were in better physical health at follow-up and their informants' reports were much more comprehensive. In one case, the warden of a sheltered housing complex had used the year to good advantage to get to know an isolated, taciturn old man and, in the other, the daughter who was interviewed at follow-up gave what seemed to us to be a more objective account than the daughter-in-law interviewed previously.

One of the two subjects whose diagnoses of mild dementia were overturned was puzzling. Her flat was crowded with rubbish, the warden of her flat initially described her as being forgetful and in need of supervision and she performed badly on testing. One year later, however, she achieved near perfect scores when tested, and the warden denied any difficulties. The reasons for her improvement remain a mystery. There was no evidence that she suffered from a functional mental disorder despite her eccentric life-style; she was in excellent physical health and she took no medication. Another subject, an elderly man, was much less anxious on review and did better on all cognitive tests. In addition, his wife, who seemed frustrated by his abject dependency when first seen, retracted her account of forgetfulness and personality change. Despite these few revisions, 97 per cent (133/137) of our diagnoses of mild, moderate and severe dementia were confirmed at follow-up.

Normal subjects' initial and follow-up MMSE scores are compared in Table 17.4 with the MMSE scores of demented subjects (CAMDEX incorporates the MMSE). Normal subjects' follow-up scores showed little change overall; only 6 per cent (20/362) showed an extreme drop of 5 points or more (two standard deviations) and another 23 showed a drop of 4 points. Without further investigation, it was impossible to distinguish between incident cases whose dementia had arisen during the course of the year; false negative cases whose dementia had been missed in error; and cases whose deterioration was due to physical illness, depression or other factors. However, there was good evidence that only four had deteriorated markedly. They were disorientated to the month or year at follow-up, they recalled no more than one of three words and they were described by the interviewers as being vague, rambling and forgetful. This suggests – but does not prove – that the number of false negative cases was relatively insubstantial.

Twenty-seven subjects who qualified for CAMDEX assessment on the basis of their low MMSE scores were diagnosed as having major depressive disorders. They were a highly select group therefore, and presented especial diagnostic difficulties as proven by the fact that, of the eighteen who survived for one year, two were judged to be demented on follow-up (O'Connor *et al.* 1990b). Both had been very disturbed initially. One was surly and abrupt and refused cognitive testing on both occasions, and the other was deluded and agitated. Their informants' initial reports of mild, variable intellectual deficits were thought to be consistent with primary depression but, when reviewed a year later, their clear physical and mental deterioration and their informants' accounts of disorientation, confusion and loss of competence in everyday tasks were strongly suggestive of progressive organic mental disorder. Neither woman justified a diagnosis of dementia initially and we chose to wait and see what would happen, just as most psychiatrists would do in clinical practice.

COMPARISON WITH OTHER STUDIES

Jorm *et al.* (1987), in a re-analysis of results pooled from twenty-seven different studies, estimated the prevalence of moderate and severe dementia at 6 per cent in age-group 75–79 years, 11 per cent in age-group 80–84 years and 21 per cent in age-group 85–89 years. Rates in Cambridge, however, were substantially lower, at 2 per cent, 6 per cent and 10 per cent respectively. Despite this apparent incongruity, the study shared a number of the methodological features found by Jorm *et al.* to be associated with lower than average rates: namely, an elderly study population, the inclusion of institutional residents, a focus on mental health problems, the use of narrow diagnostic categories (dementia as opposed to 'cognitive impairment', for example) and the use of assessment procedures sophisticated enough to distinguish between dementia sub-types. What this suggests is that surveys which focus largely or exclusively on dementia and which use sophisticated, or at least reasonably sophisticated, assessment instruments will produce lower, rather than higher, prevalence rates.

Most previous investigators studied populations aged 65 years and over, and direct comparisons are difficult because only a few stratified their findings by age-group. Cambridge rates of 5 per cent for moderate and severe dementia in a population aged 75 years and over were similar to previous reports of 5 per cent (Clarke *et al.* 1986; Li *et al.* 1989) and 7 per cent (Nielsen 1962), but lower than others of 9 per cent (Bond 1987) and 12 per cent (Campbell *et al.* 1983; Sulkava *et al.* 1985). Similarly, Cambridge rates for all cases of dementia combined (11 per cent) were

Table 17.4 Changes in mean MMSE scores of normal, minimally demented and demented subjects over one year

Initial severity rating	Initial MMSE score	Review MMSE score	Mean change (SD)	Cases	Missing cases*	Significance values**
Normal	26.3	25.4	−0.9 (2.5)	297	64	
Minimal	20.7	18.1	−2.6 (6.0)	29	1	NS
Mild	17.7	15.0	−2.7 (5.4)	67	2	$p < 0.05$
Moderate	10.7	7.6	−3.1 (6.0)	56	4	$p < 0.001$
Severe	1.2	0.5	−0.7 (1.5)	14	–	NS

* Cases excluded if any initial or follow-up items missing
** Mann-Whitney significance values, demented vs normal

similar to previous reports of 9 per cent (Hasegawa *et al.* 1986; Copeland *et al.* 1987a), 11 per cent (Engedal *et al.* 1988), 12 per cent (Copeland *et al.* 1987b) and 13 per cent (Kay *et al.* 1970) but lower than other reports of 18 per cent (Cooper 1984) and 38 per cent (Nielsen 1962).

Uniformity is reassuring but it would be rash to assume that similar prevalence rates mean that the same individuals will be classified identically by all of the wide variety of assessment procedures that have been used to date. Profoundly confused people will usually be classed as demented, no matter what procedures are employed, but the possibility exists that two studies, with identical prevalence rates, might vary so much in the sensitivities and specificities of their instruments that large proportions of respondents will be classified quite differently. In addition, only a few of the surveys listed above included institutional residents. When subjects who lived in nursing homes and hospitals are removed, prevalence in Cambridge falls from 11 per cent to 8 per cent, which is very low indeed by international standards.

Mild dementia is a particularly contentious area, and prevalence rates depend to a large degree on the methods used to diagnose it. As before, comparisons are difficult because of the frequent absence of age-stratifications, but Bond (1987) and Engedal *et al.* (1988) produced very similar rates to ours of 5.9 per cent and 6.7 per cent respectively. Figures for mild dementia in populations aged 65 years and over include 2.4 per cent (Hasegawa *et al.* 1986), 3.6 per cent (Shibayama *et al.* 1986), 5.4 per cent (Cooper 1984) and 5.7 per cent (Kay *et al.* 1964). Rates in older age-groups should be commensurately higher, and it seems therefore that CAMDEX findings, while not totally out of keeping with those from some other studies, lie very much at the lower end of the spectrum, bearing in mind that institutional residents were included.

The influence of diagnostic procedures can be mapped indirectly by comparing Cambridge findings with those of Campbell *et al.* (1983), whose rate for moderate and severe dementia of 12 per cent was considerably higher. Diagnoses in this New Zealand survey were based on scores on the Mental Status Questionnaire (MSQ) (Kahn *et al.* 1960) together with a brief informant history. Fortunately, CAMDEX includes nine of the ten MSQ items, so that approximate MSQ scores could be computed for Cambridge subjects (the missing item was replaced with an MMSE item using data kindly supplied by Professor Campbell). The MSQ, at its standard cut-point of 6/7, classified 108 of our 113 moderate and severe cases identically but 40 out of our 94 mild cases were classified as moderately or severely impaired (O'Connor *et al.* 1989b). Demarcation disputes like these, which must be very common, are inevitable when the boundaries between normality and mild dementia, mild and moderate dementia and so on are based on brief cognitive test scores rather than competence in everyday tasks and our comparison highlights the need for functional as well as cognitive assessment and also for clear, internationally acceptable criteria.

Kay *et al.* (1985) and Mowry and Burvill (1988) have demonstrated convincingly that different assessment procedures and diagnostic criteria produce markedly different numbers of mildly demented cases within the same study populations. There is no way of knowing how other investigators would rate our cases but we felt it important to check, as best we could, that our view of dementia, and of mild dementia in particular, was broadly consistent with that of others. The method adopted was to select randomly twenty CAMDEX schedules from each of its five categories (normal, minimal, mild, moderate and severe) and to score each of them blindly and in random order using the Clinical Dementia Rating (CDR) check-list (Hughes *et al.* 1982). The CDR consists of six scales of cognitive and functional capacity and uses clinical data gathered by other means to generate five categories (normal, questionable, mild, moderate and severe dementia) using simple, arithmetic rules.

CAMDEX and CDR ratings were identical in seventy-five of the 100 cases selected (Table 17.5). All of the twenty CAMDEX severe cases were graded identically, but five of moderates, six milds, six minimals and eight normals received different gradings. The disagreements were not extreme – 23 of the 25 discrepancies arose from a shift of one category from normal to minimal, minimal to mild and so on – but CAMDEX criteria and the CDR cover much the same ground and marked discrepancies were unlikely. As expected, agreement was highest for advanced dementia and lowest for normal, minimal and mild states (bearing in mind that all the normal subjects had scored 25 points or less on the MMSE and were therefore a highly select group).

Follow-up suggested that many of our minimal, and a small number of mild cases, had been diagnosed incorrectly, but this in itself cannot explain the differences in ratings which were based exclusively on data gathered in the initial CAMDEX interviews. One reason for the discrepancies might be that the CDR (in common with most other rating scales) makes no provision for deafness, blindness or dysphasia which singly, or in combination, limit subjects' ability to manage independently and to respond to cognitive tests. Physically incapacitated people were excluded in all of the CDR studies to date (Hughes *et al.* 1982; Berg *et al.* 1988; Rubin *et al.* 1989), but community researchers must take respondents as they find them and some CAMDEX ratings may have been lower because interviewers made adjustments for disabilities. This approach, though sensible and necessary, introduces a degree of speculation. We were forced to ask, 'What could this woman achieve were she not profoundly deaf or dysphasic?' and to arrive at the best answer we could. We managed to achieve a reasonable level of uniformity within our own team – CAMDEX interviewers and observers assigned identical diagnoses and severity gradings in twenty out

Table 17.5 Comparison of CAMDEX and Clinical Dementia Rating (CDR) severity gradings

CAMDEX criteria	CDR criteria					
	Normal	Questionable	Mild	Moderate	Severe	Total
Normal	12	6	2			20
Minimal	2	14	4			20
Mild			14	6		20
Moderate				15	5	20
Severe					20	20

of twenty-three joint assessments – but other researchers would possibly have drawn different conclusions in particularly difficult cases.

DISCUSSION

Study design

The project contained its share of methodological deficiencies, but there is little evidence to suggest that they impinged on our findings to any great extent. The large number of true cases required for a subsequent study of the efficacy of social interventions made it impracticable to select subjects for CAMDEX interviews from across the full range of MMSE scores. A stratified sampling technique, as described by Duncan-Jones and Henderson (1978), might have provided a clearer picture of the spread of mild dementia but this would have entailed selecting high and low scorers alike for more detailed investigation which was beyond our means. The uppermost cut-point on the MMSE of 25/26 was set too low but, even so, the proportion of subjects who were demented declined steeply from 28 per cent of those scoring 23, to 16 per cent of those scoring 24 and 10 per cent of those scoring 25 points. Extrapolating from these figures suggests that 5 per cent of subjects scoring 26 points and 2 per cent of those with 27 points were demented as well, but this would have netted only 16 extra cases, taking the prevalence rate from 10.5 per cent to 11.2 per cent (O'Connor *et al.* 1989b).

An increase of less than 1 per cent is of no practical importance but, had we used the customary cut-point of 23/24, 33 of the 119 mildly demented cases would have been missed. This important observation serves to highlight the dangers of using brief cognitive tests in community populations. Tests like the MMSE are quick and convenient, scores can be calculated easily and reliably, and hospital validation studies invariably show that they are capable of good discrimination between demented and non-demented patients. The standard MMSE cut-point, for example, derives from the observation by Folstein *et al.* (1975) that demented patients all scored 22 points or less while volunteer controls all scored 24 points or more. Unfortunately, demented patients are often so confused that they perform badly on even the simplest test while volunteers are likely to be bright, eager senior citizens with a liking for new activities. Validation studies are often biased as a consequence, and it should come as no surprise to learn that the MMSE (and every other brief test) discriminates much less well when applied in the community.

Missing data create uncertainty and diminish the impact of a study's final results, and we regret our decision not to interview the next-of-kin or other key informants of some of the people whom CAMDEX interviewers believed were fully intellectually intact. As it happened, our initial concern that telephone interviews would cause alarm was unfounded and the vast majority of relatives welcomed our approach by whatever means. We doubt very much, on the basis of our own observations, that obtaining interviews in every case would have altered our findings to any substantial degree but, even so, documented evidence would have been preferable.

The project's design had a number of features which help to offset these drawbacks. The study population was highly representative, response rates were comparatively high, and our figures suggest that demented patients were actually more likely to agree to CAMDEX assessment than normals on the grounds that refusers were younger than average and less likely to live in institutions. The accuracy and usefulness of general practice age–sex registers have been questioned (Livingston *et al.* 1990) but we doubt that this was a major difficulty in Cambridge. Virtually all British citizens are registered with a single general practitioner, regardless of whether or not they attend, and four of the six practices had checked their lists in the year before the study for other reasons. Dead or absent patients whose names had not been removed from the registers were a source of inconvenience rather than error, and the proportion of genuine patients whose names were missed in error is likely to be in the order of 2 per cent in conscientious practices which are accustomed to working with research projects (Fraser and Clayton 1981).

Diagnostic validity

CAMDEX provides a full, standardized clinical assessment, and the confirmation of 97 per cent of our diagnoses of mild, moderate and severe dementia at one-year follow-up points to a high level of clinical validity, bearing in mind that follow-up examinations were conducted by the same team using the same diagnostic instrument (post-mortem examinations will be obtained wherever possible but the numbers are very small at present). Follow-up studies are expensive and time-consuming and high mortality rates make them feasible only when the original sample was large. All of these factors have deterred most epidemiologists from attempting to validate their diagnoses and, furthermore, the findings in one of the two follow-up studies to date were disappointing.

Every one of the nine cases of dementia diagnosed in London by Copeland *et al.* (1987b) using the CARE interview were confirmed by research psychiatrists one year later but, in another study, the findings were less successful. Thirty-three elderly people examined using the Geriatric Mental State (GMS) were reviewed 20 to 131 weeks later by trainee psychiatrists who re-administered the GMS and completed an informant history in some cases (Copeland *et al.* 1986). Of the twelve cases diagnosed originally as having an organic mental disorder using a computer algorithm (AGECAT), only six were judged to be demented by the psychiatrists at follow-up, two were judged to be depressed, one had developed schizophrenia and three were non-cases. Some of the psychiatrists' intuitive diagnoses may have been incorrect, and some of the original organic diagnoses may have correctly reflected delirium which had resolved in the interim, but the latter explanation seems unlikely given the very low prevalence of delirium in the community (O'Connor *et al.* 1989b). Another explanation might be that the informant histories obtained in a proportion of the follow-up interviews indicated that subjects had not actually deteriorated from a previous level of function or that, if they had, factors other than dementia were responsible.

CAMDEX diagnoses of minimal dementia posed considerable difficulties and only a small proportion of subjects had deteriorated further when seen a year later. Some of those judged to be normal on follow-up admitted to having felt depressed when seen initially, although they had denied it at the time, but others were simply very old and frail and had a variety of disabilities which complicated their clinical presentation (O'Connor *et al.* 1990a). Rubin *et al.* (1989) reported that eleven of sixteen carefully selected clinic patients with CDR ratings of questionable dementia showed either progressive intellectual impairment over a period of several years or neuropathological evidence of Alzheimer's disease. Patients with any complicating medical, neurological or psychiatric disorders were excluded, however, and these findings cannot be generalized to community populations. Major depressive illnesses, other functional psychoses, profound deafness and aphasia occur infrequently in community populations but, when they do occur, or more usually when a number of less severe disabilities occur together, diagnostic problems are inevitable.

Physically disabled but cognitively intact old people may be labelled as demented in error if their disabilities prevent them from completing assessment procedures and, conversely, infirm old people who are also demented may be passed as normal if too much allowance is made for their blindness, deafness or other difficulties which impede communication. These difficulties can best be illustrated by reference to two particular studies. In a survey by Clarke *et al.* (1984), for example, only 1.6 per cent of subjects aged 75 years and over qualified for diagnoses of marked cognitive impairment on the basis of their low scores on a brief cognitive test. As many as 58 of the 1,203 subjects failed to complete every test item and were listed as 'unclassifiable' but, when more information became available later, 16 of the 58 'unclassifiables' were judged to be demented (Clarke *et al.* 1986). Secondly, Gurland *et al.* (1983) found that pervasive dementia was twice as common in New York as in London. However, 61 per cent of the New Yorkers were immigrants compared with 10 per cent of the Londoners, and 36 per cent had difficulty making themselves understood because of poor English, deafness, speech defects or unfavourable interview conditions, compared with 12 per cent in London. The possibility remains, therefore, that New Yorkers were rated more harshly because of the greater number of problems they experienced in completing the research interview.

Assessment procedures

Epidemiologists understandably prefer to use the shortest possible assessment procedures for reasons of economy. Brief cognitive tests like the MMSE can be administered by trained lay interviewers in a matter of minutes and can be incorporated easily into schedules which cover a wide variety of social and medical topics. The advantages are compelling, but what of the disadvantages?

Very simple tests like the Mental Status Questionnaire (Kahn *et al.* 1960), the Abbreviated Mental Test (Hodkinson 1972) and the Clifton Information-Orientation Scale (Pattie and Gilleard 1975) will detect most advanced cases (see above) but, even so, Black *et al.* (1990) have shown recently that the last-named test failed to identify six out of twenty-two 'definite' cases diagnosed using a combination of longer instruments. The MMSE, by contrast, is much more taxing and has greater sensitivity to mild degrees of cognitive impairment. Offsetting this, a higher proportion of normal elderly people 'fail' the test at its standard cut-point and will be wrongly labelled as cognitively impaired in consequence. In addition, educational attainment and social class have a considerable bearing on scores with the result that poorly educated old people are at special risk of mis-diagnosis (Anthony *et al.* 1982; Holzer *et al.* 1984). Identical effects were found in Cambridge. Respondents who had left school before their fifteenth birthdays or worked in manual occupations were significantly more likely to score 23 points or less, even when adjustments were made for age (O'Connor *et al.* 1989c). Further analyses show that these effects are not attributable to dementia, since poorly educated people from deprived backgrounds were no more likely than others to be diagnosed as demented (O'Connor *et al.* 1991).

Henderson and Huppert (1984) proposed that elderly people who have never functioned at a high level could be distinguished from those whose intellectual capacities have genuinely deteriorated as the result of the dementia by questioning a relative or other knowledgeable informant. We were aware from the outset that relatives, neighbours, friends and professional workers might view forgetfulness, inertia and other features of dementia as a normal part of the ageing process and fail to report it but, in practice, we found that this was not the case. The follow-up findings presented already suggest that informants provided misleading accounts in two cases but, otherwise, only two relatives gave descriptions that were totally at variance with our own observations, and informants' replies to questions about memory, orientation and mental function correlated to a highly statistically significant degree with subjects' scores on testing (O'Connor *et al.* 1989d). In addition, prolonged discussions with the supporters of mildly demented people made it clear that, while family members and others minimize the effects of dementia, they concede that change has taken place (Pollitt *et al.* 1989). Supporters and research psychiatrists differ, therefore, in the implications they draw from the evidence before them but our data suggest that most informants answer questions objectively and to the best of their ability.

Diagnostic criteria

The categorical view of dementia, which neatly separates 'cases' from 'non-cases', has been challenged recently by Brayne and Calloway (1988) who found, as we did, that scores on cognitive tests and measures of dependency are smoothly and continuously distributed in representative community populations. Their proposal that future research should move from the model 'Does this person have dementia?' to 'How much does he have?' is well argued, but many studies combine epidemiological interests with practical concerns and require 'cases' to examine particular questions and hypotheses. The question 'When does dementia begin?' was of particular interest in our project which was also concerned with the usefulness of identifying dementia at an early stage and of providing specially tailored help to sufferers and their families.

Dementia began, from our point of view, when specified constellations of forgetfulness, deterioration in intellectual ability, disturbances of higher cortical function and personality change became sufficient to interfere with daily function. Apraxia, agnosia and aphasia were relatively uncommon except in advanced cases or following strokes and so forgetfulness, loss of drive and interest, and a loss of practical, everyday skills formed the basis of our definition of mild dementia. This definition made good clinical sense and was closely in line with both the DSM-III (APA 1980) and ICD-10 (WHO 1987) diagnostic systems but, clearly, the dividing line between compromised and non-compromised daily function is far from straightforward. The criticism by Jorm and Henderson (1985) that the DSM-III system failed to specify how criteria should be turned into particular questions or tests has been corrected to some extent in the revised version (APA 1987) but detailed specifications of 'three out of five points on test A' or 'two out of four points on test B' require careful validation and are likely to pose difficulties when criteria developed in western countries are applied in cultures in which the majority of elderly people are illiterate.

Informant histories, in combination with a mental state examination and cognitive tests, helped us to root our definition of dementia in everyday life, and the findings presented above, together with those of Jorm and Korten (1988), show that informants' replies to questions are consistent with other, independent measures of cognitive impairment. Difficulties remain, however, in distinguishing the loss of function which accompanies dementia from the effects of physical illness and handicap. This is an important issue when dealing with very old people, many of whom suffer from multiple handicaps (O'Connor *et al.* 1989e), and it might also be that family members, and even highly trained and experienced interviewers, have lower expectations of people at the extreme end of life. Dementia of the Alzheimer's type develops insidiously, and the point at which neurological lesions express themselves in behavioural decompensation might vary considerably from one individual to another because of differences in personality, pre-morbid intelligence, physical health, environmental stimulation and perhaps many other factors. The requirement now is for longitudinal surveys of representative populations using detailed, comprehensive assessment procedures to be coupled wherever possible with post-mortem examinations.

ACKNOWLEDGEMENTS

The Hughes Hall Project for Later Life was supported by the Charles Wolfson Charitable Trust. We thank Drs J. Hyde, J. Fellowes and N. Miller and Mrs B. Jones for help with CAMDEX interviews; Drs C. Brayne and E. Gaelheer who assisted with CAMDEX reliability interviews; Mrs R. Coe for help with computing and Drs P. Brook and B. Reiss for supervision.

REFERENCES

American Psychiatric Association (1980) *Diagnostic and Statistical Manual of Mental Disorders*, third edn, Washington, DC: APA.
American Psychiatric Association (1987) *Diagnostic and Statistical Manual of Mental Disorders*, third edn, rev., Washington, DC: APA.
Anthony, J.C., LeResche, L., Niaz, U. Korff, M. von, and Folstein, M.F. (1982)

'Limits of the "Mini-Mental State" as a screening test for dementia and delirium among hospital patients', *Psychological Medicine* 12:397–408.

Berg, L., Miller, J.P., Storandt, M., Duchek, J., Morris, J.C., Rubin, E.H., Burke, W.J., and Coben, L.A. (1988) 'Mild senile dementia of the Alzheimer type: 2, longitudinal assessment', *Annals of Neurology* 23:477–84.

Black, S.E., Blessed, G., Edwardson, J.A., and Kay, D.W.K. (1990) 'Prevalence rates of dementia in an ageing population: are low rates due to the use of insensitive instruments?', *Age and Ageing* 19:84–90.

Bond, J. (1987) 'Psychiatric illness in later life: a study of prevalence in a Scottish population', *International Journal of Geriatric Psychiatry* 2:39–57.

Brayne, C. and Calloway, P. (1988) 'Normal ageing, impaired cognitive function, and senile dementia of the Alzheimer's type: a continuum?', *Lancet* i:1265–7.

Campbell, A.J., McCosh, L.M., Reinken, J., and Allan, B.C. (1983) 'Dementia in old age and the need for services', *Age and Ageing* 12:11–16.

Clarke, M., Clarke, S., Odell, A., and Jagger, C. (1984) 'The elderly at home: health and social status', *Health Trends* 16:3–7.

Clarke, M., Lowry, R., and Clarke, S. (1986) 'Cognitive impairment in the elderly – a community survey', *Age and Ageing* 15:278–84.

Cooper, B. (1984) 'Home and away: the disposition of mentally ill old people in an urban population', *Social Psychiatry* 19:187–96.

Copeland, J.R.M., Dewey, M.E., Wood, N., Searle, R., Davidson, I.A., and McWilliam, C. (1987a) 'Range of mental illness among the elderly in the community: prevalence in Liverpool using the GMS-AGECAT package', *British Journal of Psychiatry* 150:815–23.

Copeland, J.R.M., Gurland, B.J., Dewey, M.E., Kelleher, M.J., Smith, A.M.R., and Davidson, I.A (1987b) 'Is there more dementia, depression and neurosis in New York? A comparative study of the elderly in New York and London using the computer diagnosis AGECAT', *British Journal of Psychiatry* 151:466–73.

Copeland, J.R.M., McWilliam, C., Dewey, M.E., Forshaw, D.M., Shiwack, R., Abed, R., Muthu, M.S., and Wood, N. (1986) 'The early recognition of dementia in the elderly: a preliminary communication about a longitudinal study using the GMS-AGECAT package (community version)', *International Journal of Geriatric Psychiatry* 1:63–70.

Duncan-Jones, P. and Henderson, S. (1978) 'The use of a two-phase design in a prevalence survey', *Social Psychiatry* 13:231–7.

Engedal, K., Gilje, K., and Laake, K. (1988) 'Prevalence of dementia in a Norwegian sample aged 75 years and over living at home', *Comprehensive Gerontology* 2:102–6.

Folstein, M., Anthony, J.C., Parhad, I., Duffy, B., and Gruenberg, E.M. (1985) 'The meaning of cognitive impairment in the elderly', *Journal of the American Geriatric Society* 33:228–35.

Folstein, M.F., Folstein, S.E., and McHugh, P.R. (1975) '"Mini-Mental State": a practical method for grading the cognitive state of patients for the clinician', *Journal of Psychiatric Research* 12:189–98.

Fraser, R.C. and Clayton, D.G. (1981) 'The accuracy of age–sex registers, practice medical records and family practitioner committee registers', *Journal of the Royal College of General Practitioners* 31:410–19.

Gurland, B., Copeland, J., Kuriansky, J., Kelleher, M.J., Sharpe, L., and Dean, L. (1983) *The Mind and Mood of Aging*, London: Croom Helm.

Hasegawa, K., Homma, A., and Imai, Y. (1986) 'An epidemiological study of age-related dementia in the community', *International Journal of Geriatric Psychiatry* 1:45–55.

Henderson, A.S. and Huppert, F.A. (1984) 'The problem of mild dementia', *Psychological Medicine* 14:5–11.

Hodkinson, H.M. (1972) 'Evaluation of a mental test score for assessment of mental impairment in the aged', *Age and Ageing* 1:233–8.

Holzer, C.E., Tischler, G.L., Leaf, P.J., and Myers, J.K. (1984) 'An epidemiologic assessment of cognitive impairment in a community population', *Research in Community and Mental Health* 4:3–32.

Hughes, C.P., Berg, L., Danziger, W.L., Coben, L.A., and Martin, R.L. (1982) 'A new clinical scale for the staging of dementia', *British Journal of Psychiatry* 140:566–72.

Jorm, A.F. and Henderson, A.S. (1985) 'Possible improvements to the diagnostic criteria for dementia in DSM-III', *British Journal of Psychiatry* 147:394–9.

Jorm, A.F. and Korten, A.E. (1988) 'Assessment of cognitive decline in the elderly by informant interview', *British Journal of Psychiatry* 152:209–13.

Jorm, A.F., Korten, A.E., and Henderson, A.S. (1987) 'The prevalence of dementia: a quantitative integration of the literature', *Acta Psychiatrica Scandinavica* 76:465–79.

Kahn, R.L., Goldfarb, A.I., Pollack, M., and Peck, A. (1960) 'Brief objective measures for the determination of mental status in the aged', *American Journal of Psychiatry* 117:326–8.

Kay, D.W.K., Beamish, P., and Roth, M. (1964) 'Old age mental disorders in Newcastle upon Tyne. Part I: A study of prevalence', *British Journal of Psychiatry* 110:668–82.

Kay, D.W.K., Bergmann, K., Foster, E.M., McKechnie, A.A., and Roth, M. (1970) 'Mental illness and hospital usage in the elderly: a random sample followed up', *Comprehensive Psychiatry* 11:26–35.

Kay, D.W.K., Henderson, A.S., Scott, R., Wilson, J., Rickwood, D., and Grayson, D.A. (1985) 'Dementia and depression among the elderly living in the Hobart community: the effect of the diagnostic criteria on the prevalence rates', *Psychological Medicine* 15:771–88.

Li, G., Shen, Y.C., Chen, C.H., and Zhao, Y.W. (1989) 'An epidemiological survey of age-related dementia in an urban area of Beijing', *Acta Psychiatrica Scandinavica* 79:557–63.

Livingston, G., Hawkins, A., Graham, N., Blizzard, B., and Mann, A. (1990) 'The Gospel Oak study: prevalence rates of dementia, depression and activity limitation among elderly residents in inner London', *Psychological Medicine* 20:37–146.

Mowry, B.J. and Burvill, P.W. (1988) 'A study of mild dementia in the community using a wide range of diagnostic criteria', *British Journal of Psychiatry* 153:328–34.

Nielsen, J. (1962) 'Geronto-psychiatric period-prevalence investigation in a geographically delimited population', *Acta Psychiatrica Scandinavica* 38:307–30.

O'Connor, D.W., Pollitt, P.A., Treasure, F.P., Brook, C.P.B., and Reiss, B.B. (1989a) 'The reliability and validity of the Mini-Mental State in a British community survey', *Journal of Psychiatric Research* 23:87–96.

O'Connor, D.W., Pollitt, P.A., Hyde, J.B., Fellowes, J.L., Miller, N.D., Brook, C.P.B., Reiss, B.B., and Roth, M. (1989b) 'The prevalence of dementia as measured by the Cambridge Mental Disorders of the Elderly Examination', *Acta Psychiatrica Scandinavica* 79:190–8.

O'Connor, D.W., Pollitt, P.A., Hyde, J.B., Fellowes, J.L., Miller, N.D., Brook, C.P.B., and Reiss, B.B. (1989c) 'The influence of education, social class and sex on Mini-Mental State scores', *Psychological Medicine* 19:771–6.

O'Connor, D.W., Pollitt, P.A., Brook, C.P.B., and Reiss, B.B. (1989d) 'The validity of informant histories in a community study of dementia', *International Journal of Geriatric Psychiatry* 4: 203–8.

O'Connor, D.W., Pollitt, P.A., Brook, C.P.B., and Reiss, B.B. (1989e) 'A community survey of mental and physical infirmity in nonagenarians', *Age and Ageing* 18:411–14.

O'Connor, D.W., Pollitt, P.A., and Hyde, J.B. (1990a) 'A follow-up study of dementia diagnosed in the community using the Cambridge Mental Disorders of the Elderly Examination (CAMDEX)', *Acta Psychiatrica Scandinavica*, 81:78–82.

O'Connor, D.W., Pollitt, P.A., and Roth, M. (1990b) 'Coexisting depression and dementia in a community survey of the elderly', *International Psychogeriatrics*, 2:45–53

O'Connor, D.W., Pollitt, P.A., and Treasure, F.P. (1991) 'The influence of education and social class on the diagnosis of dementia in a community population', *Psychological Medicine* 21:219–24.

Office of Population Censuses and Surveys (1981) *Small Area Statistics*, London: HMSO.

Pattie, A.H. and Gilleard, C.J. (1975) 'A brief psychogeriatric assessment schedule: validation against psychiatric diagnosis and discharge from hospital', *British Journal of Psychiatry* 127:489–93.

Pollitt, P.A., O'Connor, D.W., and Anderson, I. (1989) 'Mild dementia: perceptions and problems', *Ageing and Society* 9:261–75.

Roth, M., Tym, E., Mountjoy, C.Q., Huppert, F.A., Hendrie, H., Verma, S., and Goddard, R. (1986) 'CAMDEX: a standardised instrument for the diagnosis of mental disorder in the elderly with special reference to the early detection of dementia', *British Journal of Psychiatry* 149:698–709.

Rubin, E.H., Morris, J.C., Grant, E.A., and Vendegna, T. (1989) 'Very mild senile dementia of the Alzheimer type. 1, Clinical assessment', *Archives of Neurology* 46:379–82.

Shibayama, H., Kasahara, Y., and Kobayashi, H. (1986) 'Prevalence of dementia in a Japanese elderly population', *Acta Psychiatrica Scandinavica* 74: 144–51.

Sulkava, R., Wikstrom, J., Aromaa, A., Raitasalo, R., Lehtinen, V., Lahtela, K., and Palo, J. (1985) 'Prevalence of severe dementia in Finland', *Neurology* 35:1025–9.

World Health Organization (1987) *International Classification of Diseases, ICD-10, Research Diagnostic Criteria, 1987 Draft*, WHO: Geneva.

Chapter 18

Cognitive disorders and dementia among elderly general-practice patients in a West German city

Horst Bickel

Only a small proportion of cases of dementia are potentially reversible and can at present be successfully treated. Clarfield (1988) found in a review of thirty-two published studies that the disorder remitted in only 3 per cent of cases and showed some improvement in an additional 8 per cent. In about 90 per cent of cases the prognosis is unfavourable once the illness has reached a clinically manifest degree of severity. Whether or not treatment or preventive measures in the initial stages of the illness offer better prospects of success is so far unknown, the recognition of mild or early dementia being still unreliable. The issue is an important one, since early detection and diagnosis will be an essential condition for any large-scale evaluation of therapeutic intervention.

The concept of mild or early dementia is ill defined and poorly operationalized. Although in recent years a number of scales have been developed, which permit assessment and recording of the stage of severity of dementing disorder (Hughes *et al*. 1982; Reisberg *et al*. 1982; Roth *et al*. 1986), a number of problems remain unresolved. In particular it is not yet clear to what extent these various scales, whose anchor-points are defined by relatively imprecise criteria, are directly comparable with one another. That discrepancies can result, which considerably reduce the value of the research findings, was shown by Mowry and Burvill (1988) in a study of 100 old people. Applying the widely varying criteria reported in the literature, they arrived at estimates of the frequency of mild dementia varying from 3 to 64 per cent. Equally little is known about the prognostic validity of the scales or their applicability to forms of dementing disorder other than those of typically progressive Alzheimer type.

Despite a large number of epidemiological studies, there is insufficient knowledge about the frequency, course and duration of mild dementia. Most of the studies give estimates of prevalence, but the wide variation, ranging from under 2 to over 50 per cent among over 65-year-olds, emphasizes the diagnostic problems which must be overcome before reliable estimates of the true frequency can be made. The few prospective field studies so far reported have provided evidence that cases of so-called mild dementia in the elderly population carry a much higher risk of developing clinically manifest dementia over a period of some years than do cognitively unimpaired old people (Bergmann *et al*. 1973; Copeland *et al*. 1986; Bickel and Cooper 1989; Cooper and Bickel 1989; O'Connor *et al*. 1990). It seems, however, that a very heterogeneous group of conditions is involved, whose impairments are probably diverse in nature, since only in 20 to 40 per cent of cases does the presumed state of mild dementia develop into a full-blown dementing disorder. Furthermore, most of the new cases of dementia which are identified in longitudinal studies arise in the main group of initially unimpaired persons. Questions therefore arise as to which forms of dementia are detectable at an early stage, by which specific features such progressive illnesses can be predicted and in what periods of time a population at risk must be re-examined, in order to screen effectively for those cases which are still at an early stage.

Since no useful biological markers have yet been found and the results of CT, EEG and laboratory testing are of only limited help for diagnostic screening, the focus of interest in early detection has been concentrated on the nature and extent of cognitive dysfunction. Although brief dementia scales, such as the Mini Mental State (Folstein *et al*. 1975), are too inaccurate for this purpose (Anthony *et al*. 1982), a number of research groups have succeeded in distinguishing cases of mild dementia from normal, age-related cognitive decline on the basis of objective neuropsychological testing in cross-sectional studies (Pfeffer *et al*. 1981; Storandt *et al*. 1984; Vitaliano *et al*. 1984; Flicker *et al*. 1985) as well as in predicting the further course of progressive disorders (Pfeffer *et al*. 1984; Botwinick *et al*. 1986; Rosen *et al*. 1986; Vitaliano *et al*. 1986; Wilson and Kaszniak 1986; Rubin *et al*. 1989; Storandt and Hill 1989). Despite the application of numbers of different test-batteries, the research findings have been markedly consistent. It appears that developing dementing conditions are not characterized by a general, diffuse decline in performance on all cognitive functions, but rather that certain specific functions are impaired in the earliest stages and others only later as the illness progresses. Whereas, in the initial stages of illness, decline in the different cognitive functions proceeds more or less independently, the impairment becomes gradually more generalized until in the later stages gross deficits are evident in virtually all areas of memory and cognitive functioning (Wilson and Kaszniak 1986).

This relative consistency in the pattern of progress of the illness means that the cognitive functions of most significance in differentiating mild dementia from normal old age are different from those which distinguish most clearly between mild and severe degrees of dementia. Moreover, the specific functions which contribute most to differentiating the different degrees of severity are not necessarily those most useful in predicting the further course and progress of the condition. These conclusions underline the need to cover a broad spectrum of cognitive functioning, both in differentiating between the various stages or degrees of severity of dementia, and also in trying to establish more accurate prognostic guidelines.

The deficits which are of greatest value in identifying mild and early dementia are those involving mnestic, speech and spatial-constructive functions. At this stage secondary and tertiary memory functions are chiefly affected, and there is no definite decline in primary memory performance (Ober *et al*. 1985; Huff *et al*. 1987; Botwinick *et al*. 1986; Wilson and Kaszniak 1986).

The free reproduction of meaningful verbal material, as for example in the 'logical memory' subtest of the Wechsler Memory Scale, is already significantly impaired in the early stages. The initial encoding of information and its storage and recall over a longer period appear to be affected from the onset of a dementing illness onwards (Ober *et al*. 1985; Branconnier and DeVitt 1983).

Verbal ability is affected by difficulties in finding words and in the flow of speech, which impoverish the power of expression in both its semantic and pragmatic aspects (Huff *et al*. 1987; Hart 1988; O'Donnell *et al*. 1988). Syntax and phonetics, on the other hand, remain unaffected, as does also the ability to write and read (Thompson 1987; Erkinjuntti *et al*. 1986). Comprehension of speech is affected early, though not to the same extent as expressive speech (Corkin 1982; Rosen 1983).

A variety of other functional deficits have been reported, as in orientation for time and place, in speed of motor reaction, in calculation and in drawing conclusions, but most frequently in spatial constructive abilities (Rosen 1983; Flicker *et al*. 1985; O'Donnell *et al*. 1988), as demonstrated by means of mosaic tests and the copying of geometrical figures.

Tests of secondary memory appear to be most suitable for the early detection of mild dementia (Larrabee *et al*. 1985; Berg 1988; Knopman and Ryberg 1989). Already in the early stages of the illness and in cases of so-called 'very mild dementia', performance in this area is so impaired that further monitoring of the deterioration over time may not be possible (Rubin *et al*. 1988; Storandt and Hill 1989). Other cognitive disorders are present with varying frequency in the early stages, or make their appearance only with the progress of the disorder. These, like the eliciting of primitive reflexes (Bakchine *et al*. 1989) or the presence of extrapyramidal and psychotic symptoms (Stern *et al*. 1987), can contribute to the estimation of severity and prediction of outcome, for which purposes tests of general knowledge (Storandt *et al*. 1986), recognition of objects (Vitaliano *et al*. 1986), appearance of dysphasia (Berg 1988; Faber-Langendoen *et al*. 1988), dyspraxia (Rapcsak *et al*. 1989) and disorientation (Rosen *et al*. 1986) are also of principal importance. Whether these tests are useful in the differential diagnosis of different dementing illnesses is so far uncertain (Erkinjuntti *et al*. 1986; Tierney *et al*. 1987).

The findings of the studies cited above are encouraging and have already made important contributions to the understanding of cognitive disorders in the setting of dementing processes. How far they can serve to make possible a more general approach to the early detection of dementia in practice is still unclear, since the application of such tests has been mainly confined to small, highly selected samples of the elderly. No data are yet available from the investigation of representative samples, which could provide a basis for the normative assessment of cognitive deficits in the elderly population.

Furthermore, a systematic approach to early detection calls not only for valid techniques of assessment, but also for the resolution of practical problems; in particular, how to gain access to the at-risk population and to monitor the levels of cognitive performance in individuals over a period of time. In this context the primary health-care system can occupy a key role. General medical practitioners are in contact with the great majority of the elderly population, have often known their patients for many years, see them at relatively frequent intervals and are therefore in the most favourable position to observe changes in their mental status and behaviour, and to initiate diagnostic investigation.

The importance of the general practitioner in this respect is all the greater because in most instances cognitive decline in old age does not result in referral to a medical specialist. In the Baltimore ECA Survey, for example, none of the cognitively impaired over-65-year-olds was in contact with psychiatric facilities, whereas many of them had reported their difficulties at consultations with their family doctors (German *et al.* 1985). Earlier studies, in particular that by Williamson *et al.* (1964), according to whose findings the general practitioners are aware of only 15 per cent of dementia cases among their elderly patients, have led to great scepticism concerning the general practitioners' ability to recognize such cases. Recently, however, more encouraging results have been reported, which reveal the ability of general practitioners to recognize dementing disorders in a different light. O'Connor *et al.* (1988), for example, found that general practitioners could identify half of all cases of dementia, and two-thirds of the severe cases, among over-75-year-olds in their practice populations. The assessments were generally more accurate for those patients who had consulted recently.

In a current study in Mannheim, West Germany, the possibility of early detection of dementia in general practice is being systematically explored (Cooper and Bickel 1991). The research aims are to investigate how well the practitioners can recognize dementing disorders, and to establish which cognitive functions permit a differentiation of the clinical severity, which are predictive of a progressive mental decline and which appear compatible with a normal ageing process. The order of appearance of different cognitive deficits in the course of a dementing process will be established by means of a two-year longitudinal study. With these aims in view, the practitioner is requested to make an assessment of the cognitive status of each elderly patient who consults during one month, and a stratified sample of the consulting patients is then examined with the aid of a standardized, semi-structured interview which includes a cognitive screening battery, so that the presence of cognitive impairment and its degree of severity can be reliably assessed and rated independently of the practitioner's judgement of the case. So far preliminary findings are available from the cross-sectional study in the first eleven of a total of twenty participating practices.

MATERIAL AND METHODS

1 Screening for cognitive impairments

The selection of a cognitive screening test was influenced by two main considerations. The procedure should cover a broad spectrum of cognitive functions and it should pay regard to the practical requirements: economy of time, acceptability to the elderly patients and their families and flexibility of administration. Many old people are neither willing nor able to tolerate a prolonged or demanding test procedure. Many are unable, because of motor or sensory impairments, to complete standardized psychometric test-batteries. For those who are dementing, many tests will be too difficult, so that they are constantly confronted by the evidence of their own inability. For those, on the other hand, who are mentally unimpaired, many tasks will prove too simple and may result in irritation and impatience. The interviewer must be able to adapt himself to the situation in the patient's home. Often family relatives are present, the room may be poorly lit, the patient may be confined to bed or a wheel chair or be seated behind a table. Time-limited tests, or others which call for a standardized test situation, will be impracticable under such conditions.

The decision was therefore taken to use the Hierarchic Dementia Scale, developed in Montreal by Cole *et al.* (1983) as a guide to assessment. The development of this procedure was originally based on the work of the Geneva group (Constantinidis *et al.* 1978), itself based on Piaget's theory of mental development, which postulates that the pattern of cognitive decline in dementia is a mirror-image of the order of acquisition of functional abilities in early childhood. Since then a number of other workers have provided support for this model; for example, Reisberg *et al.* (1985), who found a high agreement with their severity scale, and Nolen (1988), who applied standardized procedures for estimating the level of children's development to demented old people in long-term care and found in ten areas of functioning positive correlations between 0.58 and 0.89 with the Mini Mental State Examination.

In order to test the model of a sequential decline in performance, Cole

Table 18.1 Areas of functioning measured by the sub-tests of the augmented Hierarchic Dementia Scale

Perception	Language	Spatial-constructive abilities
Orienting	Comprehension	Construction
Looking	Denomination	Drawing
Gnosis	Reading	
	Writing	
	Similarities	

Attention and memory	*Purposive movements*	*Arithmetic ability*
		Calculation
Concentration	Ideomotor	
Registration	Ideational	
Recent memory		
Remote memory		*Primitive reflexes;*
Orientation		*motor function*
General knowledge		
(CAMDEX)		Prefrontal reflexes
Logical memory		Motor impairment of
(WMS)		CNS origin

et al. (1983) constructed twenty sub-scales, encompassing a wide range of different cognitive functions. In order to provide a more detailed information on memory functions, we augmented these twenty sub-tests of the HDS by two additional tests: the sub-scale 'General knowledge' from the CAMDEX interview (Roth *et al.* 1986) and the sub-test 'Logical memory' from the Wechsler Memory Scale. In all, the cognitive screening battery consists, therefore, of twenty-two short tests, concerned with the psychological functions of perception, memory, calculation, arithmetic, speech, purposive movement and spatial constructive ability. In addition, the presence of primitive reflexes and motor impairments of central nervous origin are also recorded.

The advantage of the HDS sub-tests consists chiefly in the possibility they afford for simple tailored testing. All the sub-scales are composed of five or ten items, giving scores between 0 and 10 points. The interviewer begins with items whose level of difficulty corresponds most closely to the overall level of functioning of each patient and then continues upwards or downwards, with more difficult or easier items, as indicated in the individual case. Whenever two successive test items can be answered correctly, the score value for the more difficult item is given. By means of this rapid form of testing, all twenty-two sub-scale ratings can be completed in from 15 to 30 minutes, without danger of over-taxing the patient, confronting him with too many failures or irritating him by over-simple questions. In addition, the flexibility of the procedure minimizes the proportion of uncompleted test-items, which otherwise can present a serious problem in testing the elderly. The test authors report an internal consistency of 0.97 for the HDS as a whole; the inter-rater agreement on independent retesting is 0.89 and the retest-reliability over a period of two weeks 0.84 (Cole 1988).

2 Research design

The design of the research project is as follows. The participating practitioners complete a form for each over-65-year-old patient who consults, or is visited by them at home, within a four-week period. This form includes, in addition to socio-demographic and diagnostic data, the practitioner's assessment of the cognitive state, based on a simple breakdown into four categories:

(a) cognitively unimpaired;
(b) mild forgetfulness or minimal cognitive deficits, which do not interfere with activities of daily living;
(c) mild dementia, resulting in slight difficulties in activities of daily living;
(d) severe or moderately severe dementia, associated with severe cognitive dysfunction and dependency on others.

In each practice, a stratified sample of twenty patients, five in each of the four categories, is drawn, together with three reserve patients in each category. In this way the whole spectrum of cognitive performance is represented and at the same time the sample is enriched by persons with a greater or lesser degree of cognitive impairment. These patients are then visited at home and examined by a physician or psychologist from the research group. The interview procedure includes, in addition to the HDS, sections dealing with physical illness and disabilities, prescribed medication and affective state, as well as a structured informant interview based on the CAMDEX procedure (Roth et al. 1986), which is to be completed in all cases where any degree of mental impairment is found. Finally, the global severity of dementia or cognitive impairment is rated on the basis of the five-point CAMDEX scale of severity and, whenever indicated, a clinical diagnosis according to the CAMDEX criteria is allocated.

The representativity of the patient collective documented in this study is qualified by the fact that it is restricted to persons consulting or being visited within a four-week period. Whereas studies of general practice in the UK and some other countries are based on registered patient populations and take advantage of the fact that almost the entire general population is registered with general practitioners, this form of sampling is not possible under the German health-care system, in which patient registration in the formal sense does not exist. Each patient with health-insurance cover (the great mass of the population) effectively renews the contract with his doctor for a three-month period when he hands over a treatment voucher covering that quarter. Membership of the health insurance system is obligatory up to a certain income level, so that the costs of medical care are covered also for low income-groups of the population. This form of health insurance applies, in particular, to the overwhelming majority of the elderly population. Only for persons in higher income-brackets is there a possibility of alternative insurance in private schemes. In practice, there is little difference between these alternatives since 'private' health care is also almost always covered by pre-paid insurance schemes, so that the cost of individual episodes of treatment are not borne directly by the patients and the filter to medical care is highly permeable for the population as a whole.

At the end of each quarter, the patient is free to change his doctor if he wishes. In general, however, most patients, and especially the elderly, tend to remain with the same doctor over long periods of time. In an earlier field study in Mannheim (Cooper 1984), more than 90 per cent of old people reported having a family doctor and more than 80 per cent having consulted him or her within the past three months. The representativity of consulting elderly patients for this age range in the population can thus be assumed to be fairly high. Inevitably, however, drawing a time-limited sample will tend to lead to an over-representation of frequent practice attenders, and also of patients living in old people's and geriatric homes, who are usually visited regularly and at short intervals by their doctors, and most of whom will therefore be registered in a four-week recording period.

In the selection of practices, care was taken to obtain a wide distribution over the city of Mannheim as a whole, so that as many as possible of the different urban areas, which vary considerably in their socio-demographic features, should be represented in the survey. Although the collaboration of a representative sample of general practitioners cannot be obtained in a research project of this kind, no evidence has so far been found to indicate that those who do participate are specially interested in psychiatry or psychiatric medicine, or tend to recruit many of their patient clientele from outside the areas in which they practise.

RESEARCH FINDINGS

1 Patient collective and practitioners' assessments

In the first eleven practices, a total of 1,972 over-65-year-old patients, with a mean age of 76.3 years, was documented. Of this collective, 70.3 per cent were women and 29.7 per cent men; 88.1 per cent lived

Table 18.2 Distribution of cognitive status ratings of elderly consulting patients, made by the general practitioners, by age-group of the patients (N = 1,972)

Cognitive status	Age-groups (yrs)						
	65–69	70–74	75–79	80–84	85–89	90+	65+
Normal; no impairment	65.3	49.0	33.2	21.0	7.9	8.1	39.0
Mild memory deficits	30.1	41.5	46.7	44.1	32.7	27.4	39.4
Mild dementia	4.2	9.0	16.1	27.4	42.4	30.6	16.5
Moderate to severe dementia	0.4	0.5	3.9	7.5	17.0	33.9	5.1
Total	100.0	100.0	100.0	100.0	100.0	100.0	100.0
No. of patients	475	390	533	347	165	62	1,972

in private households and 11.9 per cent in old people's or geriatric homes.

The practitioners rated 5.1 per cent of the patients as severely or moderately severely demented. This proportion is of about the expected order, as indicated by the earlier prevalence survey of old people in Mannheim (Cooper 1984). Rather less expected is the fact that only 39.0 per cent were judged to be cognitively quite unimpaired, whereas 39.4 per cent were rated as having minimal cognitive deficits and 16.5 per cent as being mildly demented.

A distribution by five-year age-groups gave the following picture. Below the age of 75, hardly any cases of severe dementia were found, the proportions being only 0.4 and 0.5 per cent respectively. Beyond 75 years, the proportion of demented patients rises from 3.9 per cent in the age-group 75 to 79 up to 34 per cent among those aged over 90, while conversely the proportion of fully unimpaired diminishes from 65 per cent in the youngest age-group to only 8 per cent in the two oldest age-groups. In none of the age-groups were differences in the distribution by severity found between men and women. The particularly interesting category of mild dementia also showed an age-related increase, from 4.2 per cent in the age-group 65 to 69 up to 39.2 per cent among those aged over 85 years.

Table 18.3 Drawing the interview sample

Total sample	N = 296	*Excluded*	
		Died	N = 17
		Mortally ill or in hospital	N = 9
		Moved away or changed doctor	N = 12
			N = 38
Net sample	N = 258	*Excluded*	
		Refusal or non-contact	N = 48
Interviewed	N = 210 (81.4% of net sample)		

2 Composition of the interview sample

The interview sample, stratified according to the practitioners' severity ratings, was drawn by a random number procedure from the total of 1,972 documented patients.

The number of patients selected in this way was 296, but of these 17 were found to have died, 12 to have moved away or changed doctors and 9 were too severely ill to be interviewed. Of the remaining total of 258 eligible patients, 44 refused interview, while in a further four cases the practitioner requested that no approach be made. Interviews were carried out, therefore, with 210 patients, representing 81.4 per cent of those who were eligible.

Because of the stratified sampling procedure, the interview sample differed in certain respects from the patient collective as a whole. The mean age was 78.4 years, the proportion of women 68.6 per cent and that of men 31.4 per cent; 49.5 per cent were widowed, 38.6 per cent married, 8.6 per cent single and 3.3 per cent divorced. The proportion in long-stay residental care was 20.5 per cent, the remaining 79.5 per cent living in private households.

3 Results of interview and cognitive testing

Because the interview sample was assessed in some detail, using a stand-ardized, reliable technique, it could serve as a measure of the accuracy with which the general practitioners rated the cognitive status of their elderly patients.

In Table 18.4 the practitioners' assessments are compared with the global severity ratings recorded on the basis of interview. It appears that the

Table 18.4 Distribution of interviewed patients according to cognitive status: general practitioners' ratings compared with research interview assessments (N = 210)

General practitioners' ratings	Research interview assessment (CAMDEX criteria)			
	Normal	Mild memory deficits only	Mild dementia	Moderate to severe dementia
Normal; no impairment	48	4	1	–
Mild memory deficits only	37	15	4	–
Mild dementia	5	24	16	15
Moderate to severe dementia	–	–	6	35
Total	90	43	27	50

Accuracy of GPs' ratings (normal or mild memory deficits vs mild to severe dementia):

Sensitivity = 93.5%; Positive predictive value = 71.3%

Specificity = 78.2%; Negative predictive value = 96.3%

practitioners and the research interviewers were in full agreement in 54.3 per cent; that the practitioners under-estimated the cognitive impairments in 11.4 per cent and that they over-rated them in 34.3 per cent. Contrary to expectation, therefore, the Mannheim practitioners tended to report cognitive decline and dementia in their elderly patients too frequently, rather than too seldom. In general, however, the level of agreement is remarkably high. Taking mild and severe cases of dementia together, the practitioners identified 72 of 77 cases correctly (93.5 per cent) and, conversely, excluded a dementing condition correctly in 104 out of 133 patients (78.2 per cent).

These research findings indicate that, in epidemiological terms, the general practitioners' ratings provide a method of screening for dementia which is highly sensitive and also has a high negative predictive value. On the other hand, the specificity and positive predictive value of this method of screening is distinctly lower, because of the overall tendency of the doctors to over-estimate the frequency of such impairments.

If the results of comparison between the practitioner ratings and interviewer judgements are extrapolated onto the whole collective of 1,972 consulting patients, we get the distribution shown in Table 18.5. Although the observed case frequency among the patients cannot be taken as representative for the elderly population in general, it does not appear that the consulting patients are at a notably increased risk for a dementing illness.

Table 18.5 Extrapolation of severity ratings onto the whole patient collective, by correction of the GPs' assessments (N = 1,972)

General practitioners' ratings	Expected numbers according to CAMDEX criteria			
	Normal	Mild memory deficits only	Mild dementia	Moderate to severe dementia
Normal; no impairment	697	58	14	–
Mild memory deficits only	514	208	56	–
Mild dementia	27	130	87	81
Moderate to severe dementia	–	–	15	85
Total (100%)	1,238 (62.8%)	396 (20.1%)	172 (8.7%)	166 (8.4%)

A proportion of 8.4 per cent with severe or moderately severe dementia is not above chance expectation, given that the patient collective has a higher mean age than the Mannheim elderly population as a whole (76.3 years vs 74.4 years) and, moreover, that persons in residential care are over-represented (11.9 per cent vs around 5 per cent). The same point is valid for the estimate of 8.7 per cent for persons with mild forms of dementia. Minimal cognitive deficits are present in an estimated 20.1 per cent, while the remaining 62.8 per cent are rated as cognitively unimpaired. Whether these proportions correspond to the distribution in the elderly population as a whole cannot be determined, as the necessary investigations have not yet been undertaken. More important, however, than the precise frequencies is the general conclusion that general practitioners are able to recognize the great majority of dementia cases among their patients, whether these are severe or mild in degree.

How far the early detection of dementia can be improved by measurement of cognitive functions, and for which suspected cases identified on screening a further diagnostic investigation is indicated, must await findings of the planned longitudinal study. That the general practitioner can make a fairly reliable assessment of cognitive status is to some extent confirmed by comparison of his ratings with the profiles obtained using the test battery (cf. Figure 18.1).

The profiles shown in Figure 18.1 are based on the twenty sub-scales of the Hierarchic Dementia Scale, augmented by the two additional scales of general knowledge and logical memory. On all twenty-two sub-scales,

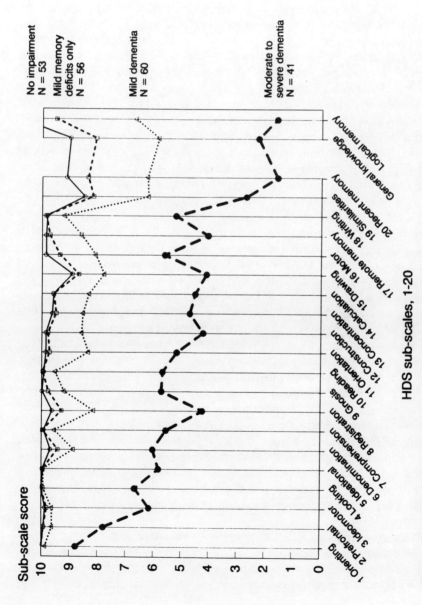

Figure 18.1 Mean test scores on augmented Hierarchic Dementia Scale, according to general practitioners' rating of cognitive impairment

highly significant group differences were found, using the Kruskall–Wallis rank variance analysis (Conover 1971). The performance of patients whom the practitioners assessed as severely or moderately severely demented are clearly reduced on all sub-tests. Lower mean performance levels are also evident for patients classed as mildly demented, whereas the groups classed as cognitively normal and minimally impaired show no significant differences in test performance.

Figure 18.2 shows the sub-test profiles for four different grades of clinical severity, as assessed by the interviewers on the basis of CAMDEX criteria. The severely impaired show a generalized decline in all cognitive functions. Moderately severely demented patients can also be clearly distinguished from the remaining groups. Here, the most pronounced impairments are of short- and long-term memory (8, 17, 20 and logical memory), in orientation (11), in constructive abilities (12), in verbal abstraction (19) and in general knowledge. Whereas in the group of mild dementia cases also it is chiefly the memory functions, constructive abilities, verbal abstraction and general knowledge that are impaired, a comparison with the cognitively normal group also shows highly significant differences with respect to concentration and arithmetic ability. Ideomotor function, understanding of speech, naming of objects, drawing, writing and reading, on the other hand, do not seem to be significantly affected at this stage.

In Figure 18.3 the cumulative distributions of total unweighted HDS scores for the four severity grades 'severe dementia', 'moderate dementia', 'mild dementia' and 'no dementia' have been plotted. With a maximum total score of 200, none of the unimpaired patients scores less than 165 points; 85 per cent achieved 185 or more points. The total scores for the mildly demented also varied within a narrow range of from 130 to 190 points; most members of the group achieved over 160 points.

Cases of mild dementia can be differentiated quite well from unimpaired persons by these test scores, the distributions overlapping with one another to only a small extent. Patients with clinically manifest degrees of dementia, on the other hand, are distributed over almost the whole range of scores. As expected, they can be differentiated quite well from the unimpaired patients, whereas their scores overlap to a considerable extent with those of the mildly demented group. These findings confirm that the transitions from one severity grade to another are flowing and that in representative samples of the elderly population no discontinuities in the distribution of total scores can be expected: in other words, clinical dementia appears to be part of a continuous spectrum of cognitive decline (Brayne and Calloway 1988).

In general, the objective assessment of cognitive performance should make possible a better differentiation of the stages of dementia and closer comparability of research findings from different groups. The aim of neuropsychological testing can, however, be fulfilled only if the observed

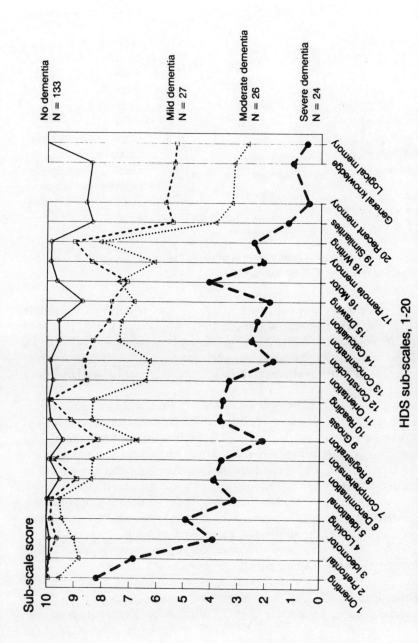

Sub-scale score

No dementia
N = 133

Mild dementia
N = 27

Moderate dementia
N = 26

Severe dementia
N = 24

1 Orienting
2 Prefrontal
3 Ideomotor
4 Looking
5 Ideational
6 Denomination
7 Comprehension
8 Registration
9 Gnosis
10 Reading
11 Orientation
12 Construction
13 Concentration
14 Calculation
15 Drawing
16 Motor
17 Remote memory
18 Writing
19 Similarities
20 Recent memory
General knowledge
Logical memory

HDS sub-scales, 1-20

Figure 18.2 Mean test scores on augmented Hierarchic Dementia Scale, according
to severity of dementia (CAMDEX criteria)

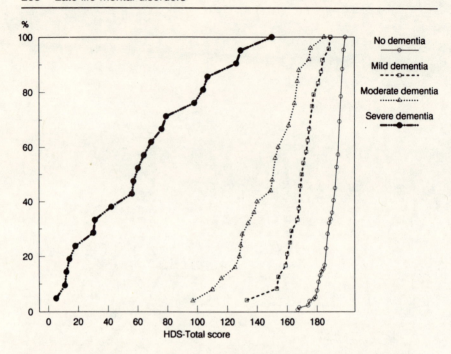

Figure 18.3 Cumulative distribution of Hierarchic Dementia Scale total scores, according to severity of dementia (CAMDEX criteria)

level of performance is actually pathognomonic for dementia and not simply due to the influence of age, sex, social class or educational level (Gurland 1981; O'Connor *et al.* 1989). This issue cannot be satisfactorily resolved by means of cross-sectional studies; one can, however, establish how much of the variance in scores is attributable to severity of dementia and how much is due to such confounding variables.

Table 18.6 sets out the simple correlations of the HDS sub-scale scores with age, sex, social class and educational attainment. Global severity and age correlate significantly with all the test scores without exception. The relatively close association between age and test scores is accounted for by the fact that the cognitively impaired patients are concentrated in the higher age-groups, whereas the majority of those with no impairment are in the younger age-groups. This built-in correlation does not apply to the other variables, whose associations with the test scores are generally weak and in only a few of the sub-tests statistically significant.

In order to separate the influence of clinical severity from these confounding effects, an analysis of co-variance was carried out in which clinical severity, age, sex and social class were included as independent variables. Educational level was not included because it is highly correlated with social class and extremely unevenly distributed. The findings set out

Table 18.6 Correlation of augmented HDS sub-scale scores with severity of dementia and socio-demographic characteristics

Sub-scale	Severity of dementia[1]	Age[2]	Sex[2]	Social class[1]	Education[1]
Orienting	−.44***	−.27***	−.04	.06	.08
Prefrontal	−.48***	−.32***	.01	−.02	.10
Ideomotor	−.50***	−.39***	−.11	.06	.05
Looking	−.47***	−.34***	−.06	−.02	.03
Ideational	−.48***	−.35***	−.10	.08	.09
Denomination	−.52***	−.35***	−.11	.04	.07
Comprehension	−.55***	−.38***	−.09	.11	.10
Registration	−.63***	−.47***	.02	.08	.02
Gnosis	−.62***	−.45***	−.09	.05	.05
Reading	−.54***	−.39***	−.02	.03	.09
Orientation	−.71***	−.46***	−.11	.11	.11
Construction	−.66***	−.45***	−.03	.07	.03
Concentration	−.59***	−.42***	−.07	.01	.11
Calculation	−.66***	−.47***	−.05	.10	.12
Drawing	−.54***	−.50***	−.14	.19**	.21**
Motor	−.57***	−.39***	.06	−.03	.04
Remote memory	−.74***	−.47***	−.04	−.08	.10
Writing	−.61***	−.41***	.00	.06	.07
Similarities	−.54***	−.48***	−.17**	.17**	.18**
Recent memory	−.70***	−.50***	.06	.04	.07
HDS – total	−.76***	−.49***	−.06	.11*	.13*
General knowledge	−.66***	−.58***	−.19**	.16**	.19**
Logical memory	−.63***	−.46***	−.03	.13*	.16**

[1] Rank correlation (Kendall's tau)   * p<0.05
[2] Pearson or biserial correlations   ** p<0.01
                                        *** p<0.001

in Table 18.7 are based on the proportion of the total variance which is explained by these different variables, given that the main effect is significant. Unexplained variance may be due to the unreliability of the test procedure or to other factors; for instance, the irrelevance of the test for dementia-related cognitive decline. It can be seen that the global severity of dementia explained the variance in sub-test scores to an extent ranging from 36.9 per cent (Orienting) to 79.1 per cent (Remote memory). In all, 84 per cent of the total variance could be explained in terms of the severity of dementia. Age, sex and social class exercise a significant influence on the performance of individual sub-tests, but the proportion of total variance they explain is so low as to be negligible. It is therefore safe to assume that the HDS test scores are not influenced to any significant extent by age, sex, or social class and that they can for practical purposes be regarded as specific for decline or impairment in cognitive ability.

Table 18.7 Influence of severity of dementia, age, sex and social class on the augmented HDS sub-scale scores: results of analysis of co-variance

Sub-scale	Mean	(SD)	Severity of dementia	Age	Sex	Social class
			Proportion of variance explained[1]			
Orienting	9.7	(1.0)	36.9	–	–	–
Prefrontal	9.4	(1.5)	39.7	–	–	–
Ideomotor	9.1	(2.2)	62.4	–	1.2	–
Looking	9.4	(2.0)	57.3	–	–	–
Ideational	9.2	(2.5)	67.4	–	–	–
Denomination	8.7	(2.5)	47.0	–	1.4	–
Comprehension	9.0	(2.4)	62.1	–	–	–
Registration	8.0	(2.8)	71.5	–	–	–
Gnosis	8.9	(2.3)	68.5	0.6	–	–
Reading	9.0	(2.5)	59.7	–	–	–
Orientation	8.5	(2.5)	74.9	–	1.7	–
Construction	8.4	(3.1)	68.8	–	–	–
Concentration	8.3	(2.6)	71.9	–	0.6	–
Calculation	8.2	(2.8)	67.7	–	–	–
Drawing	7.7	(2.5)	66.3	–	2.3	–
Motor	8.4	(2.6)	48.8	–	–	–
Remote memory	8.3	(2.9)	79.1	–	–	1.2
Writing	8.8	(2.6)	67.4	–	–	–
Similarities	6.6	(3.9)	42.8	1.5	3.5	3.3
Recent memory	6.6	(3.6)	69.2	–	–	–
HDS Total score	170.9	(42.8)	84.0	–	0.5	–
General knowledge	6.6	(3.4)	65.5	1.4	4.1	4.6
Logical memory	7.6	(4.9)	58.5	–	–	2.4

[1] Percentage given only for those variables where the main effect is significant at the 5% level

DISCUSSION

These preliminary findings from eleven practices give support to the view that general practitioners can play an important part in the identification both of clinically manifest dementia and of milder or earlier forms of cognitive impairment among old people in the community. All those patients who according to the research criteria suffered from severe or moderately severe dementing illness had been correctly classified by the practitioners. Of the milder forms of cognitive disorder, only 18.5 per cent had been missed. Although the proportion of 'false positives' (21.8 per cent) was relatively high, closer examination showed that this inaccuracy was due mainly to an over-rating of the severity of minor cognitive and memory deficits. Only 5.5 per cent of the patients who had no or only minimal impairments were incorrectly classified as cases of 'mild dementia' and none as cases of moderate or severe dementia. This finding is all the more striking, in that the guidelines supplied to the practitioners were for practical reasons shorter and simpler than the severity rating scale which the research group used as criterion in making their assessments at interview. Moreover, in some instances the home interview could be carried out only after a delay of several months, and although in these cases the practitioners were asked to reconsider their initial assessments in the light of further developments, comparison between the two ratings was then unavoidably less direct. Taking into account these potential sources of error and disagreement, one must conclude that the overall standard of case-identification by the general practitioner is now considerably higher than has been assumed on the basis of earlier reports.

This suggests that general practice represents a promising setting for applied research, the principal difficulty now residing, as O'Connor *et al.* (1988) have emphasized, less in an inadequate recognition of old-age mental disorders by the primary-care physician, than in the absence of clear guidelines for diagnostic and therapeutic intervention following on this recognition. A closer co-operation between primary health care and specialist services will be necessary to equip the practising physician with the knowledge and guidelines which will enable him to participate more effectively in coping with what has become one of the commonest and most serious forms of illness found in the elderly population.

It would, however, be premature to conclude simply from the good agreement between the practitioners' assessment and those of the research team, that the early detection of dementia in this setting now has high validity and predictive power, or can be readily incorporated into daily practice. For one thing, the research findings to date are based on a cross-sectional study. Only on the basis of longitudinal data will it be possible to establish what proportion of developing dementias can actually be recognized at an early stage, and how many of the minor cognitive impairments are attributable to benign age-related changes or reversible conditions. Moreover, it is not known how far the standard of case-recognition observed in these practices during one month could be replicated in other practices and maintained over prolonged periods.

The simple, hierarchical classification used by the practitioners in this study does not permit any differentiation of patients according to the clinical prognosis; for example, between reversible disorders, persisting mild cognitive impairments and chronic, progressive dementing conditions. Since peripheral biological markers for dementia are not yet available, one must in practice rely on psychological or neuropsychological tests, which have the important advantage that they can supplement the medical assessment of each patient by a standardized, reliable procedure.

The augmented Hierarchic Dementia Scale, which served this purpose in the present study, consists of twenty-two simple, rapidly administered sub-tests, and was found to be eminently practicable for use with a random sample drawn from an unselected group of elderly consulting patients. Its flexible method of application makes it particularly suitable in a situation in which both cognitively unimpaired and demented patients have to be examined and assessed by a single instrument and with a procedure acceptable to both. Only occasionally was it necessary to omit individual sub-tests; for example, in interviewing old people with severe sensory impairments.

The results of examination using the augmented HDS correspond in great measure to clinical experience, to model stereotypes of the 'stages' of dementia and to the results of more intensive neuropsychological investigation. It is not possible, from cross-sectional data alone, to draw any firm conclusions about the order in which different psychological impairments develop in the course of a dementing illness. One can, however, draw some inferences from the differing profiles of impairment which appear to be characteristic for different grades of clinical and sub-clinical severity, with regard both to the sequence of events and the tempo of change in dementing illness.

From this viewpoint, it seems that severe ideomotor and ideational apraxias, as well as nominal aphasia and impairment of visual perception, are not manifest until a fairly late stage, since they are found only in association with severe dementia. One must, however, remember that these differences between the severity grades may be a function of the relative difficulty of completion of each sub-test, as well as of the specific underlying impairments. With test items making greater demands than those contained in the HDS sub-scales, it might well be possible even in the earliest stages of a dementing process to identify deficits which this procedure does not detect. The present findings, in short, are subject to the limitations unavoidable in reliance on a single test procedure.

Among those abnormalities already detectable in the earlier stages of a developing dementia appear to be disturbances in concentration and orientation, impaired capacity for verbal abstraction, acalculia and constructive apraxia, together with disturbances of secondary and long-term memory. Some of these functions probably deteriorate steadily with the further progression of the disease. Others, however, such as 'logical' memory, verbal abstraction, calculation and concentration, show indications of a stepwise progression, in that the impairments remain for some time at a stable level and then grow more severe in the later stages.

A number of impairments – agnosia, alexia, agraphia and loss of two-dimensional constructive ability – are detectable in the earlier stages but nevertheless do not serve to distinguish between mild and moderately severe degrees of dementia. More definitely associated with the onset of the moderately severe stage are the appearance of primitive reflexes and difficulties in the understanding of speech and language.

To what extent the various cognitive impairments should be regarded as pathognomonic for dementing illness is still unclear. From the analysis of co-variance, it seems highly unlikely that they are due simply to the influence of age, sex or social class on patients' test performance. Only prospective longitudinal research, however, will show which disorders of psychological part-function are of prognostic importance and whether the early detection of developing dementing conditions can be accurate enough to provide prognostic guidance in the individual case.

ACKNOWLEDGEMENT

This study is supported by a grant from the Federal Ministry of Science and Technology. It is conducted under the supervision of Professor B. Cooper (Head of the Department of Epidemiological Psychiatry). I would like to thank Dr M. Arneburg, Dr H. Sandholzer, M. Schäufele and Dr A. Zintl-Wiegand for their help in data collection.

REFERENCES

Anthony, J.C., LeResche, L., Niaz, U., Korff, M.R. von, and Folstein, M.F. (1982) 'Limits of the "Mini-Mental State" as a screening test for dementia and delirium among hospital patients', *Psychological Medicine* 12:397–408.

Bakchine, S., Lacomblez, L., Palisson, E., Laurent, M., and Derouesne, C. (1989) 'Relationship between primitive reflexes, extra-pyramidal signs, reflective apraxia and severity of cognitive impairment in dementia of the Alzheimer type', *Acta Neurologica Scandinavica* 79:38–46.

Berg, L. (1988) 'Mild senile dementia of the Alzheimer type: diagnostic criteria and natural history', *Mount Sinai Journal of Medicine* 55:87–96.

Bergmann, K., Kay, D.W.K., Foster, E.M., McKechnie, A.A., and Roth, M. (1973) 'A follow-up study of randomly selected community residents to assess the effects of chronic brain syndrome and cerebrovascular disease', in R. de la Fuente and M.N. Weisman (eds) *Proceedings of the V World Congress of Psychiatry*, Mexico, 1971, *Excerpta Medica*, Amsterdam, pp. 856–65.

Bickel, H. and Cooper, B. (1989) 'Incidence of dementing illness among persons aged over 65 years in an urban population', in B. Cooper and T. Helgason (eds) *Epidemiology and the Prevention of Mental Disorders*, London: Routledge, pp. 59–76.

Botwinick, J., Storandt, M., and Berg, L. (1986) 'A longitudinal, behavioral study of senile dementia of the Alzheimer type', *Archives of Neurology* 43:1124–7.

Branconnier, R.J. and DeVitt, D.R. (1983) 'Early detection of incipient Alzheimer's disease: some methodological considerations on computerized diagnosis', in B. Reisberg (ed.) *Alzheimer's Disease*, New York: Free Press, pp. 214–27.

Brayne, C. and Calloway, P. (1988) 'Normal ageing, impaired cognitive functioning and senile dementia of the Alzheimer type: a continuum?', *Lancet* i:1265–6.

Clarfield, A.M. (1988) 'The reversible dementias: do they reverse?', *Annals of Internal Medicine* 109:476–86.

Cole, M.G. (1988) 'Measuring levels of disability – an hierarchical approach', in J. Wattis and I. Hindmarch (eds) *Psychological Assessment of the Elderly*, New York: Livingston, pp. 81–91.

Cole, M.G., Dastoor, D.P., and Koszycki, D. (1983) 'The Hierarchic Dementia Scale', *Journal of Clinical and Experimental Gerontology* 5:219–34.

Conover, W.J. (1971) *Practical Nonparametric Statistics*, New York: Wiley.

Constantinidis, J., Richard, J., and de Ajuriaguerra, J. (1978) 'Dementias with senile plaques and neurofibrillary changes', in A.J. Isaacs and F. Post (eds) *Studies in Geriatric Psychiatry*, New York: Wiley, pp. 119–52.

Cooper, B. (1984) 'Home and away: the disposition of mentally ill old people in an urban population', *Social Psychiatry* 19:187–96.

Cooper, B. and Bickel, H. (1989) 'Prävalenz und Inzidenz von Demenzer-krankungen in der Altenbevölkerung. Ergebnisse einer populationsbezogenen Längsschnittstudie in Mannheim', *Nervenarzt* 60:472–82.

Cooper, B. and Bickel, H. (1991) 'Early detection of dementia in the primary care setting', in D. Goldberg and D. Tantam (eds) *The Public Health Impact of Mental Disorder*, Göttingen: Hogrefe & Huber.

Copeland, J.R.M., McWilliam, C., Dewey, M.E., Forshaw, D., Shiwach R., Abed, R.T., Muthu, M.S., and Wood, N. (1986) 'The early recognition of dementia in the elderly: a preliminary communication about a longitudinal study using the GMS-AGECAT package (community version)', *International Journal of Geriatric Psychiatry* 1:63–70.

Corkin, S. (1982) 'Some relationships between global amnesias and the memory impairments in Alzheimer's disease', in S. Corkin (ed.) *Alzheimer's Disease: a Report of Progress*, New York: Raven Press, pp. 149–64.

Erkinjuntti, T., Laaksonen, R., Sulkava, R., Syrjaelaeinen, R., and Palo, J. (1986) 'Neuropsychological differentiation between normal aging, Alzheimer's disease and vascular dementia', *Acta Neurologica Scandinavica* 74:393–403.

Faber-Langendoen, K., Morris, J.C., Knesevich, J.W., LaBarge, E., Miller, J.P., and Berg, L. (1988) 'Aphasia in senile dementia of the Alzheimer type', *Annals of Neurology* 23:365–70.

Flicker, C., Ferris, S.H., Crook, T., Bartus, R.T., and Reisberg, B. (1985) 'Cognitive function in normal aging and early dementia', in J. Traber and W.H. Gispen (eds) *Senile Dementia of the Alzheimer Type*, Heidelberg: Springer, pp. 2–17.

Folstein, M.F., Folstein, S.E., and McHugh, R. (1975) '"Mini-Mental State": a practical method for grading the cognitive state of patients for the clinician', *Journal of Psychiatric Research* 12:189–98.

German, P.S., Shapiro, S., and Skinner, E.A. (1985) 'Mental health of the elderly: use of health and mental health services', *Journal of the American Geriatric Society* 33:246–52.

Gurland, B.J. (1981) 'The borderlands of dementia: the influence of sociocultural characteristics on rates of dementia occurring in the senium', in N.E. Miller and G.D. Cohen (eds) *Clinical Aspects of Alzheimer's Disease and Senile Dementia*, New York: Raven Press, pp. 61–80.

Hart, S. (1988) 'Language and dementia: a review', *Psychological Medicine* 18:99–112.

Huff, F.J., Becker, J.T., Belle, S.H., Nebes, R.D., Holland, A.L., and Boller, F. (1987) 'Cognitive deficits and clinical diagnosis of Alzheimer's disease', *Neurology* 37:1119–24.

Hughes, C.P., Berg, L., Danziger, W.L., Coben, L.A., and Martin, R.L. (1982)

'A new clinical scale for the staging of dementia', *British Journal of Psychiatry* 140:566–72.

Knopman, D.S. and Ryberg, S. (1989) 'A verbal memory test with high predictive accuracy for dementia of the Alzheimer type', *Archives of Neurology* 46:141–5.

Larrabee, G.J., Largen, J.W., and Levin, H.S. (1985) 'Sensitivity of age-decline resistant ("hold") WAIS subtests to Alzheimer's disease', *Journal of Clinical Experimental Neuropsychology* 7:497–504.

Mowry, B.J. and Burvill, P.W. (1988) 'A study of mild dementia in the community using a wide range of diagnostic criteria', *British Journal of Psychiatry* 153:328–34.

Nolen, N.R. (1988) 'Functional skill regression in late-stage dementias', *American Journal of Occupational Therapy* 42:666–9.

Ober, B.A., Koss, E., Friedland, R.P., and Delis, D.C. (1985) 'Processes of verbal memory failure in Alzheimer-type dementia', *Brain and Cognition* 4:90–103.

O'Connor, D.W., Pollitt, P.A., Hyde, J.B., Brook, C.P.B., Reiss, B.B., and Roth, M. (1988) 'Do general practitioners miss dementia in elderly patients?', *British Medical Journal* 297:1107–10.

O'Connor, D.W., Pollitt, P.A., Hyde, J.B., Fellows, J.L., Miller, N.D., and Roth, M. (1990) 'A follow-up study of dementia diagnosed in the community using the Cambridge Mental Disorders of the Elderly Examination', *Acta Psychiatrica Scandinavica* 81:78–82.

O'Connor, D.W., Pollitt, P.A., Treasure, F.P., Brook, C.P.B., and Reiss, B.B. (1989) 'The influence of education, social class and sex on Mini-Mental State scores', *Psychological Medicine* 19:771–6.

O'Donnell, B.F., Drachman, D.A., Lew, R.A., and Swearer, J.M. (1988) 'Measuring dementia: assessment of multiple deficit domains', *Journal of Clinical Psychology* 44:916–23.

Pfeffer, R.I., Kurosaki, T.T., Chance, J.M., Filos, S., and Bates, D. (1984) 'Use of the mental function index in older adults: reliability, validity, and measurement of change over time', *American Journal of Epidemiology* 120:922–35.

Pfeffer, R.I., Kurosaki, T.T., Harrah, C.H., Chance, J.M., Bates, D., Detels, R., Filos, S., and Butzke, C. (1981) 'A survey diagnostic tool for senile dementia', *American Journal of Epidemiology* 114:515–27.

Rapcsak, S.Z., Croswell, S.C., and Rubens, A.B. (1989) 'Apraxia in Alzheimer's disease', *Neurology* 39:664–8.

Reisberg, B., Ferris, S.H., and DeLeon, M.J. (1985) 'Senile dementia of the Alzheimer type: diagnostic and differential diagnostic features with special reference to functional assessment staging', in J. Traber and W.H. Gispen (eds) *Senile Dementia of the Alzheimer Type*, Berlin: Springer, pp. 18–37.

Reisberg, B., Ferris, S.H., DeLeon, M.J., and Crook, T. (1982) 'The Global Deterioration Scale for assessment of primary degenerative dementia', *American Journal of Psychiatry* 139:1136–9.

Rosen, W.G. (1983) 'Clinical and neuropsychological assessment of Alzheimer's disease', in R. Mayeux and W.G. Rosen (eds) *The Dementias*, New York: Raven Press, pp. 51–63.

Rosen, W.G., Mohs, R.C., and Davis, K.L. (1986) 'Longitudinal changes: cognitive, behavioral, and affective patterns in Alzheimer's disease', in L.W. Poon (ed.) *Handbook for Clinical Memory Assessment of Older Adults*, Washington, DC: APA, pp. 294–301.

Roth, M., Tym, E., Mountjoy, Q., Huppert, F.A., Hendrie, H., Verma, S., and Goddard, R. (1986) 'CAMDEX: a standardised instrument for the diagnosis of mental disorder in the elderly with special reference to the early detection of dementia', *British Journal of Psychiatry* 149:698–709.

Rubin, E.H., Drevets, W.C., and Burke, W.J. (1988) 'The nature of psychotic symptoms in senile dementia of the Alzheimer type', *Journal of Geriatric Psychiatry and Neurology* 1:16–20.

Rubin, E.H., Morris, J.C., Grant, E.A., and Vendegna, T. (1989) 'Very mild senile dementia of the Alzheimer type. I. Clinical assessment', *Archives of Neurology* 46:379–82.

Stern, Y., Mayeux, R., Sano, M., Hauser, W.A., and Bush, T. (1987) 'Predictors of disease course in patients with probable Alzheimer's disease', *Neurology* 37:1649–53.

Storandt, M., Botwinick, J., and Danziger, W.L. (1986) 'Longitudinal changes: patients with mild SDAT and matched healthy controls', in L.W. Poon (ed.) *Handbook for Clinical Memory Assessment of Older Adults*, Washington, DC: APA, pp. 277–84.

Storandt, M., Botwinick, J., Danziger, W.L., Berg, L., and Hughes, C.P. (1984) 'Psychometric differentiation of mild senile dementia of the Alzheimer type', *Archives of Neurology* 41:497–9.

Storandt, M. and Hill, R.D. (1989) 'Very mild senile dementia of the Alzheimer type. II. Psychometric test performance', *Archives of Neurology* 46:383–6.

Thompson, I.M. (1987) 'Language in dementia. Part I: a review', *International Journal of Geriatric Psychiatry* 2:145–61.

Tierney, M.C., Snow, W.G., Reid, D.W., Zorzitto, M.L., and Fisher, R.H. (1987) 'Psychometric differentiation of dementia: replication and extension of the findings of Storandt and coworkers', *Archives of Neurology* 44:720– 2.

Vitaliano, P.P., Breen, A.R., Albert, M.S., Russo, J., and Prinz, P.N. (1984) 'Memory, attention, and functional status in community-residing Alzheimer type dementia patients and optimally healthy aged individuals', *Journal of Gerontology* 39:58–64.

Vitaliano, P.P., Russo, J., Breen, A.R., Vitiello, M.V., and Prinz, P.N. (1986) 'Functional decline in the early stages of Alzheimer's disease', *Journal of Psychology and Aging* 1:41–6.

Williamson, J., Stokoe, I.H., Gray, S., Fisher, M., Smith, A., McGhee, A., and Stephenson, E. (1964) 'Old people at home: their unreported needs', *Lancet* 1:1117–20.

Wilson, R.S. and Kaszniak, A.W. (1986) 'Longitudinal changes: progressive idiopathic dementia', in L.W. Poon (ed.) *Handbook for Clinical Memory Assessment of Older Adults*, Washington, DC: APA, pp. 285–93.

Chapter 19

Dementia: case ascertainment and health service utilization in a rural US community

Mary Ganguli, Lewis H. Kuller, Steven Belle, Graham Ratcliff, F. Jacob Huff and Katherine M. Detre

In 1986, the National Institute on Aging funded six Alzheimer's Disease Patient Registries (ADPRs) across the United States (NIA 1986). The overall objectives of the ADPR programme were to establish model registries which would create an ongoing data base for etiological research, and establish a clinical information system to facilitate clinical trials for Alzheimer's disease. One such ADPR was funded at the University of Pittsburgh, in Pittsburgh, Pennsylvania. This chapter reports preliminary results from the Pittsburgh ADPR, with specific reference to the use of health and human services by persons with dementing disorders.

In addition to the stated goals of NIA's ADPR programme, it appeared to us that a population-based registry could serve additional, perhaps more tangible, goals for communities. Knowledge of how many and what types of dementias are prevalent in a given community would help providers and policy-makers plan adequate and appropriate services for these individuals. However, not all affected individuals will spontaneously seek out and use these services. Knowledge of who the affected individuals are, how they may be tracked down and identified, what services they currently use, and whether they have been recognized as demented by their clinicians, will also be of great value in assessing the utilization of services. If patterns of utilization of services by the cognitively impaired and demented can be defined, it may be possible to establish a case-finding strategy based on service use. Further, if the registry is ongoing, the use and effectiveness of services can be monitored along with time trends in prevalence, incidence and duration of the disease.

In the United States, the absence of a national health programme makes it difficult either to establish a case registry or to study the use of health and human services on the basis of general practice lists. Potential subjects must be identified by other means, such as by survey, referral, or advertisement, or through the active, voluntary participation of one or more health care providers. Although persons aged 65 years and older have better health insurance through Medicare than many younger US citizens, coverage of different services is variable. Subjects who agree to participate in a study may or may not have a regular health-care provider (for example, a clinic or private physician). Further, those who do may choose to permit the investigators to gain access to their medical or social service records, but the provider is under no obligation to supply the investigators with useful, or any, information. With health services as well as record-keeping being less than uniform, the data gathered from providers alone are likely to be insufficient for the establishment of case registries. This scenario probably varies across countries, and could lead to comparisons of successful case-ascertainment strategies under different health insurance systems. This chapter describes our experience in one rural American population.

The current structure of the health-insurance system for older Americans may be summarized briefly as follows. All persons with annual personal incomes close to (in Pennsylvania, at or below 120 per cent of) the designated poverty level are covered by Medical Assistance (Medicaid), which reimburses their health-care services and prescribed medication costs. All others aged 65 years and over, if they contributed to (or were dependants of persons who contributed to) Social Security while they were employed, are covered by Medicare. Medicare has two parts, A and B, both of which require the patient to pay an annual 'deductible' amount either out of pocket or through another insurance plan (*Medicare Handbook* 1989). Medicare Part A covers costs of in-patient hospitalization, and also some skilled nursing home care, home health care and hospice care. There are fairly stringent restrictions on the diagnoses for which hospitalization is covered, and on the maximum reimbursable length of hospital stay for these diagnoses. Medicare Part B covers 80 per cent of out-patient (ambulatory) costs, including visits to participating physicians (who have agreed to accept payment at the levels allowed by Medicare) and most laboratory tests. Additional coverage varies across states. Most patients purchase supplementary insurance from private insurance companies, to cover the remaining 20 per cent after the payment of an annual deductible amount ($75 in Pennsylvania). There are additional restrictions on payment for out-patient psychiatric care, but in Pennsylvania visits related to dementia are exempt from any reimbursement 'ceiling' after the deductible amount is paid. Home health care, such as the services of visiting nurses, is covered 100 per cent for certain time-limited, skilled nursing services in the home. Social services are covered in conjunction with hospital and home health-care services. The cost of prescribed medication is not covered, except by Medicaid, unless the person subscribes to a private plan. In Pennsylvania, persons below a certain income level benefit from a programme which uses state lottery proceeds to subsidize medication costs for the elderly. Additionally, psychiatric patients below a certain income level may have their psychotropic drugs paid for by their county's mental health programme. In general, the process of keeping track of these complex and changing regulations, of payments and benefits, and, in particular, of the 'paperwork', is quite difficult and burdensome for the elderly consumer as well as for the providers of health services.

Goldman (1984) estimated that, in the USA, individuals over the age of 65 years make up 11 per cent of the general population but use 18 per cent of the ambulatory care, 22 per cent of the acute hospital admissions, 34 per cent of hospital days and 90 per cent of nursing home beds. The use of health and human services by elderly Americans, and specifically by the cognitively impaired elderly in the community, has been studied in the East Baltimore part of the Epidemiological Catchment Area (ECA) programme (Eaton et al. 1981). Older persons in this population were found to be very unlikely to have received specialty mental health care, and only slightly more likely to have received care for mental problems within the general medical sector. The cognitively impaired elderly received no specialty mental health care, and only a very small proportion of these cases had 'mental health content' in their visits to private medical practitioners (German et al. 1985). Cognitively impaired subjects had a significantly lower probability of receiving any health services than did unimpaired subjects, although the range and types of services used did not differ significantly (Frank et al. 1988).

The University of Pittsburgh's ADPR was set up as a model population-based registry of all cases of dementia in a defined population. For practical reasons, this population was defined as an age-stratified random sample of persons aged 65 and older in a circumscribed geographical area. The registry was based on an epidemiological survey of this population, which then served as the 'gold standard' for case ascertainment. Simultaneously, surveillance of the health and social service records in this area allowed the identification of cases who had been noted as demented by the providers of these services. Data from all sources would then be used to help determine the ideal case-ascertainment strategy for any community, given its demographic structure and its health and human service resources.

The Pittsburgh ADPR is linked to the University of Pittsburgh Alzheimer's Disease Research Center (ADRC). It also participates in the NIA-funded Consortium to Establish a Registry for Alzheimer's Disease (CERAD) (Morris et al. 1989). This is a multicentre project which pools standardized assessment data from several ADRCs; by using its protocol we are able to ensure greater comparability for our own data, as well as provide CERAD with population 'norms' on its neuropsychological battery from our community sample. The project is known locally as the Monongahela Valley Independent Elders Survey (MoVIES), a title chosen to give it a more positive and less threatening image than that of a survey for dementia.

MATERIALS AND METHODS

Study site and population

Registry establishment was based on a survey of the elderly residents of the communities of the mid-Monongahela Valley of south western Pennsylvania, an area approximately 25 miles south of Pittsburgh. This is a rural area, formerly home to the now defunct steel industry. The population is largely blue-collar, of low income and education levels, of mostly European descent, with low rates of in- and out-migration. This population was selected partly because its health and social services are provided within a circumscribed area.

Sampling

As we lacked the resources to conduct our own census, and US Census data were seven years old by the project's starting time, we used a sampling frame primarily based on the voter registration list for the two counties. The electoral roll includes all subjects who have ever voted; we were therefore not too concerned about systematic bias resulting from the low probability that the aged and infirm had voted in recent elections. This list was supplemented by 'senior citizen' lists obtained from the local health centre, in an effort to include elderly persons who may have never voted in the area, but may have been in contact with a health or human services agency.

From the master sampling frame, a 1:13 stratified random sample was drawn within the 65–74 and 75+ age groups. The 75+ group was relatively oversampled because of its known higher risk of dementia. The sampled individuals were then contacted to determine eligibility, and to obtain consent to participate.

Eligibility criteria were as follows. First, age 65 or over, which is the most common definition of 'elderly' in the USA, and the age criterion in most studies of dementia. We recognized that this would preclude the identification of most cases of early onset or 'pre-senile' dementia in the sample, but also that the yield of such cases from the 55–65 age-group in a population survey would not be cost-effective. We also assumed that early onset dementias are a small but highly visible group which is more likely to seek and receive medical attention, and therefore be easier to identify through service providers, than the older cases.

Second, independent community living – that is, not institutionalized in a long-term-care facility at the time the sample was drawn (Goldman 1984). It is well known that dementia is often the cause of such institutionalization,

Table 19.1 MoVIES cognitive screening battery

1 Mini Mental State Exam (MMSE)*
2 Story, immediate and delayed recall
3 Word list, immediate recall*
4 Word list, delayed recall*
5 Word list, delayed recognition*
6 Verbal fluency, letters P and S
7 Verbal fluency, fruits and animals*
8 Boston Naming Test (CERAD version)*
9 Temporal orientation
10 Praxis (circle, diamond, cube, and cross)*
11 Clock drawing
12 Trail-making A
13 Trail-making B

* CERAD neuropsychological battery; CERAD = Consortium to Establish a Registry for Alzheimer's Disease, NIA 1986–present

and that a large proportion of institutionalized elderly are demented. However, they are also a group that has already sought and obtained services, and can be easily identified if need be.

Third, fluency in English, which was an eligibility criterion necessitated by the difficultly of interpreting the results of standard English-language neuropsychological tests in those not fluent in English.

Fourth, at least 6th grade education, a criterion also imposed because of the difficulty of interpreting cognitive test data in subjects with low levels of education. The education requirement was waived in the case of persons currently aged 85 and older (a cohort which had had very limited educational opportunities in its youth) as it would have excluded too many potential subjects.

Case ascertainment

Case ascertainment in the MoVIES project is a multistage survey process, comprised of cognitive screening, initial clinical evaluation and final diagnostic assessment of progressively smaller groups of eligible subjects.

1 Cognitive screening

Cognitive screening is carried out in the subject's home, using a battery of tests described below. Data are also gathered on demographic characteristics, health-services utilization, medication use, functional ability and social supports. Consent is sought to review medical, social-service, home-health and any recent hospital records.

The MoVIES cognitive screening battery was constituted to cover all testable cognitive domains, as we currently understand them, in a concise and portable form usable in the field. It includes the CERAD neuropsychological battery and some additional tests, as shown in Table 19.1. The battery includes the MMSE (Folstein *et al.* 1975) which is a widely used and validated cognitive screening tool, and would therefore allow easy comparability with other studies.

Definition of cognitive impairment

Our main concern was that operational criteria be derived from the study population itself, rather than from 'standard', fixed cut-off scores derived from non-comparable experimental or clinical populations. The criteria for cognitive impairment used in the MoVIES study represent an attempt to synthesize two current sets of diagnostic criteria: (1) the DSM-III (APA 1980) criteria for dementia, which stipulate global cognitive impairment, defined as impairment in several domains, including memory, in the presence of clear consciousness, and (2) the NINCDS–ADRDA Work Group (McKhann *et al.* 1984) criteria for the clinical diagnosis of Alzheimer's disease, which specify impairment in at least two cognitive domains. Impairment is defined as performance at or below the fifth percentile of controls; we extended the definition of 'controls' in this case to include the entire population sample, so as to make it more truly normative. The hypothesis is that most demented members of a population would be found in the lowest fifth percentile of that population on cognitive testing. In pilot testing, we found cut-off scores at the fifth percentile of the sample to identify as impaired fewer subjects than we had anticipated. To ensure adequate sensitivity, we established the following operational criteria for cognitive impairment for the MoVIES study:

(a) total score at or below the 10th percentile of the population on the MMSE (a score of 24/30); and/or
(b) scores at or below the 10th percentile of the population on at least one memory test and one other test; and/or
(c) independent rating of impairment by the project neuropsychiatrist.

2   Initial clinical evaluation

On subjects designated as cognitively impaired by the above criteria, initial clinical evaluation is carried out according to the standardized CERAD protocol. It includes a history, physical and detailed neurological examination. A family member or other responsible care-giver is interviewed whenever

Table 19.2 Demographic composition by cognitive impairment: random sample
(MoVIES N = 1,261)

Variables	Impaired ≤10th percentile (N = 259)	Intact >10th percentile (N = 1,002)
Mean age	76.7 ± 6.2	71.9 ± 5.3
Sex ratio F:M	42:58	58:42
Median education	6–9th grade	High-school graduate
Currently married	141 (54%)	412 (41%)
Living alone	85 (33%)	308 (31%)

possible. Medical, social-service and home-health records, and also the physicians' responses to letters are reviewed for additional information of diagnostic relevance.

A determination is made as to whether the subject meets DSM-III diagnostic criteria for dementia (APA 1980). If so, the dementia is rated for severity on the Clinical Dementia Rating Scale (CDR) (Hughes *et al.* 1982). A score of 0 reflects no dementia; a score of 0.5 reflects possible/doubtful dementia; scores of 1 or greater reflect definite dementia of increasing severity.

3   Final diagnostic evaluation

Subjects with CDR scores of 0.5 or more are requested to undergo the complete diagnostic evaluation ('dementia workup'), preferably at the University of Pittsburgh Alzheimer's Disease Research Center. Differential diagnostic data are not part of the current presentation.

RESULTS

Because the study is still in progress at the time of writing, the data presented here are of a preliminary nature.

Sample composition

The main demographic characteristics of the random sample as it currently stands (N = 1,261) are as follows: the mean age is 73 years, and the median educational level is high-school graduate. The female-to-male ratio is 54:46; 58 per cent are currently married and 31 per cent live alone.

Table 19.3 Health-service utilization by cognitive impairment
(MoVIES N = 1,261)

Variables	Impaired ≤ 10th percentile (N = 259)		Intact > 10th percentile (N = 1,002)	
	N	%	N	%
≥1 'usual' source of health care	249	96	941	94
≥2 sources of health care	114	44	413	41
Mental health services	7	2.7	24	2.4
Social services	17	6.6	16	1.6
Home health care	25	9.6	38	3.8
Hospitalized in the past 6 months	43	16.6	93	9.3

Cognitive impairment

Applying the 'tenth percentile' criteria for cognitive impairment, 259 subjects (20.5 per cent) have thus far been classified as cognitively impaired. Table 19.2 shows the demographic characteristics of the impaired and unimpaired (intact) groups.

It should be noted that, looked at cross-sectionally, cognitive impairment is measured only by scores on neuropsychological tests. It is therefore important to be sensitive to characteristics other than dementia which are associated with the standard of performance on such tests. Age, sex, and educational level are known to be such characteristics (for example, Holzer *et al.* 1984; Kittner *et al.* 1986) and, in our data, appear to be associated with 'cognitive impairment', as will be seen subsequently (Table 19.4).

Use of health and human services

Table 19.3 shows the patterns of health-service utilization in the two groups. The categories are not mutually exclusive, in that subjects could have used more than one service; but there is no overlap among them, in that the same service is not classified under more than one heading. The first item, 'at least one usual source of health care', represents the subjects' responses to the question 'What is your usual source of health care?' (To

Table 19.4 Health and social-services utilization and cognitive impairment
          (MoVIES N = 1,261)

Independent variables		Odds ratio	95% confidence interval
Age	(1) 70–74 vs < 70	2.6	(1.6, 4.1)
	(2) ≥ 70 vs < 70	5.8	(3.7, 9.0)
Educational level	< HS vs ≥ HS	3.0	(2.2, 4.0)
Sex	Male vs female	2.2	(1.6, 2.9)
Social services contact		2.9	(1.3, 6.1)
Hospitalized in past 6 months		1.7	(1.1, 2.7)

Stepwise logistic regression
Dependent variable: Cognitive impairment by 10th percentile criterion

some extent, the responses are subjective, in that they reflect the subjects'
interpretations of what is 'usual'. There are further questions about the
frequency of visits and date of most recent visit, which are not presented
here.) The choices are: 'no doctor'; 'private doctor', clinic or out-patient
department of hospital' (either of which could be a general practitioner
or specialist); 'emergency room', and 'other professional' (which could
include, for example, chiropractors and holistic health practitioners, but
rarely did; it excludes nurses, social workers and so on). It is possible,
for example, for a cardiologist also to function as a subject's primary
physician if his or her health problems are largely cardiovascular. In this
table, responses to this question were dichotomized as 'no doctor' and all
other responses.

The second item in Table 19.3 refers to subjects having two or more
'usual' sources of health care, and is based on responses to the question,
'Do you see any other doctors, specialists or therapists?' Responses are
limited to practitioners seen in the last five years, classified as 'yes' or 'no',
and more detailed information is then obtained. The practitioners named
in response to this question are also likely to be physicians, more likely to
be specialists; very rarely, for example, physiotherapists. Psychiatrists are
classified separately in this table under 'mental health services', along
with psychologists, counsellors and so on.

'Social services' in this table include not only the services provided by
social workers and caseworkers but also programmes such as 'Meals on
wheels' and 'Adult day care'. 'Home health care' refers to visiting nurses,
health aides, physiotherapists and others who provide care for home-bound
subjects under a physician's orders. 'Hospitalized in the past six months'
refers to in-patient stays of any duration in acute-care facilities (that is,
not day hospitals, nursing homes or hospices, which were inquired about
separately and were not used by this cohort at baseline).

Table 19.5 Demographics: intact, impaired and demented groups
(MoVIES N = 601)

Variables	Cognitively intact (N = 493)	Cognitively impaired (N = 108)		
		Not demented (N = 53)	Possibly demented (N = 32)	Definitely demented (N = 23)
Mean age	71.3 ± 5	74 ± 7	76 ± 6	78 ± 4
F:M	58:42	34:66	31:69	65:35
Median education	High-school graduate	9–11	6–8	6–8
Married (%)	63	57	47	48
Living alone (%)	28	28	38	35

Table 19.4 shows the results of a preliminary attempt to examine the association of cognitive impairment, as defined earlier, with health and human service utilization. A stepwise logistic regression analysis was performed with cognitive impairment as the dependent variable, and the health-service variables (listed in Table 19.3) as independent variables. This procedure yields adjusted odds ratios (ORs) which are estimates of the relative risk of cognitive impairment associated with each independent variable, after adjusting for the effects of all the other independent variables in the model. Age, sex and educational level were included as independent variables; it should be noted that greater age, male sex and lower level of education were all associated with the presence of 'cognitive impairment' or, at least, with poor cognitive test performance. In this mode, the ORs associated with each of these variables suggest that, after controlling for age, sex, and education, only the use of social services (OR = 2.9) and of hospitalization in the past six months (OR = 1.7) were associated with the presence of cognitive impairment.

Dementia

Out of the first 601 subjects in the random sample, 108 were declared 'cognitively impaired' and have undergone the clinical investigation. Twenty-three of them have been diagnosed as 'definitely demented', with a CDR score of 1 or more; a further thirty-two have been diagnosed as 'possibly demented' and given a CDR score of 0.5. The demographic characteristics and health-service use patterns of these groups, compared with those of the cognitively intact (unimpaired) and 'impaired but not demented' groups, are shown in Tables 19.5 and 19.6.

Table 19.7 shows the results of two stepwise logistic regression analyses,

Table 19.6 Health-service utilization: intact, impaired and demented groups (MoVIES N = 601)

Variables	Cognitively intact (N = 493)		Cognitively impaired (N = 108)		
			Not demented (N = 53)	Possibly demented (N = 32)	Definitely demented (N = 23)
≥1 usual source of health care	459	(93%)	49 (93%)	32 (100%)	23 (100%)
≥2 usual sources of health care	209	(42%)	22 (42%)	17 (53%)	9 (39%)
Mental health services	15	(3%)	2 (4%)	0 (0%)	3 (13%)
Social services	4	(0.8%)	1 (2%)	3 (9%)	3 (13%)
Home health care	18	(4%)	2 (4%)	3 (9%)	5 (22%)
Hospitalized in the past 6 months	52	(11%)	4 (8%)	6 (19%)	5 (22%)

similar to that described above. With 'possible or definite dementia' as the dependent variable, the use of social services carried an OR of 9.3, and hospitalization in the last 6 months an OR of 2.3. With only 'definite dementia' as the dependent variable, however, the use of home health-care and mental health services carried ORs of 4.3 and 8.6, respectively. These data in particular should be interpreted with caution because several cognitively impaired subjects have yet to undergo clinical evaluation to determine the presence or absence of dementia.

DISCUSSION

Most subjects in this study thus far appear to have a regular source of primary health care in the form of a private practitioner, and this variable does not distinguish the cognitively impaired and demented from the unimpaired. Although the frequency of the use of home health, social and mental health services is not high, their use is strongly associated with the presence of impairment and/or dementia; furthermore, the records maintained by these care providers appear thus far to be more standardized and consistent than physicians' office records and hospital records, with regard to documenting the presence of cognitive impairment and dementia. The selective use of health and human services by cognitively impaired and demented members of the community may therefore be a useful but largely untapped resource for case ascertainment.

Table 19.7 Health-service utilization and dementia (MoVIES N = 601)

1. POSSIBLE OR DEFINITE DEMENTIA

Independent variables		Odds ratio	95% confidence interval
Age	(1) 70 – 74 vs < 70	3.1	(1.2, 8.32)
	(2) ≥ 70 vs < 70	7.4	(3.0, 18.4)
Education	< HS vs≥ HS	3.3	(1.75, 6.27)
Social services		9.3	(2.2, 39.7)
Hospitalization in the past 6 months		2.3	(1.06, 4.87)

Stepwise logistic regression
Dependent variable: '*Possible or definite dementia*' (CDR ≥ 0.5)

2. DEFINITE DEMENTIA

Independent variables		Odds ratio	95% confidence interval
Age	(1) 70 – 74 vs < 70	6.1	(0.7, 52.1)
	(2) ≥ 70 vs < 70	18.4	(2.3, 146.8)
Education	<HS vs ≥ HS	2.2	(0.8, 5.9)
Home health care		4.3	(1.3, 14.1)
Mental health services		8.6	(2.1, 35.9)

Stepwise logistic regression
Dependent variable: '*Definite dementia*' (CDR ≥ 1)

REFERENCES

American Psychiatric Association (1980) *Diagnostic and Statistical Manual of Mental Disorders*, third edn (DSM-III), Washington, DC: APA.

Eaton, W.W., Regier, D.A, Locke, B.Z., and Taube, C.A. (1981) 'The Epidemiologic Catchment Area Program of the National Institute of Health', *Public Health Reports* 96:319–25.

Folstein, M.F., Folstein, D.E., and McHugh, P.R. (1975) 'Mini-Mental State: a practical method for grading the cognitive state of patients by the clinician', *Journal of Psychiatric Research* 12:189–98.

Frank, R.G., German, P.S., Burns, B.J., Johnson, W., and Miller, N. (1988) 'Use of services by cognitively impaired elderly persons residing in the community', *Hospital and Community Psychiatry* 38:555–7.

German, P.S., Shapiro, S., and Skinner, E.A. (1985) 'Mental health of the elderly: use of health and mental health services', *Journal of the American Geriatric Society* 33:246–52.

Goldman, R. (1984) 'Biosocial aspects of ageing: impact of mental and physical disabilities of the aged on society', in D.W.K. Kay and G.D. Burrows (eds) *Handbook of Studies on Psychiatry and Old Age*, Amsterdam: Elsevier.

Holzer, C.E., Tischler, G.L., Leaf, P. J., and Myers, J.K. (1984) 'An epidemiological assessment of cognitive impairment in a community population', *Research in Community Mental Health* 4:3–32.

Hughes, C.P., Berg, L., Danziger, W.L., Coben, L.A., and Martin, R.L. (1982) 'A new clinical scale for the staging of dementia', *British Journal of Psychiatry* 140:556–72.

Kittner, S.J., White, L.R., Farmer, M.E., Wolz, M., Kaplan, E., Moes, E., Brody, J.A., and Feinleib, M. (1986) 'Methodological issues in screening for dementia: the problem of education adjustment', *Journal of Chronic Disease* 39:163–70.

McKhann, G., Drachman, O., Folstein, M., Katzman, R., Price, D., and Stadlan, E.M. (1984) 'Clinical diagnosis of Alzheimer's disease: report of the NINCDS–ADRDA Work Group', *Neurology* 34:939–44.

Medicare Handbook (1989) Publication No. HCFA 10050, US Department of Health and Human Services, Baltimore, MD.

Morris, J.C., Heyman, A., Mohs, R.C., Hughes, J.P., van Belle, G., Fillenbaum, G., Mellits, E.D., and Clark, C. (1989) 'The Consortium to Establish a Registry for Alzheimer's Disease (CERAD). Part I. Clinical and neuropsychological assessment of Alzheimer's disease', *Neurology* 39:1159–65.

National Institute on Aging (1986) Request for co-operative agreement applications: RFA. Alzheimer Disease Patient Registry (ADPR): authorized by US Congress PL 99–158: 'Health Research Extension Act of 1985'.

Part V

Problems of method: case-finding, classification and taxonomy

Chapter 20

Identification of psychiatric cases in primary health-care settings
The utility of two-phase screening designs

Patrick E. Shrout

Screening in medicine generally refers to the application of a systematic procedure for identifying persons who are at high risk of having an otherwise unrecognized disorder. While the usual examples of screening procedures are often technologically complex, such as mammography examinations for breast cancer, or enzyme-linked immunosorbent assays (ELISA) for HIV infection, even simple medical history questions can be considered to be screens. When an individual is positive on a screen, the clinician goes on to collect additional information that will establish or rule out specific diagnoses, and starts appropriate therapeutic treatment for those who appear to have a disorder. Individuals who are negative on a screen tend not to have additional follow-up. In general, the most satisfactory screening procedures are ones that can feasibly be administered to large numbers of persons, produce relatively few false negatives, and have few enough false positives so as not to be a burden on the medical facilities or on the patients themselves.

Williams (1986) reviewed screening in the context of mental illness and primary care. In his review, he followed Sackett and Holland (1975) in distinguishing three applications of screening techniques. One is the identification of persons from the general population who might benefit from a specific treatment. A second application is the diagnosis of a person who has consulted a primary-care provider for some apparent medical problem. A third is the estimation of the proportion of a population that is affected by a specific disorder. In his review, Williams concluded that psychiatry needs better assessment and treatment methods before the use of screening procedures can be widely recommended in general populations. He expressed optimism, however, that psychiatric screening measures might be useful for case-finding in primary-care settings. He called for continued development of sophisticated screening measures for psychiatry, and for outcome studies of treatments initiated on persons identified through screening and case-finding procedures.

An exceedingly important issue in primary-care research and clinical practice is how much the knowledge and methods developed in psychiatric clinical research generalize to primary-care populations. Although it is obvious that the prevalence of psychiatric disorders will be much lower in primary-care populations than in psychiatric hospitals and clinics, it is much less obvious that assessment and diagnosis in primary-care populations will be more difficult, that the course of the disorder may be different, and that the responsiveness to treatment may vary considerably from what one would expect of a psychiatric patient. Some of these differences are the result of statistical mechanisms, while others are attributable to the fact that psychiatric patients have undergone a selection process to get to mental health institutions.

The statistical problems that emerge when one moves from psychiatric to primary-care populations almost all arise from the fact that the prevalence of many specific disorders is low or very low. When actual cases are rare, the effect of a few false positive classifications can be startling. Measures that were reliable in the psychiatric settings may no longer be reliable in the new population (see Shrout, Spitzer and Fleiss 1987), cases identified for research may contain a large proportion of persons without the actual disorder of interest, and resources allocated for treating persons with the disorder may be spent more on persons falsely diagnosed as positive than on persons who actually have the disorder. These implications have been discussed more in detail by Shrout and Fleiss (1981). The essential point is that diagnostic methods that work well in settings with moderate to high base rates of disorder may not work well when imported to settings with low rates of psychiatric disorder.

A mathematical analysis of the effect of base rate on the reliability and the predictive power of a psychiatric measurement procedure can be done if one makes assumptions about the sensitivity (the proportion of true cases diagnosed correctly) and specificity (the proportion of true non-cases diagnosed correctly) of the procedure. This analysis, however, will be misleading if one simply assumes that the sensitivity and specificity obtained in psychiatric clinical populations generalize to primary-care or community populations. Although sensitivity and specificity values do not depend mathematically on base rates, they are very much affected by the types of true cases and non-cases used in validity studies. Compared to the persons with mental disorder detected in primary-care settings, cases recruited in psychiatric settings are likely to have more severe symptoms, to be more impaired by their symptoms, and to have more co-morbidity. Moreover, as a result of their interactions with mental health professionals, they are also likely to be more sophisticated in describing their psychopathology, and to have accepted their roles as psychiatric patients. These differences will tend to make the sensitivity of diagnostic procedures higher in psychiatric settings than in other settings, since true cases will provide ample evidence of their disorder. However, the specificity of the diagnostic procedures is often lower in psychiatric populations. True non-cases of one disorder may have another psychiatric disorder that can be confused in the diagnostic process. Very few of the non-cases found in a psychiatric setting will actually be healthy, happy individuals. This latter type of person, of course, is easiest to diagnose correctly as a non-case, and is typically found in moderate to large numbers in the general population or in a population of persons receiving general medical care.

In the light of the statistical effects of base-rate changes, and because results on diagnostic validity cannot be extended from psychiatric to primary-care settings, Williams's (1986) call for more research on screening, case-identification and treatment in primary care is especially apt. Even before screening programmes for case-management can be contemplated, one needs to have good empirical data on the prevalence of disorders in different primary-care populations, and also on the utility of screening measures and diagnostic procedures in these populations.

In an effort to facilitate research both on psychiatric morbidity in primary-care populations and on methodology for identifying undetected psychiatric cases in such populations, I examine in this chapter statistical issues arising from the design and analysis of two-phase assessment procedures. All three of Sackett and Holland's (1975) applications of a screen and follow-up assessment are examples of two-phase designs, but I will focus on case-finding for research and epidemiological surveys. The first phase assessment (traditionally referred to as 'the screen') is assumed to classify persons into two groups, one containing those who probably have the disorder under study $(S+)$ and one containing those unlikely to have it $(S-)$ according to the screen. The second phase assessment is assumed to be a diagnostic procedure which yields an operationally defined diagnostic criterion. In this chapter I assume that the diagnostic distinction of interest is binary; either the respondent is a case $(D+)$ or he is not a case $(D-)$. This diagnostic criterion will invariably be costly relative to the screen.

For both the estimation of rates of disorders and the identification of confirmed cases for clinical research, the investigator must determine (1) what screening rule should be used, (2) who among the $S+$ and $S-$ patients are to be followed with a second-phase assessment, and (3) whether a two-phase design is in fact an improvement over a simple one-phase procedure. I consider first the design of an epidemiologic survey for estimating the prevalence of a disorder, and then a case-identification exercise.

ASSESSMENT OF THE PREVALENCE OF A DISORDER IN A PRIMARY-CARE POPULATION

Although primary-care practitioners may have a rough idea of the proportion of their patient population who are experiencing a psychiatric disorder, these informal estimates may be quite biased (see, for example, Cohen and

Table 20.1 Schematic layout of expected results from a two-phase survey

First-phase assessment	Second-phase assessment			
	Case	Non-case	Not evaluated	Total
Screen positive $(S+)$	$\lambda_1 f_1 \pi N$	$(1-\lambda_1)f_1 \pi N$	$(1-f_1)\pi N$	πN
Screen negative $(S-)$	$\lambda_2 f_2 (1-\pi)N$	$(1-\lambda_2)f_2(1-\pi)N$	$(1-f_2)(1-\pi)N$	$(1-\pi)N$
				N

where λ_1 is the rate of the disorder among screen positives,
λ_2 is the rate of the disorder among screen negatives,
π is the proportion expected to be positive on screening,
f_1 is the proportion of $S+$ assessed in the second phase, and
f_2 is the proportion of $S-$ assessed in the second phase

The prevalence estimate is $p = \lambda_1\pi + \lambda_2(1-\pi)$

Cohen 1984). If the disorder is indeed rare in a population, the systematic examination of a large series of patients by a mental health professional will be costly and perhaps inefficient. As has been described by several statisticians (Cochran 1977; Deming 1977; Neyman 1938; Tenenbein 1970), an alternative design for estimating the prevalence of a disorder is the two-phase design, in which an inexpensive screen is administered to a large sample of persons, and the more expensive diagnosis is made on a smaller sample of persons from the screened positive $(S+)$ and screened negative $(S-)$ groups.

Unlike the usual medical screening or case-identification procedures that require that only persons from the $S+$ group be given further assessment, the prevalence-estimation procedure requires that samples of both $S+$ and $S-$ be diagnosed. Let f_1 be the fraction of the screened positives who are followed in the second phase and f_2 be the fraction of the screened negatives who are followed in the second phase. These fractions must be determined in advance, and the sample of each group to be followed must be drawn randomly. I shall review the choices of f_1 and f_2 that produce the smallest standard error for the estimate of p for a given budget.

The sample of persons positive on the screen who are included in the second phase allows the prevalence of the disorder in the $S+$ group to be estimated. I will call this prevalence λ_1. Similarly, λ_2 is the prevalence in the $S-$ group. Let π be the proportion of the total first phase sample who are in the $S+$ group. Using this notation, a 2-by-3 table with the expected results of the two-phase design is laid out schematically in Table 20.1. The prevalence (p) in the total population is a weighted average of λ_1 and λ_2: $p = \lambda_1\pi + \lambda_2(1-\pi)$.

The values of f_1 and f_2 ideally are chosen so that the estimate of the prevalence is as precise as possible, given the resources available to the investigator. The relative costs of the screening and follow-up assessments will influence the choice of values for f_1 and f_2. Let us first consider the case in which resources are needed both to pay someone to administer and score the screen, and to pay expert diagnosticians for the second-stage assessment. Later, I will comment on how our results apply to the case in which the administration of the screen is to be done by existing staff at minimal or no expense to the researcher. When both the screen and the follow-up diagnosis involve expense, the size of the sample screened will affect the resources available for follow-up, and vice versa. The larger the values of f_1 and f_2, the larger the sample included in the second phase, and the smaller the size of the sample that can be screened. As shown in Cochran (1977) and Shrout and Newman (1989), the squared standard error of $\hat{p}$ (the estimate of p) is a function of f_1 and f_2 and other parameters:

$$V(\hat{p}) = \frac{1}{N} \left[\frac{\pi\lambda_1(1 - \lambda_1)}{f_1} + \frac{(1 - \pi)\lambda_2(1 - \lambda_2)}{f_2} + \pi(1 - \pi)(\lambda_1 - \lambda_2)^2 \right]. \quad (1)$$

The values of f_1 and f_2 that minimize this expression are,

$$f_1^* = \sqrt{\frac{\lambda_1(1 - \lambda_1)}{(\lambda_1 - \lambda_2)^2\pi(1 - \pi)} \frac{c_S}{c_D}}$$

and $\qquad\qquad\qquad\qquad\qquad\qquad\qquad\qquad\qquad\qquad\qquad\qquad$ (2)

$$f_2^* = \sqrt{\frac{\lambda_2(1 - \lambda_2)}{(\lambda_1 - \lambda_2)^2\pi(1 - \pi)} \frac{c_S}{c_D}},$$

where C_S and C_D are respectively the costs of administering the screen and of administering the diagnostic procedure. The values of f_1^* and f_2^* are assumed to be between 0 and 1, but Shrout and Newman (1989) have pointed out that when p is small the obtained values may go beyond that range, especially for f_1^*. When f_1^* is larger than 1, they recommend setting f_1 to 1.0 exactly, and using the following to find f_2:

$$f_2^{**} = \sqrt{\frac{\lambda_2(1 - \lambda_2)(\pi + c_S/c_D)}{\pi\lambda_1(1 - \lambda_1) + \pi(1 - \pi)(\lambda_1 - \lambda_2)^2}}. \quad (3)$$

If f_2^{**} is also greater than 1.0, one can conclude that a two-phase design is not efficient.

When the investigators know approximately the values of the sensitivity (S_e) and specificity (S_p), but not of λ_1 or λ_2, they can use Bayes' formula (see Fleiss 1981:2–6) to calculate

$$\lambda_1 = pS_e/[pS_e + (1 - p)(1 - S_p)]$$

and

$$\lambda_2 = p(1 - S_e)/[(1 - p)S_p + p(1 - S_e)].$$

Because these formulae depend on p, the value to be estimated in the two-phase design, one should try a range of plausible values to determine the stability of the planned values for f_1 and f_2.

We previously raised the possibility that in some settings there may be virtually no cost involved in administering and coding the screen, and that all resources can be allocated to the second phase assessment. In such a case, the equations in (2) do not apply, since their derivation assumes that $C_S/C_D > 0$. The question still remains, however, as to what proportion of those followed in the second phase should come from the screened positive and the screened negative groups. Fortunately, equation (3) gives the answer. The ratio of $S+$ to $S-$ patients included in the follow-up should be $1:f_2$**. The variance of the prevalence estimate will be,

$$V(\hat{p}) = \left[\frac{\pi\lambda_1(1 - \lambda_1)}{n_1} + \frac{(1 - \pi)\lambda_2(1 - \lambda_2)}{n_2} + \frac{\pi(1 - \pi)(\lambda_1 - \lambda_2)^2}{N} \right]$$

where n_1 and n_2 are the numbers assessed in the second phase from the $S+$ and $S-$ groups. The total number of patients administered the screen, N, should be large enough to make the third term negligible.

Let us return to the situation in which there is some cost associated with the administration of the screen, and consider a numerical example to illustrate the use of the equations described above. Suppose that in a given primary-care population about 5 per cent of patients have a depressive disorder and a two-phase survey is planned to establish that fact. Suppose also that there exists a screening scale with moderate validity that can be administered economically, but at some real expense. We might consider two cutpoints on the scale, one that classifies about 18 per cent of the patients into $S+$ with a sensitivity of .75 and a specificity of .85, and a lower cutpoint that classifies about 28 per cent into $S+$ with a sensitivity of .85 and a specificity of .75. From equation 4 we can determine that only about 21 per cent of the $S+$ group defined with the higher cutpoint will truly have a depressive disorder; this figure is often called the positive predictive value of the screen (Fleiss 1981). Using the lower cutpoint, the positive predictive value will be about 15 per cent. From equation 5 we estimate that the rates of depression in the $S-$ patients are 1.5 per cent and 1.0 per cent respectively for the higher and lower cutpoints. If one subtracts λ_2 from

Table 20.2 Planning a two-phase prevalence estimation procedure:
a hypothetical numerical example

	High cutpoint	Low cutpoint
Assume		
Prevalence *(p)*	.05	.05
Sensitivity *(S_e)*	.75	.85
Specificity *(S_p)*	.85	.75
Cost Ratio *(C_S/C_D)*	.10	.10
Resources *(B)*	200	200
Calculate		
Proportion screened positive	.18	.28
($\pi = p\,S_e + (1-p)\,S_p$)		
Rate in *S+* (λ_1: equation 4)	.2083	.1518
Rate in *S−* (λ_2: equation 5)	.0152	.0101
Design parameters		
f_1^* (equation 2)	1.73	1.79
f_2^* (equation 2)	.52	.51
f_1^{**} (equation 3)	1.00	1.00
f_2^{**} (equation 3)	.35	.31
Number screened (equation 6)	355	331
Standard error (equation 1)	.0141	.0139
Cost ratio for which one- and two-phase designs are equally efficient (equation 7)	.21	.24

unity, one obtains the negative predictive value; that is, the proportion of those screened negative who are truly without the disorder.

To push the example further, let us suppose that the second phase assessment involves the administration of a semi-structured diagnostic interview by a psychiatrist, and that this costs about ten times what it costs to administer and score the screen (that is, $C_S/C_D = .10$). Given this cost ratio and the estimated λ_1, λ_2 and π values, we can calculate the proportions of the $S+$ and $S-$ groups that should be included in the second-phase assessment. Let us consider first the screening rule defined by the higher cutpoint. When we apply the formula for f_1^* from equations 2, we obtain a value for f_1 which exceeds 1.00, the logical maximum for a proportion. Following Shrout and Newman (1989), we set f_1 to 1.0 (that is, we plan to include all of the screened positive patients in the second-phase assessment) and apply equation 3 to get .35, the proportion of the $S-$ group to be followed. These calculations are summarized in Table 20.2 for both the high and low cutpoints on the hypothetical screen. For the low cutpoint, the two-phase design that minimizes the standard error of the prevalence estimate is one that calls for including all of the $S+$ group and 31 per cent of the $S-$ group.

Note that the screening rules defined by the two cutpoints may produce different numbers of persons in the first and second phases, assuming that the financial resources are fixed. To characterize the amount of resources in a scale-free form, let $B = Resources/C_D$, the number of diagnoses that could be afforded if no screening assessments were made. If f_1 and f_2 are constants, the number of persons to be screened is given by

The actual number of persons given the diagnostic assessment is equal to, $N_d = N_s[\pi f_1 + (1-\pi)f_2]$. When resources are to be allocated between two phases of case-finding using the higher cutpoint, 164 diagnostic assessments and 355 first-phase screening assessments would be budgeted for. With the lower cutpoint, 167 persons would be given diagnostic assessment, and the number to be screened initially could be reduced to 331. When the cost ratio is as small as .10, slight changes in the number of persons given diagnostic assessments can have a moderate to large impact on project costs, and hence possibly on the resources available for screening.

Perhaps the most important question that can be addressed by these calculations is which of the two cutpoints produces the smaller standard error for the prevalence estimate. In our example, the expected standard error (the square root of the result from equation 1) is .0139 for the lower cutpoint, and .0141 for the higher cutpoint. While these values are very close, it appears that the improvement in sensitivity associated with the lower cutpoint is somewhat more important than the loss in specificity resulting from screening more persons into the $S+$ group.

Another design comparison of great interest is that between a simple one-phase design and an optimal two-phase design. The one-phase design would involve the assessment of a fixed sample of patients with the best diagnostic method available. Continuing with our numerical example, the standard error of a prevalence estimate based on a sample of size 200 when the true prevalence is .05 would be $\sqrt{p(1-p)/N} = \sqrt{(.05)(.95)/200} = .0154$. Because this is larger than either of the standard errors considered from the two-phase design, we conclude that in this instance the two-phase design is more efficient.

The relative efficiency of the two-phase design compared to a simple diagnostic survey depends heavily on the cost ratio of the screen to the diagnostic assessment. In general, the lower this ratio, the more efficient a two-phase design will be. A question addressed by Shrout and Newman (1989) is how close the cost of the screen can be to the cost of diagnosis before the two-phase survey is no longer efficient. Assuming that f_1 is set to 1.0 and that f_2 is determined using equation 3, they determined that the cost ratio, $C_S/C_D = C$, for which the two designs produce exactly the same standard error, is given by,

$$C = \frac{[\sqrt{p(1 - p)} - (1 - \pi) \sqrt{\lambda_2(1 - \lambda_2)}]^2}{\pi[\lambda_1(1 - \lambda_1) + (1 - \pi)(\lambda_1 - \lambda_2)^2]} - \pi. \tag{7}$$

This can be solved as a function of Se and Sp using equations 4 and 5. When the anticipated ratio of the cost of screening to diagnostic assessment is less than C, the two-phase design will be more efficient than the simple one-stage survey design. For example, for the higher cutpoint in Table 20.2 the two-phase procedure would be more efficient if the cost of the screen was less than 21 per cent of the cost of diagnosis. For the lower cutpoint, the cost ratio could approach 24 per cent before the one-phase design became more efficient.

Shrout and Newman (1989) and Shrout (1990) have provided evaluations of equation 7 in tabular form for various choices of p, Se and Sp. Figure 20.1 shows these same results graphically for $p = .05$. One can see from this figure that, except for very high levels of sensitivity, the two-phase design will only surpass the one-phase design in efficiency if the cost of screening is one-third or less than that of the diagnostic assessment. It is also apparent that changes in sensitivity have a somewhat larger effect on C than changes in specificity, as was observed in the numerical example given above.

When reviewing the circumstances in which a two-phase design is more efficient than a one-phase diagnostic survey, it is important to remember that we have assumed that all patients in $S+$ would be given a diagnostic assessment, and that f_2 has been chosen to minimize the standard error of the estimate. If f_2 is set arbitrarily, rather than using equation 3, the efficiency of the two-stage procedure can suffer considerably. For example, suppose that an investigator who planned to use the lower cutpoint in the example shown in Table 20.2 insisted on setting f_2 to 10 per cent rather than the optimal 31 per cent. Such a decision may be based on intuitive unease from the realization that of the 167 persons to be given the diagnostic assessment, nearly 45 per cent will be from the $S-$ group according to the optimal design, and that few of these $S-$ assessments will yield cases of disorder. The standard error of the prevalence estimate from the modified design would be expected to be 0.0161, which is not only larger than the value of .0139 expected from the optimal two-phase design, but also larger than that of .0154 expected in the simple one-stage survey. The potential efficiency of the two-phase design is lost by submitting too few persons in $S-$ to a diagnostic assessment.

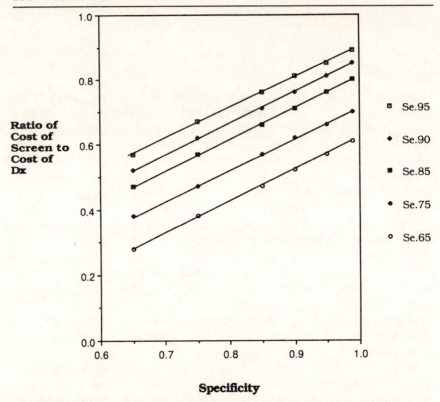

Ratio of
Cost of
Screen to
Cost of
Dx

□ Se.95

♦ Se.90

■ Se.85

♦ Se.75

○ Se.65

Specificity

Figure 20.1 Cost ratio of screen to diagnosis for which one- and two-phase designs are equally efficient for prevalence estimation when prevalence is .05

FINDING CONFIRMED CASES OF A DISORDER IN A PRIMARY-CARE POPULATION

If the purpose of the screening procedure is to identify a sample of patients from a primary-care population who have a specific disorder, then the optimal two-phase prevalence design will indeed be unappealing. Assuming that the screen is related to the diagnostic outcome, the probability of finding a true case in the $S-$ group is a fraction of that in the $S+$ group, and hence the most efficient strategy of finding cases will be to fix $f_1 = 1.0$ and $f_2 = 0$.

If all those screened as positive are given the diagnostic assessment, while none of the screened as negative are assessed in the second phase, the expected number of confirmed cases out of N_s persons screened is $\pi\lambda_1 N_s$. From equation 6, we know that $N_s = B/(\pi + C)$, where as before, B represents the resources in terms of the number of diagnostic interviews that could be conducted if no screen were used, and C is the cost ratio of the first-phase assessment to the second-stage assessment. Thus, for a two-phase study with fixed resources B, the expected number of cases that can be identified is $\pi \lambda_1 B/(\pi + C)$. In contrast, the number of confirmed cases that are expected from a single-phase case-identification procedure in which B persons are given only the diagnostic assessment is pB. As in the previous section, we can determine what the value of C will be when the two-phase design is equal in efficiency to the one-phase design. This will occur when

$$C = (1\text{-}p)\ (S_e + S_p - 1)$$

Returning to our numerical example in Table 20.2, we can apply equation 8 to see that a two-phase design will be more efficient than a one-phase design in identifying cases if the cost of the screening procedure is less than 57 per cent the cost of the diagnostic procedure. Note that this value is more than twice the value of C needed to make the two-phase design more efficient than the one-phase survey for prevalence estimation. Note also that the two screening rules illustrated in Table 20.2 produce the same value of C when equation 8 is evaluated, since the sum of S_e and S_p is the same for the two rules. This means that neither sensitivity nor specificity is more important as the efficiency of the two-phase procedure approaches that of the one-phase design. When the cost ratio is very low, as in the Table 20.2 example, the two screening rules do differ somewhat. The expected number of cases to be identified by the rule with the higher cutpoint is twenty-six, whereas for the lower cutpoint it is twenty-two. A one-stage survey could expect to identify ten cases.

Shrout (1990) has tabulated values of C from equation 8 as a function of sensitivity, specificity and prevalence. Figure 20.2 shows a graphic representation of those results for the prevalence of .05. When the ratio of the costs of a screen to a diagnostic assessment is less than the values of C shown in the figure, the two-phase design will be more efficient than the one-phase design. A comparison of Figures 20.1 and 20.2 reveals that, like the numerical example, two-phase designs are likely to be more efficient for case-identification than for prevalence estimation. Even if the cost of the screening procedures approaches the cost of diagnosis, the two-phase design may still be preferable to a one-stage design for case identification.

An important fact that should be kept in mind when considering a two-phase design for case-identification is that the cases obtained are not a simple random sample of the population. Identified cases will tend to be persons who are willing to admit symptoms, or who otherwise make themselves conspicuous during the screening process. Although the sampling bias may not be serious for treatment studies, such bias could be especially detrimental to risk-factor research.

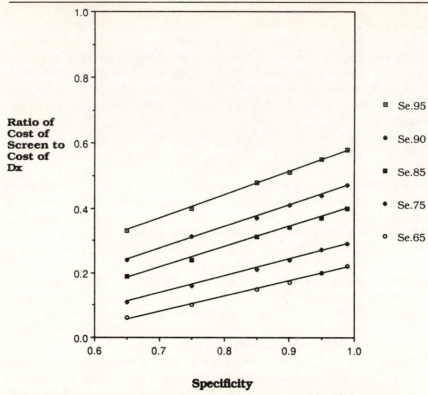

Figure 20.2 Cost ratio of screen to diagnosis for which one- and two-phase designs are equally efficient for case-identification when prevalence is .05

CONCLUSION

Two-phase designs may be useful for research in primary-care settings, even if the time is not yet ripe for prescriptive screening programmes to identify persons in primary care who might be treated for mental disorders. The effectiveness of psychiatric screening programmes in primary-care settings will turn in part on the availability of efficient assessment procedures for patients in these populations, the existence of evidence that interventions are effective among patients who have not themselves sought treatment for mental disorders, and the ability of mental health service planners to determine the prevalence rates of target disorders. Only systematic research in primary-care settings will provide these tools and this information.

Two-phase designs are not necessarily preferable to simple one-phase surveys. Not only are they more complicated logistically, but they may also be less efficient in producing estimates of prevalence or in identifying confirmed cases of disorder. The efficiency of the procedure is dependent both on the quality of the screening measure, and on the relative cost of the screen to the diagnostic procedure.

In this chapter I have attempted to provide rules for determining whether two-phase designs are likely to be worth their considerable effort. An example was given to illustrate how these rules might be applied in practice to compare different screening rules. Numerical evaluations of other two-phase designs can be calculated fairly easily using 'spreadsheet' programs that are available for personal computers. The assumptions about a screen's sensitivity, specificity and the expected prevalence can be entered as constants and the formulae corresponding to the equations in this chapter can be entered in a series of cells. When the constants are changed, most programs automatically recalculate the relevant results. Those considering adopting a two-phase design are encouraged to work out their own numerical examples that mimic their application in order to see how sensitive the design is to the assumptions made.

In formulating the rules for this chapter, I assumed that the two-phase procedures were designed to be optimal for a given purpose. An important fact that emerged is that a design that is optimal for one purpose may be far from optimal for another purpose. This fact has also been discussed by Hand (1987). If a non-optimal design is adopted, the investigator may compromise the efficiency and utility of a two-phase procedure.

The two-phase designs discussed in this chapter were kept relatively simple. I assumed that the screen yielded a binary result, that the screening rule was well defined (in terms of cutpoints or algorithms), and that a single binary outcome could be specified. Other authors have addressed some of the problems that were avoided by my assumptions. Duncan-Jones and Henderson (1978) have described and evaluated screening rules that make use of more than two screening categories. Murphy *et al.* (1987) have described how signal-detection methods can be used to choose among many possible screening rules. A problem not addressed in this chapter or in the literature is the design of a two-phase screen for multiple outcomes. If two or more different disorders are of interest, it is possible that a given screening rule and two-phase design will be efficient for studying one disorder but inefficient for the others. Solutions to this problem will require information not only about the sensitivity and specificity of the different disorders, but also about rates of co-morbidity and the degree to which failures of specificity for one disorder are actually true positives for another disorder.

REFERENCES

Cochran, W. G. (1977) *Sampling Techniques*, third edn, New York: Wiley.

Cohen, P. and Cohen, J. (1984) 'The clinician's illusion', *Archives of General Psychiatry* 41:1178–82.

Deming, W. E. (1977) 'An essay on screening, or on two-phase sampling, applied to surveys of a community', *International Statistical Review* 45:29–37.

Duncan-Jones, P. and Henderson, S. (1978) 'The use of a two-stage design in a prevalence study', *Social Psychiatry* 13:231–7.

Fleiss, J. L. (1981) *Statistical Methods for Rates and Proportions*, second edn, New York: Wiley.

Hand, D. J. (1987) 'Screening vs prevalence estimation', *Applied Statistics* 36:1–7.

Murphy, J. M., Berwick, D. M., Weinstein, M. C., Borus, J. F., Budman, S.H., and Klerman, G. L. (1987) 'Performance of screening and diagnostic tests: application of receiver operating characteristics analysis', *Archives of General Psychiatry* 44:550–5.

Neyman, J. (1938) 'Contributions to the theory of sampling human populations', *Journal of the American Statistical Association* 33:101–16.

Sackett, D. L. and Holland, W. W. (1975) 'Controversy in the detection of disease', *Lancet* ii:357–9.

Shrout, P. E. (1990) 'Statistical design of screening procedures', in C. Attkisson and J. Zich (eds) *Screening for Depression in Primary Care*, New York: Routledge, Chapman and Hall, pp. 84–97.

Shrout, P. E. and Fleiss, J. L. (1981) 'Reliability and case detection', in J. Wing, P. Bebbington and L.N. Robins (eds) *What is a Case? the Problem of Definition in Psychiatric Community Surveys*, London: Grant McIntyre, pp. 117–28.

Shrout, P. E. and Newman, S. (1989) 'Design of two-phase prevalence surveys of rare disorders', *Biometrics* 45:549–55.

Shrout, P. E., Spitzer, R. L., and Fleiss, J. L. (1987) 'Quantification of agreement in psychiatric diagnosis revisited', *Archives of General Psychiatry* 44:172–7.

Tenenbein, A. (1970) 'A double sampling scheme for estimating from binomial data with misclassification', *Journal of the American Statistical Association* 65:1350–61.

Williams, P. (1986) 'Mental illness and primary care: screening', in M. Shepherd, G. Wilkinson, and P. Williams (eds) *Mental Illness in Primary Care Settings*, London: Tavistock.

Chapter 21

The latent structure of anxiety and depression in treated and untreated samples of two US populations

William W. Eaton and Howard D. Chilcoat

The terms 'anxiety' and 'depression' encompass a very broad range of symptoms which tend to co-vary together. One major nosologic question has been the relationship of the symptoms of anxiety to the symptoms of depression (for example, Mendels *et al.* 1972; Prusoff and Klerman 1974). In its most simplistic form this question resolves into the question as to whether there exist one or two syndromes: the 'lumper' versus 'splitter' debate. Prior to the 1980 publication of the American Psychiatric Association's Diagnostic and Statistical Manual (DSM-III), many disorders relevant to these two general rubrics were included in the category of neurosis. The DSM-III split them into the two groups, anxiety disorders and affective disorders. The wisdom of this decision is still being debated (Tyrer 1985; Stavrakaki and Vargo 1986).

It is evident that primary-care physicians play a critical role in the detection and treatment of mental disorders, particularly in light of the evidence that more individuals treated for mental disorders receive care exclusively from primary care than from psychiatric services (Regier *et al.* 1978; Eastwood 1975; Goldberg 1979). Other studies have shown that the standard of identification of psychiatric disturbances by primary-care providers has generally been poor (Hankin and Oktay 1979). In one study, about half the individuals meeting criteria for a psychiatric diagnosis (according to the DIS/DSM-III system) were identified as having an emotional problem by the primary-care practitioner (von Korff *et al.* 1987). A question arises as to whether this failure in identification is a result of the insensitivity of primary-care providers to patients' mental health disturbances; or whether those individuals who receive care in the primary-care sector have a milder and less noticeable form of symptomatology.

The symptoms of anxiety and depression are frequent enough to appear often in primary-care settings. Anxiety and depression are also often mild enough for a primary-care physician to consider treating them without specialist referral. It is unclear whether the nosologic structure of DSM-III, which has evolved out of the clinical practice of psychiatry, is applicable to primary care, where many individuals with anxiety and depression are treated.

Data from the Epidemiologic Catchment Area (ECA) Programme have been analysed with new numerical taxonomic techniques (Bartholomew 1987; McCutcheon 1987) in order to shed light on this issue. These data have three advantages, unique in combination, for such an analysis. First, the data include reported symptoms which can be organized so as to duplicate exactly the structure of DSM-III disorders. This characteristic is not unusual in samples which originate in clinical populations, but it is unusual in samples which originate from the general population. Second, it is derived from a general population sample – that is, the sample is not selected from persons in either psychiatric or general medical treatment. Third, the sample sizes are large, so that enough cases are generated to be statistically informative.

The results of analyses of co-variation in symptoms of anxiety and depression in the ECA samples have been described elsewhere (Eaton and Bohrnstedt 1989). The structure which was revealed conformed neither to the DSM-III symptom structure, nor to the kind of simple structure which would be expected if a single disorder were causing the co-variation. Thus, the general applicability of the DSM-III classification, which arose out of clinical psychiatric experience, was not confirmed when it was tested empirically on a sample drawn from the general population.

The analyses in this chapter integrate earlier taxonomic work on anxiety and depression with the theme of primary care. The question of interest is: does the co-variation in symptoms of anxiety and depression form patterns in the primary-care sector which are similar to those found in psychiatric patients; and are these patterns similar to those found in the population of individuals who receive no health care?

To address this question we:

1 estimate the use of primary-care and psychiatric specialist services in the ECA sites selected for analysis;
2 examine the latent structure of anxiety and depression when the latent structure for all sectors of care is constrained to be equal; and
3 develop a latent class model which efficiently explains the observed associations among symptoms, and differences in these associations across health-care sectors.

METHODS

The Epidemiologic Catchment Area (ECA) Programme is a series of epidemiologic surveys conducted by university-based researchers in five community mental health centre catchment-area populations (Eaton *et al.* 1981). At each site interviews were conducted with probability samples of approximately 3,000 individuals living in private households and approximately 500 individuals living in institutions. The research design is described in Eaton *et al.* (1981) and Eaton and Kessler (1985).

The section of the interview on psychopathology common to all the ECA sites was drawn from the NIMH Diagnostic Interview Schedule (DIS). This is a highly structured interview designed to resemble a typical psychiatric interview and to yield similar results in terms of specific mental-disorder diagnoses. A study of inter-rater agreement conducted with a sample of patients in a clinical setting produced moderately good concordance for diagnoses (Robins *et al.* 1981).

Symptoms elicited by answers to questions in the DIS can be organized into the following four diagnostic categories related to anxiety and depression: Panic Disorder (Questions 61–2); Phobic Disorder, including the subtypes of Agoraphobia, Social Phobia and Simple Phobia (Questions 68a–n); Major Depressive Disorder (Questions 72–9); and Dysthymia (Questions 73–9). Several other questions in the DIS are relevant to these general areas of psychopathology but are not necessarily related to specific disorders: four questions on potential somatic aspects of anxiety (Questions 44–7), two questions on mood, not explicitly related to Depression by the DIS/DSM-III algorithm (Questions 57–8), and a question on general nervousness (Question 61). Positive answers to these questions are followed by probes to determine whether they meet pre-determined criteria of severity and to ensure that they are not caused by influences unrelated to psychopathology, such as physical illness or injury, medication, drugs or alcohol. A self-reported behaviour or complaint which fulfils these criteria is considered to be a probable psychiatric symptom. A final question determines when the symptom was most recently experienced, according to the method of von Korff and Anthony (1982). Here we analyse symptoms which pass the severity threshold, which are not explained by medication, drugs, alcohol, physical illness or injury, and which occurred during the month prior to the interview.

The data for these analyses are derived from two sites of the ECA Programme: Baltimore, Maryland (Johns Hopkins) and Piedmont, North Carolina (Duke). These sites were chosen because they have important methodological and socio-cultural similarities. Both used the recency probes on the first wave of data collection, which were crucial for the taxonomic analysis. In both Baltimore and Piedmont the samples consisted of roughly one-third black and two-thirds white respondents. The first wave of interviewing yielded 3,481 completed interviews in Baltimore, a response rate of 78 per cent, and 3,921 interviews in Piedmont, a response rate of 77 per cent. Even though initial analyses of data on non-response (von Korff *et al.* 1985; Cottler *et al.* 1987) do not reveal strong biases among socio-demographic or psychopathologic variables according to non-response status, differences in sample composition and response rate led to our decision to omit data from Los Angeles, the only other ECA site to use the recency probes.

Latent class analysis attempts to identify an unobserved latent variable which explains the association among a set of observed variables. Latent class analysis has been described as a categorical data analogue to factor analysis. Factor analysis assumes that the observed variables are normally distributed, whereas latent class analysis makes no assumptions regarding distributional form, other than the constraint that the observed variables are categorical in nature. A successful latent variable reduces the association among the observed variables to insignificance within each level, or class, of the latent variable. The deviation of the expected proportions, generated by the latent class model, from the observed proportions can be evaluated through the use of a chi-square statistic.

Two sets of parameters are generated from the latent class analysis. The first set is the prevalence of the sample in each of the latent classes. In these analyses, we are interested in the proportion of the sample in each latent class for each sector of medical care. Another set of parameters is the conditional probabilities – the proportion of individuals with or without a specific symptom, given that they are in a specific latent class. The conditional probabilities for a specific symptom must sum to one over each latent class.

Latent class analysis can be used to test hypotheses in addition to the generation of parameters. This can be done by comparing the fit of a series of hierarchical models, in which restrictions on the models are relaxed or increased. A likelihood ratio test can be performed by referencing the difference in the chi-square statistic of both models to a chi-square distribution with the degrees of freedom equal to the difference in the degrees of freedom between the hierarchical models. Through this procedure, a model can be developed which most efficiently explains the observed associations.

RESULTS

Consistent with earlier results from the ECA Programme (Shapiro *et al.* 1984), nearly 60 per cent of the population, in both Baltimore and Durham, reported having received some form of health treatment in the six months prior to the interview, as Table 21.1 shows. Only about 3 per cent had received care from a psychiatrist, psychologist, social worker, mental health clinic, drug or alcohol clinic, or some other form of professional treatment for psychological problems. About 55 per cent had received care from a general practitioner or other primary-care source, while the remainder of the population had not used health-care services at all during the six months prior to interview. These categories are hierarchical and mutually exclusive, so that an individual using primary-care health services *and* visiting a psychiatrist would be classified in the psychiatric sector only.

Table 21.1 Use of primary health care and psychiatric specialist services: Baltimore and Durham ECA sites

	Utilization of medical services in the six months preceding interview		
Care sector utilized	Baltimore (%)	Durham (%)	Total
No health services used	40.3	41.9	3,045
Primary care only	56.2	55.3	4,122
Psychiatric sector	3.5	2.8	232
Total	100.0	100.0	7,399
	(3,481)	(3,918)	
Missing data	0	3	

Three-sector equality model

Three latent classes are sufficient to explain the co-variation in symptoms of anxiety and depression in the total population (Table 21.2). The conditional probabilities in Table 21.2 arise from a model which requires the latent structure to be identical in each sector of treatment. Although this condition is a very strong constraint on the data, the fit is fairly good, with a chi-square of 575.2 on 736 degrees of freedom. These probabilities are virtually identical to those obtained in earlier analyses which did not divide the sample into three sectors of treatment (Eaton *et al.* 1989). The adequacy of fit of this three-sector equality model further supports the general robustness of the latent structure underlying co-variation between symptoms of anxiety and depression.

Class I in Table 21.2 consists of individuals who are relatively free of symptoms (about 77 per cent of the population). Class II consists of individuals who report being nervous, having phobias and problems with sleep and weight or appetite, but show relatively little dysphoria. We have tentatively dubbed this class 'distressed', and it has an estimated prevalence of almost 20 per cent. Class III includes individuals who report symptoms suggesting major depressive disorder, as well as phobias, and who perceive themselves as nervous persons. It is noteworthy that the occurrence of panic attacks is more closely related to this third class (conditional probability of 0.22), which has a heavy loading of symptoms of depression, than to the second class (conditional probability of 0.04), where dysphoria, psychomotor retardation and suicidal ideation are also absent. We have tentatively dubbed this class 'Major Depression with Anxiety', and it has a prevalence of about 3 per cent.

The proportions of individuals in the three classes differs strongly by sector of care, as Table 21.3 shows, even though the latent structure is identical to that presented in Table 21.2.

Table 21.2 Latent class model with all sectors constrained to be equal

| Symptom group | Conditional probability of a positive response for members of class: | | |
	Class I	Class II	Class III
Dysphoria	0.00	0.08	0.79
Somatic depression	0.06	0.50	0.97
Psychomotor retardation	0.00	0.13	0.56
Suicidal ideas	0.00	0.02	0.40
Somatic anxiety	0.00	0.07	0.18
Phobias	0.13	0.38	0.66
Panic attacks	0.00	0.04	0.22
Nervous person	0.14	0.53	0.81
Estimated prevalence	77.0%	19.7%	3.3%

Among persons receiving no medical treatment, Class I (those with few or no symptoms) predominates (85 per cent). Of the untreated group 12 per cent have the symptom constellation which puts them into Class II, and less than 2 per cent are in Class III. Nearly one-quarter of those treated in the primary-care sector fall into the 'distressed' category, but less than 4 per cent of those in the primary medical-care settings are in Class III. It is only in the psychiatric sector that Class III forms a significant proportion (17 per cent). Nearly half of those persons in contact with psychiatric services in the previous six months were in the 'distressed' category.

Two-sector equality model

These results are informative and intriguing, but one must be cautious interpreting the test of fit. The assumptions necessary for the chi-square statistic are violated in this analysis because so many of the 768 cells in the cross-tabulation for the latent class analysis had expected frequencies less than five. In effect, even though the sample was very large, the estimate of degrees of freedom is inflated because of the sparsity of the data, and the chi-square test loses power to reject the model. We therefore adopted a series of strategies to improve the fit of the model as efficiently as possible, as shown in Table 21.4.

In latent class analysis, the chi-square statistics are additive if the models are hierarchical, and likelihood ratio tests are thereby obtained by comparing models. In general, unless specifically noted, we compare each of the models in Table 21.4 to the three-sector equality model, so that the resulting tests demonstrate whether there has been a statistically significant improvement in fit. These comparative tests do not suffer from the effect of sparsity of data noted above.

Table 21.3 Distributions of three latent classes according to utilization of
Medicare care: three-sector equality model

	No medical treatment in last 6 months (%)	Primary medical care only (%)	Psychiatric specialist care (%)
Class I	85.8	73.0	33.0
Class II	12.3	23.4	49.7
Class III	1.9	3.6	17.3
	100.0	100.0	100.0

One strategy to improve the fit of the three-sector equality model is to
relax the constraint that the three sectors have identical latent structures.
The 'two-sector equality' model requires that the latent structure be identical in the two treatment sectors (psychiatric and primary care); in effect,
releasing the sample of persons who have not used any form of health-care
service to have a different taxonomic structure. This strategy produces an
improvement in fit (likelihood chi square of 50 on 20 degrees of freedom),
but it is not as impressive as the improvement produced by requiring the
untreated sector to be identical to the primary-care sector (labelled 'unrestricted psychiatric'); in effect, releasing the psychiatric sector (likelihood
chi square of 78 on 19 degrees of freedom). A further improvement in fit
is obtained if we do not constrain the taxonomic structure at all, but leave
all sectors unrestricted.

Symptom-based model improvement

A further strategy for improving the fit of the three-sector equality model
is to relax the constraint of equality on certain carefully chosen symptoms.
By examining differences in conditional probabilities in model 4 (all sectors
unrestricted), we can generate hypotheses about which symptoms will
produce the greatest improvement in fit. The conditional probabilities in
model 4 are presented in Table 21.5. For example, in the unconstrained
model, the conditional probability for dysphoria in Class III was 1.00 in
the psychiatric sector, and nearly as high (0.92) in the primary-care sector;
but only 0.69 among the group with no medical treatment. The conditional
probability for this symptom was allowed to vary across sectors, producing
6 degrees of freedom but only a small improvement in fit (chi square of 8.2).
Similarly, the conditional probabilities for panic varied considerably across
sectors (Table 21.5), so it was released, again with little effect (model 6).

The only symptom which produced a strong improvement in fit by itself,
was the perception of oneself as a nervous person. Table 21.5 shows that, in
the unconstrained model, this probability varied considerably across sectors

Table 21.4 Statistics for selected latent class models

Model	Overall chi square	Degrees of freedom	Likelihood ratio test	Degrees of freedom	P
Sector-based models					
1 Three-sector equality	575.2	736	–	–	–
2 Two-sector equality	524.8	716	50.4	20	<.001
3 Unrestricted psychiatric	496.9	717	78.3	19	<.001
4 All sectors unrestricted	452.1	696	44.8*	21	<.005
Symptom-based models					
5 Unrestricted dysphoria	567.0	730	8.2	6	<.2
6 Unrestricted panic	566.5	731	8.7	5	<.2
7 Unrestricted nervousness	520.3	730	54.9	6	<.001
Sector by symptom models, Psychiatric sector					
8 Nervousness	532.5	733	42.7	3	<.001
9 Panic (II–III)	569.9	734	5.3	2	<.1
10 8 + 9	526.4	731	48.8	5	<.001
11 Psychomotor retardation	525.3	730	49.9	6	<.001
Other sectors					
12 10 + Dysphoria, unrestricted	518.1	725	57.1	11	<.001
13 12 + 11	515.4	724	59.8	12	<.001
14 3 + Dysphoria (III)	496.5	716	78.7	20	<.001
15 14 + Panic (III)	494.8	715	80.4	21	<.001
16 Selected symptoms, unrestricted	515.7	727	59.5	9	<.001

* Comparison is to model 3

in Classes II and III. The improvement in fit is notable, with a chi square of 54.9 on only 6 degrees of freedom.

Close examination of Table 21.5 reveals certain symptoms that have unusually low or high conditional probabilities in one particular sector of care. The most efficient strategy for improving fit may be to release a set of single coefficients. Generally, these 'outlier' probabilities are found in the psychiatric sector. In Table 21.5 an asterisk is placed by every probability that differs from its corresponding value in other sectors by more than .20, or by a factor of four. There are nine asterisks in the table, and seven of the nine are in the psychiatric sector. In some situations we hypothesized it might be efficient to release probabilities in only one or two latent classes; the chi-square value in Table 21.4 for model 9 shows that this strategy is ineffective for panic attacks, which is released in Classes II and III in the psychiatric sector only, with only a marginal improvement in fit.

The bottom section of Table 21.4 shows models that are increasingly less general, being based more on the data as revealed in Table 21.5. None of these models is markedly successful in explaining the observed distributions. Many other models were attempted but it was difficult to improve the fit beyond model 3. In model 16 ('selected symptoms unrestricted'), for example, all nine probabilities with an asterisk in Table 21.5 were unconstrained, losing 9 degrees of freedom and a chi square of 59.60; a significant improvement in fit. This model is not hierarchical with model 3, so that a precise statistical comparison is not available, but model 3 fits better overall and is much more concise in description and understanding.

DISCUSSION

The similarity in taxonomic structures across sectors of care is more impressive than the differences. A single latent class structure based on eight symptoms and three classes was fitted simultaneously to all three sectors of service use. The remarkable thing may be, much as with the proverbial dancing bear, that this large set of data, whose potential for complexity of structure is so great, could be fitted to so simple a structure with the degree of success shown here.

Differences between the sectors may be informative, nevertheless (Table 21.5). The psychiatrist will have an easier time recognizing distressed individuals (Class II), since they are more likely to manifest dysphoria, somatic anxiety and panic attacks, and to report being nervous, than those meeting criteria for Class II in the primary-care sector. In this regard the stability of somatic symptoms of depression across sectors of care may be important. These symptoms, which consist of weight loss or gain, poor appetite, sleep disturbance and fatigue, should perhaps be thought of as the 'core' symptoms of distress when they occur with mood

Table 21.5 Latent class model with all sectors and symptoms unconstrained

Symptom group and sector	Conditional probability of a positive response for members of class		
	Class I	Class II	Class III
Dysphoria			
Untreated	.00	.13	.69
Primary care	.00	.11	.92
Psychiatric	.01	.36*	1.00
Somatic depression			
Untreated	.04	.57	1.00
Primary care	.08	.64	.95
Psychiatric	.16*	.71	1.00*
Psychomotor retardation			
Untreated	.00	.14	.51
Primary care	.00	.20	.58
Psychiatric	.03	.18	.94*
Suicidal ideas			
Untreated	.00	.02	.47
Primary care	.00	.03	.50
Psychiatric	.01	.07	.56
Somatic anxiety			
Untreated	.00	.05	.11
Primary care	.00	.12	.20*
Psychiatric	.00	.30*	.00
Phobias			
Untreated	.13	.36	.70
Primary care	.15	.43	.73
Psychiatric	.22	.43	.55
Nervous person			
Untreated	.14	.42	.90
Primary care	.18	.59	.78
Psychiatric	.44*	1.00*	.89
Panic attacks			
Untreated	.00	.05	.14
Primary care	.00	.04	.24
Psychiatric	.00	.26*	.30

* The conditional probability for this symptom differs from its value in one of the other sectors by a factor of four; or, by a difference of .20

disturbance. The concept of a core group of symptoms might facilitate communication between primary-care doctors and psychiatric specialists, much as the concept of 'core' symptoms of schizophrenia has facilitated communication about schizophrenia in different cultures.

In Class III, which is closest to Major Depressive Disorder, individuals in the psychiatric sector are much more likely to manifest psychomotor retardation or agitation (conditional probability of .94 in Table 21.5). Primary-care practitioners do not always have the benefit of these conspicuous features to aid them in recognizing the disorder (conditional probability of .58 in Table 21.5). This fact may explain some of the failure of primary-care doctors to recognize depression. Training courses in primary health care could benefit by paying greater attention to the difficulties in diagnosing depression in the absence of psychomotor retardation.

REFERENCES

Bartholomew, D.J. (1987) *Latent Variable Models and Factor Analysis*, London: Oxford University Press.

Cottler, L.B., Zipp, J.F., Robins, L.N., and Spitznagel, E.L. (1987) 'Difficult-to-recruit respondents and their effect on prevalence estimates in an epidemiologic survey', *American Journal of Epidemiology* 125:329–39.

Eastwood, M.R. (1975) *The Relation between Physical and Mental Illness*, Toronto: Toronto University Press.

Eaton, W.W. and Kessler, L.G. (eds) (1985) *Epidemiologic Field Methods in Psychiatry: the NIMH Epidemiologic Catchment Area Program*, New York: Academic Press.

Eaton, W.W., Regier, D.A., Locke, B.Z., and Taube, C.A. (1981) 'The Epidemiologic Catchment Area Program of the National Institute of Mental Health', *Public Health Reports* 96:319–25.

Eaton, W.W. and Bohrnstedt, G.W. (eds) (1989) 'Latent variable models for dichotomous outcomes: applications to data from the NIMH Epidemiologic Catchment Area Program', *Sociological Methods and Research* (Special issue).

Goldberg, D.P. (1979) 'Detection and assessment of emotional disorders in primary care', *International Journal of Mental Health* 8:30–48.

Hankin, J. and Oktay, J.S. (1979) *Mental Disorder and Primary Medical Care: an Analytical Review of the Literature*, US Department of Health, Education, and Welfare publication (ADM) 78–661, Bethesda, MD: National Institute of Mental Health.

Korff, M.R. von, and Anthony, J.C. (1982) 'The NIMH Diagnostic Interview Schedule modified to record current mental status', *Journal of Affective Disorders* 4:365–71.

Korff, M.R. von, Cottler, L., George, L.K., Eaton, W.W., Leaf, P.J., and Burnam, A. (1985) 'Non-response and non-response bias in the ECA surveys', in W.W. Eaton and L.G. Kessler (eds) *Epidemiologic Field Methods in Psychiatry: the NIMH Epidemiologic Catchment Area Program*, New York: Academic Press, pp. 85–98.

Korff, M.R. von, Shapiro, S., Burke, J.D., Teitlebaum, M., Skinner, E.A., German, P., Turner, R.W., Klein, L., and Burns, B. (1987) 'Anxiety and depression in a primary care clinic: comparison of diagnostic interview schedule, general health questionnaire, and practitioner assessments', *Archives of General Psychiatry* 44:152–6.

McCutcheon, A. (1987) *Latent Class Analysis*, Beverly Hills: Sage Publications.

Mendels, J., Weinstein, N., and Cochrane, C. (1972) 'The relationship between depression and anxiety', *Archives of General Psychiatry* 27:649–53.

Prusoff, B. and Klerman, G.L. (1974) 'Differentiating depressed from anxious neurotic outpatients', *Archives of General Psychiatry* 30:302–8.

Regier, D.A., Goldberg, I.D., and Taube, C.A. (1978) 'The de facto US mental health services system: a public health perspective', *Archives of General Psychiatry* 38:685–93.

Robins, L.N., Helzer, J.E., Croughan, J., and Ratcliff, K.S. (1981) 'National Institute of Mental Health Diagnostic Interview Schedule: its history, characteristics, and validity', *Archives of General Psychiatry* 38:381–9.

Shapiro, S., Skinner, E.A., Kessler, L.G., Korff, M.R. von, German, P.G., Tischler, G.L., Leaf, P.J., Benham, L., Cottler, L., and Regier, D.A. (1984) 'Utilization of health and mental health services: three epidemiologic catchment area sites', *Archives of General Psychiatry* 41:971–8.

Stavrakaki, C. and Vargo, B. (1986) 'The relationship of anxiety and depression: a review of the literature', *British Journal of Psychiatry* 149:7–16.

Tyrer, P. (1985) 'Neurosis divisible?', *Lancet* i: 685–8.

Chapter 22

Psychiatric syndromes among persons in contact with general medical and psychiatric services in eastern Baltimore

James C. Anthony, Alan J. Romanoski, Gerald Nestadt, Daniel E. Ford and Morton Kramer

The point of departure for this chapter is a filter model for the pathway to psychiatric care, first used by Fink *et al.* (1969) and then refined by Goldberg and Huxley (1980). This model concerns the selection processes that determine whether, where, and how mentally disordered individuals receive treatment: matters of considerable importance in the planning, organization and delivery of primary care and specialty psychiatric services (Hollingshead and Redlich 1958; Shepherd *et al.* 1966; Shepherd and Wilkinson 1988). For example, during a specified interval of time, some community residents receive services from a specialist in psychiatry; others do not. According to the filter model, the variation is influenced to some extent by characteristics of the patient, and to some extent by other factors such as organization of medical services. Similar influences affect whether patients decide to visit a primary-care doctor for help with psychiatric problems, whether primary-care doctors discuss these problems with their patients, and whether patients receive treatment for these problems (Fink *et al.* 1969; Goldberg and Huxley 1980; Goldberg and Gask, this volume).

The filter model leads to a set of testable propositions about the nature and type of disorders that serve as determinants of psychiatric care. It seems likely that cases with the more severe psychiatric disorders pass through each filter more readily. Alternately, in some treatment systems the cases with severe disorders might bypass the filter corresponding to primary medical care and directly enter psychiatric services (Goldberg and Huxley 1980). The implication is that over time the concentration of these problems becomes greater on one side of each filter as compared to the other side. The differential concentration can be expressed in terms of prevalence: for example, the prevalence of severe problems will be greater among medical patients who have received specialty psychiatric care within a given span of time, as compared to those not receiving care. Of course, effective treatment can change these prevalence relationships.

A few prospective studies have produced evidence pertinent to the filter model. For example, studying a cohort of Icelanders, Helgason (1964) found that those developing schizophrenia had a substantially higher chance of being admitted to psychiatric beds, as compared to those with neurosis. Analysing prospectively gathered interview data from a cross-sectional sample of adults in eastern Baltimore, Shapiro *et al.* (1986) found that need for mental health services measured in a baseline interview had a strong association with subsequent mental health visits to general medical and psychiatric care services.

In other contexts, evidence concerning these propositions has been developed when prevalence of psychiatric disorders among treated individuals has been compared to prevalence among untreated individuals (for instance, Cooper 1966; Leaf *et al.* 1985; Kessler *et al.* 1987), or as compared to community samples (Wing *et al.* 1981). However, in theory, these relative prevalence comparisons face a problem of possible confounding. For example, if depressed mood were found to be more common among medical-service users, this might be because women are more likely than men to use medical services and also more likely to have depressed mood. Moreover, if a fairly non-specific complaint such as worrying proves to be more common among psychiatric-service users as compared to general-medical-service users, this might be because cases with schizophrenic or other psychoses are more likely to worry, not because worrying has any direct or independent influence on who receives care from psychiatric specialists. Confounding can be examined and taken into account by means of statistical manoeuvres such as stratification when samples are quite large; multivariable models are useful when the sample size is more limited (for instance, Kleinbaum and Kupper 1978), as illustrated in several studies (Tessler *et al.* 1976; Leaf *et al.* 1985).

The study here reported includes a prevalence analysis designed to identify specific types of psychiatric syndrome occurring more commonly among community residents with recent use of general medical services, as compared to those with no recent use of these services. The study also includes a prevalence analysis designed to identify types of psychiatric syndrome occurring more commonly among community residents with recent use of psychiatric services, as compared to those receiving general medical services but no specialty psychiatric care. In these analyses, multiple logistic regression and discriminant function techniques have been used to hold constant or adjust for potentially confounding socio-demographic variables and also the co-occurrence of psychiatric syndromes.

The central issue in this study is whether specific types of psychiatric syndrome are associated with receipt of general medical services and psychiatric care. We can shed light on the public health significance of this issue by considering what we can expect to find and what contrary findings might mean. To the extent that community residents visit their primary-care doctors and other general medical care providers for treatment of worrying, depressed mood, and other so-called 'minor' psychiatric illnesses, one should expect the associated syndromes to be more common among general medical service users than among community residents without recent use of these services. According to the filter model, syndromes characteristic of schizophrenic conditions and other severe psychiatric disorders should be associated more strongly with use of specialty psychiatric services than with use of general medical services (Goldberg and Huxley 1980). If these predictions are not met, then we must seek out factors or processes that might be dampening the strength of the observed associations. The presence of a superbly effective and efficient treatment system would seem an implausible explanation. More likely, for specific types of psychiatric disturbance, the community cases face obstacles to receipt of medical and psychiatric care in greater number and variety than other community residents. If our public-health work is to be complete, the known obstacles that block effective treatment and control of these psychiatric disturbances must be removed (APHA 1962).

MATERIALS AND METHODS

Subjects for the study were recruited for the Baltimore segment of the Epidemiologic Catchment Area Program, sponsored by the National Institute of Mental Health. These survey respondents were sampled in 1981 as adult residents of households in eastern Baltimore City, an area inhabited by 268,000 persons. Since the survey sample and study methods have been described in detail elsewhere (Kramer et al. 1985; Shapiro et al. 1984; Eaton et al. 1984; Anthony et al. 1985; Folstein et al. 1985; Shapiro et al. 1986; Ford et al. 1989), only a brief summary is included here.

In Baltimore, the survey involved a two-stage design. In Stage One, trained lay interviewers administered the Diagnostic Interview Schedule (DIS) and supplementary questions on related topics, including recent psychiatric care and use of other health services. A total of 3,481 respondents were interviewed, approximately 78 per cent of the probability sample designated for the first stage of work.

From among the 3,481 Stage One respondents, 527 were selected at random for Stage Two psychiatric examinations; an additional 559 were selected because their Stage One interviews revealed evidence of current psychiatric disturbances (such as a low score on the Mini-Mental State Examination, or a high score on a twenty-item interview version of the General Health Questionnaire). One of the four participating psychiatrists saw each Stage Two participant and in the course of a 60–120-minute standardized psychiatric examination made ratings of the present mental state and observed behaviour, as well as the history of past psychiatric disturbances. The psychiatrists used the entire 140-item Present State Examination, 9th edition (Wing et al. 1974) and made additional ratings as well. Characteristics of the examination, including reliability of diagnostic ratings, have been described by Romanoski *et al*. (1988). The study psychiatrists examined 810 persons at Stage Two (74.6 per cent), usually within three weeks of the Stage One interview. The completion rate for persons selected on the basis of psychiatric disturbances was approximately equal to that for randomly selected subjects (*ca*. 75 per cent).

A key issue in the data analyses involved differences in the prevalence of specific psychiatric syndromes among individuals with and without recent use of general medical and specialty psychiatric services, as compared to other persons. Recent use of general medical and psychiatric services was identified from affirmative responses to Stage One questions concerning services used in the 6 months prior to that interview. The definitions of general medical and psychiatric services conform to prior usage in reports on the Epidemiologic Catchment Area surveys (Shapiro *et al*. 1984; Shapiro *et al*. 1986; Ford *et al*. 1989).

The presence of psychiatric syndromes in the month prior to Stage Two was determined by Present State Examination (PSE) symptom ratings made by the Stage Two psychiatrist-examiner. These psychiatrists were given no data on participants' responses to Stage One questions; moreover, they did not know which persons were selected at random and which because of their responses. The PSE-Catego computer program was used to derive individual PSE 'syndromes' from groups of related symptoms as described by Wing *et al*. (1974; 1981), and to characterize psychiatric disturbances of individuals in relation to these syndromes. Here, following Wing *et al*., the term 'syndrome' means a symptom group or cluster defined on clinical grounds and made operational via the PSE-Catego system, not an inference about morbid states drawn on the basis of a combination of symptoms and signs. Some PSE syndromes represent relatively homogeneous clinical units with diagnostic specificity and meaning. For example, 'nuclear syndrome' is defined in terms of individual symptom ratings for eight 'first-rank' features of schizophrenia, including thought broadcast and delusions of control. Other PSE syndromes have been described as 'rag bags' (Wing *et al*. 1974). For example, 'non-specific psychosis' is defined in relation to a heterogeneous collection of fifteen PSE symptom ratings, including clouding of consciousness or stupor, suspicion, bizarre appearance, evasiveness concerning delusions, and heightened or changed perception.

Statistical analysis began with the estimation of prevalence, followed by multiple logistic regression and discriminant function analyses. In the multivariate analyses, the dependent variables were use of general medical services and use of psychiatric services in the 6 months prior to interview (coded 0/1). PSE syndrome variables were set to zero when the corresponding Catego score was zero; otherwise, the PSE variable equalled 1, unless the Catego score was a missing value (for example, all symptom ratings coded 8 for 'not known' or 9 for 'not applicable'). Dummy-coded

(0/1) indicators also were used to explore whether associations between syndromes and use of services were confounded by socio-demographic factors (sex, age, ethnicity and years of schooling) and to provide statistical control over these factors. When appropriate, the regression models were specified to include one or more variables reflecting which persons were selected at random and which because of their responses to the Stage One interview. Quite deliberately, the models were not enlarged to include medication use, sick-leave and physical illness or disability. These variables might be secondary to the presence of psychiatric syndromes; by holding them constant we might distort the associations we wished to estimate.

Multiple logistic regression analyses were used to obtain the odds ratio estimate for degree of association between use of health services and each individual PSE syndrome. Because only small numbers were involved, the discriminant function was used to identify linear combinations of PSE syndromes which correlated with being a user of services. The discriminant function does not yield odds ratio estimates of association and is subject to normality assumptions and several other constraints not imposed with multiple logistic regression. Even so, the discriminant function approach can be used to identify statistically significant correlations within a regression framework (Press and Wilson 1978).

Unless noted explicitly, all statistical analyses have involved sampling weights or regression terms to account for differences in the probability of sample selection for Stage One and Stage Two assessments. In keeping with the exploratory nature of this research, all observed p-values at or below 0.10 have been reported; they are provisional estimates based on Statistical Analysis System procedures (CATMOD, STEPDISC, FREQ). No Bonferroni tests or other adjustments have been made to compensate for multiple comparisons; neither has there been any attempt to estimate survey design effects (Eaton et al. 1984).

RESULTS

1 Prevalence estimation

Table 22.1 shows selected characteristics of the 810 respondents for whom Present State Examination ratings were made during the Stage Two examinations. The survey completion rate at Stage One was higher for women. In consequence, 65 per cent of the participants were female. Reflecting the adult household population of eastern Baltimore, about 40 per cent of the respondents were blacks, with a small number in other ethnic or racial groups (such as American Indian).

Almost 30 per cent of the sample were aged 65 years or older. This was a consequence of an intentional over-sampling of elderly residents in Stage

Table 22.1 Selected characteristics of the Stage Two segment of the household sample (N = 810), Eastern Baltimore Mental Health Survey Baltimore, MD, 1981

Characteristics	Number of respondents	Per cent distribution
All persons	810	100
Sex		
Male	286	35
Female	524	65
Race-ethnicity		
White	463	57
Non-white	347	43
Age (yrs)		
18–44	396	49
45–64	186	23
65+	228	28
Schooling (in years)		
0–8	287	35
9–11	201	25
12 or more	322	40
Use of medical services		
Not within past 6 months	265	33
Within past 6 months ('recent')	545	67
Use of specialty psychiatric services among those with recent medical care		
Not within past 6 months	494	91
Within past 6 months	51	9

One (Kramer *et al.* 1985); that is, deliberately increasing the probability of sample selection for older people. To some extent, the over-sampling of elderly people also accounted for the percentage distribution for years of schooling, more than one-third of the sample having completed fewer than nine years of schooling. Table 22.1 also shows the number and percentage of persons in the sample who reported use of ambulatory general medical services. In the 6 months prior to interview, 265 Stage Two subjects (33 per cent) did not make any contact with these services and 545 (67 per cent) did so. Among the latter, 51 (9.4 per cent) also reported use of out-patient services in the specialty mental health sector (for example, treatment at a mental health centre or by a psychiatrist). There were eleven persons reporting recent out-patient contact with the specialty mental health sector, while in the same period they had no contact with general medical services (data not shown in a table). The survey data do not reveal whether these respondents entered into psychiatric care via earlier referrals from general medical providers, or whether they were examples of the 'American bypass' around the primary-care filter (Goldberg and Huxley 1980). Due to the uncertainty, these eleven respondents were included in analyses to estimate community prevalence, but not in subsequent analyses.

Table 22.2 shows the unweighted number and percentage of Stage Two subjects with individual PSE syndromes, as well as syndrome prevalence estimates for the adult household population under study. It also shows PSE syndrome prevalence estimates for area residents who had received no recent general medical care and for those with recent use of general medical services. For these estimates we used weighting procedures to compensate for variation in probability of sample selection (for instance, the elderly over-sample) as well as survey non-response (Eaton *et al.* 1984; Anthony *et al.* 1985).

In order of frequency, the most commonly rated PSE syndromes in the Stage Two sample were the worrying syndrome (28 per cent), situational anxiety (22 per cent), tension (18 per cent), simple depression or depressed mood (16 per cent) and irritability (14 per cent). Based on estimates weighted to represent the area's adult household population, these also were the most prevalent syndromes among persons with and without recent health services use (columns 4 and 5 of Table 22.2). Although the estimates for PSE syndrome prevalence based on our community survey were somewhat lower than estimates from earlier surveys, this set of five PSE syndromes has been found to be prevalent in two other field-study populations: in Camberwell, London, and in two Ugandan villages (Wing *et al.* 1981).

A comparison of estimates in columns 4 and 5 of Table 22.2 indicated that 'other symptoms of depression' (such as somatic complaints such as early waking, loss of libido or appetite) and few other PSE syndromes were more prevalent among recent users of general medical services than among non-users. In fact, for a number of syndromes there was evidence of *lower* prevalence among the users of general medical services. This assessment of relative prevalence was based not only on the size of the prevalence estimate for each group, but also on a test of statistical significance using unweighted sample data.

The PSE syndromes with apparently lower prevalence among medical service users included several potentially indicative of schizophrenia: the nuclear syndrome (for example, thought intrusion, primary delusions), the residual syndrome (for instance, behaves as if hallucinated, hears muttering or whispering), and delusions of reference, as well as others: organic impairment (such as of memory), self-neglect, sexual and fantastic delusions, overactivity (gross excitement, inappropriate or embarrassing behaviour) and the PSE symptom group termed 'non-specific psychosis'. In addition, recent medical service users were less likely to be rated as

Table 22.2 Estimated prevalence of PSE syndromes found in the community and among recent users of medical and psychiatric services: data from Stage Two of the Eastern Baltimore, Mental Health Survey, Baltimore MD, 1981

PSE syndrome	Unweighted number in sample (N = 810)	Unweighted percentage in sample	Weighted community prevalence	Estimated prevalence among:		
				Persons with no recent medical care contacts (N = 265)	General medical service users (N = 545)	Specialty psychiatric service users (N = 51)
Nuclear schizophrenic syndrome	8	1.0	<0.5	0.5	0.2	2.7
Catatonic syndrome	2	<0.5	<0.5	0.2	0.0	0.0
Incoherent speech	2	<0.5	<0.5	0.1	0.0	0.0
Residual schizophrenic syndrome	10	1.2	<0.5	0.6	0.2	1.7
Depressive delusions & hallucinations	2	<1.0	<0.5	0.0	0.1	0.0
Simple depression	127	15.7	7.3	6.9	7.6	22.8
Obsessional syndrome	20	2.5	1.5	2.3	1.1	5.3
General anxiety	42	5.2	3.4	5.4	2.4	6.2
Situational anxiety	179	22.1	18.9	17.0	19.8	21.5
Hysteria	42	5.2	3.0	3.4	2.8	18.0
Affective flattening	12	1.5	<0.5	0.5	0.4	6.2
Hypomania	14	1.7	1.6	1.5	1.7	4.7
Auditory hallucinations	9	1.1	<0.5	0.4	0.3	4.2
Delusions of persecution	7	0.9	<0.5	0.3	0.1	2.1
Delusions of reference	6	0.7	<0.5	0.4	0.1	1.1
Grandiose and religious delusions	3	<0.5	<0.5	0.1	<0.1	1.1
Sexual and fantastic delusions	8	1.0	<0.5	0.4	0.2	2.2
Visual hallucinations	7	0.9	<0.5	0.1	0.3	4.5
Olfactory hallucinations	7	0.9	0.6	1.2	0.2	1.7
Overactivity	6	0.7	<0.5	0.4	0.2	0.0
Slowness	22	2.7	1.0	0.9	1.0	8.3
Non-specific psychosis	44	5.4	3.6	3.7	3.5	6.6

Table 22.2 (cont'd)

Depersonalization	7	0.9	<0.5	0.0	0.5	7.8
Special features of depression	23	2.8	1.5	1.2	1.6	17.8
Agitation	7	0.9	1.5	0.3	0.2	0.0
Self-neglect	25	3.1	1.3	2.2	1.0	0.0
Ideas of reference	29	3.6	2.0	2.7	1.7	7.3
Tension	143	17.7	10.3	10.9	10.0	34.3
Lack of energy	26	3.2	1.4	1.4	1.4	6.3
Worrying, etc.	229	28.3	15.4	14.6	15.8	31.3
Irritability	110	13.6	7.5	6.5	8.0	16.8
Social unease	59	7.3	4.5	4.8	4.3	11.2
Loss of interest and concentration	73	9.0	4.1	3.3	4.4	22.6
Hypochondriasis	13	1.6	0.6	1.0	0.4	2.7
Other symptoms of depression	67	8.3	8.3	2.2	6.9	11.4
Organic impairment	48	5.9	2.0	2.3	1.9	0.0
Subcultural delusions or hallucinations	2	0.2	<0.5	0.2	0.0	0.0

providing information of doubtful reliability on the basis of misleading answers from the subject or difficulty in obtaining responses needed to make PSE ratings.

Column 6 in Table 22.2 shows the prevalence of each PSE syndrome among recent users of both general medical services and specialty psychiatric services. When compared with data on all general medical service users (column 5), the syndromes found to be more prevalent among recent users of specialty psychiatric services ($p<0.10$) were: the nuclear and residual syndromes potentially indicative of schizophrenia, simple depression, hysteria (for example, conversion symptoms), affective flattening, hypomania, auditory hallucinations, delusions of persecution, delusions of reference, grandiose and religious delusions, visual hallucinations, depersonalization, special features of depression (such as pathological guilt), ideas of reference, tension (such as tension pains, restlessness), lack of energy (namely, subjective anergia), worrying, irritability, social unease, loss of interest and concentration, hypochondriasis, other (somatic) symptoms of depression and 'non-specific psychosis'. It is notable that the Stage One interview recorded no recent use of specialty mental health services for forty-eight subjects with organic impairment, twenty-five subjects with self-neglect, seven subjects with agitation, or six subjects with overactivity (Table 22.2, column 6).

2 Syndromes associated with recent general medical care

Up to this point, our study of PSE syndromes in relation to medical and psychiatric service usage has failed to consider possible confounding effects. Our preparatory analyses showed that recent users of general medical services were more likely to be women, and to have received at least nine years of schooling, while recent use of specialty mental health services varied with age, as well as with sex and years of schooling. To the extent that these characteristics also were associated with the presence of PSE syndromes, the direct comparison of prevalence estimates might give a distorted view of syndromes associated with entry into general medical care or psychiatric care.

We used a sequence of logistic regression models to examine associations between use of services and each PSE syndrome individually, while holding constant the suspected confounding variables. In these models, we used regression terms instead of weighting procedures to account for differences in sample selection probabilities. We also used a regression term to hold constant whether the respondent was rated as a reliable informant, since this characteristic had an inverse association with use of general medical services. The indicator for each PSE syndrome was coded so that persons rated as 'syndrome absent' served as a reference category. Accordingly, a statistically significant odds ratio (OR) estimate above 1.0 served to

Table 22.3 Estimated odds ratios showing PSE syndromes associated with recent use of general medical services: data from the Eastern Baltimore Mental Health Survey, Baltimore, MD, 1981 (N = 545 users of general medical services and 265 non-users)

PSE syndromes	Unadjusted[1] odds ratio estimate	p-value	Initial[2] adjusted odds ratio estimate	p-value	Final[3] adjusted odds ratio estimate	p-value
Those having a positive association						
Other symptoms of depression	1.9	0.03	1.9	0.03	1.9	0.05
Situational anxiety	1.5	0.02	1.5	0.02	1.5	0.05
Worrying, etc.	1.4	0.07	1.4	0.05	1.3	0.11
Social unease	2.0	0.04	2.0	0.04	2.0	0.04
Tension	1.9	0.04	1.9	<0.01	1.9	<0.01
Those having an inverse association						
Self-neglect	0.3	0.05	0.3	0.05	0.4	0.01
Non-specific psychosis	0.6	0.07	0.6	0.07	0.3	0.02
Organic impairment	0.6	0.10	0.6	0.10	0.6	0.10
Residual syndrome	0.3	0.08	0.3	0.09	0.3	0.08
Nuclear syndrome	0.3	0.09	0.3	0.09	0.3	0.09
Delusions of reference	0.2	0.10	0.2	0.09	0.3	0.13
Sexual and fantastic delusions	0.3	0.09	0.3	0.10	0.3	0.14
Overactivity	0.2	0.10	0.2	0.10	0.2	0.11

[1] Odds ratio estimates and p-values from logistic regression models with no other variables held constant
[2] Odds ratio estimates and p-values from logistic regression models, holding sample selection constant
[3] Odds ratio estimates and p-values from logistic regression models, holding constant sample selection, sex (female), schooling (9–11 years), and an assessment of the respondent's reliability. For the syndromes of non-specific psychosis and self-neglect, the estimates in this column are for subjects sampled at random

indicate a reasonably stable positive association between presence of a PSE syndrome and recent use of services; odds ratio estimates below 1.0 to indicate the inverse associations. If a given PSE syndrome had no association with use of services, or had an inverse association, then the evidence was not consistent with greater syndrome prevalence among users of services. Under such circumstances, it becomes difficult to maintain that the syndrome has promoted recent use of services.

The unadjusted odds ratio estimates in Table 22.3 showed statistically significant and positive associations between recent use of general medical services and presence of the following PSE syndromes: 'other' symptoms of depression (namely, somatic symptoms), situational anxiety (such as specific phobias) and worrying syndrome. When we used the logistic model to hold constant sample selection and potential confounding variables, there was no appreciable change in the odds ratio estimates, though levels of statistical significance were affected. According to this evidence, recent users of general medical services were 1.9 times as likely to have somatic symptoms of depression as non-users. They were 1.5 times as likely as non-users to have specific phobias or other symptoms comprising the situational anxiety syndrome. Under the multivariable logistic regression model, the degree of association between worrying and recent use of medical services was small (OR = 1.3).

The multivariable analyses indicated that recent users of general medical services were less likely than non-users to manifest self-neglect syndrome, and there were a number of other PSE syndromes associated inversely, as shown in Table 22.3. Tests for interaction produced some evidence that the degree of association varied in relation to the sampling procedure. Self-neglect had a moderately inverse association when present among respondents selected at random (OR = 0.4); the association was stronger but still inverse among respondents sampled on the basis of information from the Stage One interview (OR = 0.2). The symptoms grouped under the heading of 'non-specific psychosis' had a strongly inverse association when present among respondents chosen at random (OR = 0.3), but a weakly positive association among respondents sampled because of Stage One information (OR = 1.06).

The logistic regression models also pointed toward associations involving the PSE syndromes of social unease and tension. Specifically, recent users of medical services were about twice as likely as non-users to manifest the PSE syndromes of social unease and tension. Comparison of prevalence estimates in Table 22.2 did not disclose such associations.

In order to explore mutual confounding among PSE syndromes, we used stepwise discriminant function analyses to identify PSE syndromes which have independent correlations with being a recent user of general medical services. The results showed independent correlations involving the syndromes of tension and self-neglect. However, once the discriminant

Table 22.4 Estimated odds ratios showing PSE syndromes associated with recent use of specialty psychiatric services, among recent users of general medical services; unweighted data from the Eastern Baltimore Mental Health Survey, Baltimore, Maryland, 1981 (N =51 psychiatric service users and 494 with general medical contacts only)

PSE syndrome	Unadjusted odds ratio estimate	p-value	Initial[1] adjusted odds ratio estimate	p-value	Final[2] adjusted odds ratio estimate	p-value
Visual hallucinations	15.4	<0.01	13.2	<0.01	52.1	<0.01
Affective flattening	17.8	<0.01	17.4	<0.01	19.8	<0.01
Auditory hallucinations	15.4	<0.01	13.2	<0.01	19.8	<0.01
Delusions of persecution	13.9	<0.01	25.2	0.01	17.3	0.03
Nuclear schizophrenic syndrome	20.4	0.02	15.0	0.03	12.5	0.01
Residual schizophrenic syndrome	10.0	0.02	13.2	0.01	10.0	0.03
Depersonalization	13.9	<0.01	11.5	<0.01	8.3	<0.01
Special features of depression	7.0	<0.01	6.2	<0.01	7.9	<0.01
Hypomania	5.9	<0.01	6.4	<0.01	5.3	0.01
Hypochondriasis	5.1	0.02	4.3	<0.05	5.3	0.05
Hysteria	5.5	<0.01	4.8	<0.01	4.5	<0.01
Loss of interest and concentration	4.2	<0.01	3.7	<0.01	4.3	<0.01
Non-specific psychosis	3.5	0.01	3.0	0.03	3.2	0.02
Lack of energy	3.5	0.02	3.1	0.04	3.3	0.04
Ideas of reference	3.5	0.02	3.2	0.03	3.1	0.05
Tension	3.8	<0.01	3.3	<0.01	2.9	<0.01
Simple depression	1.1	0.01	2.0	0.05	2.3	0.02
Social unease	2.6	0.02	2.4	0.04	2.2	0.06
Worrying, etc.	2.4	<0.01	2.1	0.02	2.0	0.03
Other (somatic) symptoms of depression	2.2	0.05	2.0	0.08	1.9	0.13
Irritability	3.5	0.02	1.7	0.13	1.4	0.38

[1] The unadjusted estimates for the odds ratio and p-values are based on models in which no other variables were held constant. The initial adjusted estimates are from models in which sample selection was held constant

[2] The subsequent adjusted estimates are from models in which sample selection and the following potential confounding variables were held constant: gender, age (2 dummy-coded terms), and years of schooling

Table 22.5 Present State Examination syndromes that were retained in the stepwise discriminant function analyses to discriminate recent users of general medical services from non-users and to discriminate recent users of specialty psychiatric services from non-users: unweighted data from the Eastern Baltimore Mental Health Survey, Baltimore, MD, 1981

Present State Examination syndrome	Syndromes retained in models on recent medical service use*	Syndromes retained in models on recent use of specialty psychiatric services*
Tension	Yes (p = 0.011)	Yes (p = 0.096)
Self-neglect	Yes (p = 0.089)	No
Social unease	No	No
Situational anxiety	No	No
Worrying, etc.	No	No
Non-specific psychosis	No	No
Other (somatic) symptoms of depression	No	No
Visual hallucinations	No	Yes (p < 0.001)
Affective flattening	No	Yes (p < 0.001)
Loss of interest and concentration	No	Yes (p < 0.001)
Hysteria	No	Yes (p < 0.001)
Special features of depression (e.g., guilt)	No	Yes (p < 0.002)
Hypomania	No	Yes (p = 0.008)
Residual syndrome	No	Yes (p = 0.038)
Depersonalization	No	Yes (p = 0.038)

* Unless a p-value is shown, the corresponding PSE syndrome did little to improve the performance of the discriminant functions (p>0.10). The discriminant function for medical service use included terms for sample selection, gender, schooling and the assessment of the respondent's reliability; no others qualified for inclusion. The discriminant function for mental health service use among medical service users included terms for sample selection, gender, age, and schooling, as described in Table 22.4. Other suspected confounders under study did not improve the discriminant functions

function included these PSE variables as well as others to reflect sample selection, sex, schooling and respondent reliability, no other PSE syndromes qualified for entry into the discriminant function: the evidence did not indicate independent correlations between recent use of general medical services and the other PSE syndromes listed in Table 22.3.

3 Syndromes associated with recent psychiatric care

Table 22.4 shows odds ratio estimates for the degree of association between specific PSE syndromes and use of specialty mental health services, among persons with recent use of general medical services. In contrast to the findings on recent general medical care, these results indicated a number of associations that were both strong and statistically significant, even when potential confounding was taken into account. The associations were strongest for PSE syndromes characteristic of the schizophrenic or other psychoses, such as the nuclear syndrome, the residual syndrome, hallucinations, affective flattening, delusions of persecution, and for depersonalization. Strong associations were also found for syndromes characteristic of affective disorders (for example, pathological guilt and other special features of depression, or hypomania). Syndromes with weak to moderate associations included hypochondriasis and hysteria, loss of interest and concentration, lack of energy, ideas of reference, tension, simple depression, social unease, worrying syndrome and 'non-specific psychosis'. Once potentially confounding variables were taken into account, other (somatic) symptoms of depression and irritability had a fairly low degree of association with recent use of specialty psychiatric services, for which the level of significance exceeded 10 per cent (Table 22.4).

The logistic models with interaction terms showed a tendency towards variation in the strength of association, depending upon how respondents were sampled for psychiatric examination. For example, the odds ratio estimate for special features of depression (pathological guilt) was 12.1 when this syndrome was present among those sampled at random for Stage Two; it was only 3.3 for those sampled because of Stage One responses indicating current psychiatric disturbances. We mention this as a lead for future inquiry, while noting that these exploratory results might be due to chance alone or could be misleading artefacts.

No use of specialty services was reported by subjects who qualified for the syndromes of self-neglect, agitation, overactivity or organic impairment. This is evidence of strongly inverse associations, but because of the small numbers of respondents manifesting these syndromes, no logistic regression models were used to estimate odds ratios.

Finally, stepwise discriminant function analyses were used to test for mutual confounding among PSE syndromes. These analyses showed that recent use of specialty psychiatric services was correlated independently with eight of the sixteen PSE syndromes found to have had statistically significant associations in our final logistic regression models, as shown in Table 22.5. After forced entry of key co-variates listed in the footnote to Table 22.5 the order of syndrome entry determined by the stepwise analysis was as follows: affective flattening, visual hallucinations, loss of interest and concentration, hysteria, special features of depression (such as pathological guilt), hypomania, the residual syndrome often associated with schizophrenia, depersonalization and tension. Each of these syndromes helped to discriminate recent psychiatric service users from non-users, even after the discriminating value of the other listed syndromes was taken into account. Once these syndromes were included in the model, the others did not seem to add new information discriminating psychiatric service users from others in contact with general medical services.

DISCUSSION

According to results from this two-stage procedure, twelve PSE syndromes had an estimated prevalence in the survey community of 2 per cent or greater. These were simple depression, general (free-floating) anxiety, situational anxiety, hysteria, tension, worrying, irritability, social unease, loss of interest and concentration, other (somatic) symptoms of depression, organic impairment and the 'non-specific psychosis' symptom group. In general, the prevalence of these syndromes was at the 2 per-cent level or was higher among recent users of general medical services and also among persons with recent use of both general medical services and specialty psychiatric services. The exception was the syndrome of organic impairment. Apparently, none of the persons with organic impairment had received recent specialty psychiatric services. This finding may be a simple reflection of a problem in recall or reporting of health services utilization by such persons. Alternately, it also might indicate that individuals with organic impairment seldom receive specialty psychiatric care (cf. German *et al.* 1985; Cooper, this volume).

For the most part, the multivariate analyses on recent use of psychiatric services were in accordance with the filter model of the pathway to care described by Goldberg and Huxley (1980). These results upheld an expectation based on the idea that individuals with the more severe disorders pass more readily into psychiatric care, at least to the extent that many of the PSE syndromes found to be associated specifically with psychiatric service use are characteristic of schizophrenic or other psychoses, and the more severe affective disorders. For non-specific syndromes associated with a broad range of disorders (for example, tension, worrying), the degree of association was smaller or was absent. However, the discriminant function analyses indicated that being a recent user of specialty psychiatric services correlated with eight of these PSE syndromes. This pattern of results could mean that the determinants of psychiatric care include something more specific or distinctive than a general clinical severity factor or trait. Unless the syndrome correlations in the final discriminant function analyses were the result of a single general factor, specific types of psychiatric syndromes must have been more prevalent among recent users of specialty psychiatric services.

It is noteworthy that being a recent user of general medical services had positive associations only with social unease, the tension syndrome, situational anxiety and the other (somatic) symptoms of depression. The tension syndrome, made up from ratings of tension pains, muscular tension and restlessness, helped discriminate respondents with and without recent medical service contact, but no other syndrome had an independent positive correlation once tension and the background co-variates were taken into account. The only other syndrome that seemed to aid in the discrimination was self-neglect, which was correlated inversely.

Two explanations can be offered. The first requires that we think of the tension syndrome and the self-neglect syndrome as specific and distinctive determinants of general medical service use. That is, the tension syndrome by itself might determine who uses medical services. It certainly is plausible that tension pains and muscular tension promote visits to the doctor, and the initial associations with social unease, anxiety and somatic depression might have occurred only because patients with these syndromes also suffered from tension. Similarly, the self-neglect syndrome by itself is a plausible inverse determinant of general medical service use in that not going to the doctor can be a manifestation of self-neglect. The inverse association may be telling us no more than this.

As an alternate explanation, it is conceivable that associations involving tension and self-neglect arise because these two syndromes serve as manifest indicators for two more general latent factors that determine recent use of general medical services. For example, presence of the tension syndrome may indicate a more general factor (such as severity of non-specific psychiatric distress) that also accounts for associations involving worry, somatic symptoms of depression, social unease, situational anxiety and even the 'non-specific psychosis' symptom group. Presence of the self-neglect syndrome may indicate a separate general factor (for example deterioration in social adaptation) that also accounts for inverse associations involving the nuclear and residual syndrome (such as of schizophrenia), delusions and inappropriate or embarrassing behaviour, as well as behaviours during the Stage Two examination that lead the examiner to have questions about the respondent's reliability.

The present analysis did not provide information needed to assess whether tension should be regarded as a specific and distinctive determinant of medical service use or as a manifest indicator of a more general factor such as non-specific psychiatric distress. However, the discriminant function analysis indicated that even after accounting for the doubtful reliability assessment, the self-neglect syndrome helped discriminate recent general medical service users from non-users. Thus, being a user of general medical services was found to vary in relation to self-neglect, quite apart from what the self-neglect ratings shared with the assessment of respondent reliability. The null relationships observed for other PSE syndromes suggested that presence of these syndromes was not promoting visits to the primary-care physician or other general medical care providers.

There are, of course, several limitations that must be considered in relation to these findings. Given the dynamic, prospective character of hypotheses developed under the filter model, it is important to note that these results were based on interview data from a cross-sectional field survey. We chose to treat recent use of services as a dependent variable, and to express variation in recent use of services as function of current psychiatric syndromes. This approach has been used in previous Epidemiologic Catchment Area analyses using diagnostic data from the Diagnostic Interview Schedule (for example, Shapiro *et al*. 1984; German *et al*. 1985). To us, it has seemed that the degree of association between recent use of services and current psychiatric syndromes would be influenced more by psychiatric syndromes leading to usage of services than the reverse. However, we note that the odds ratio estimates of association obtained in these analyses might have been attenuated to the extent that general medical care providers or specialists in psychiatric care had treated their recent patients effectively.

We also acknowledge that observed inverse associations might have developed because psychiatric syndromes can interfere with the accurate and complete recall and reporting of health services use, on which this study has relied. Interference of this type, mentioned above in relation to organic impairment, also could account for inverse associations involving other psychiatric syndromes, including self-neglect and other syndromes characteristic of the schizophrenic and other psychoses, as well as associations involving the assessment of respondent reliability.

It also is possible that the odds ratio estimates for association were elevated spuriously to the extent that patients receiving treatment from psychiatric specialists gave more complete and accurate reports about their symptoms than patients under treatment. Further, although the study design kept the Stage Two examiners blind to results from the Stage One interviews, the format of the PSE allowed the examiners to ask suggested questions about recent use of medical and psychiatric services. Appearance of these questions prior to the PSE ratings creates an opportunity for a diagnostic suspicion bias whereby responses to the early questions can influence later diagnostic ratings (for instance, when an examiner feels obliged to rate certain symptoms once the subject reports recent psychiatric treatment).

Finally, some caution must be expressed in relation to the nature and size of the sample for these analyses. This was a large-scale epidemiologic field survey with a two-stage design for direct psychiatric examination of a random sub-sample, in addition to a sub-sample based on Stage One evidence of psychiatric disturbance. Even so, there were too few subjects for multiple logistic regression analyses to evaluate interactions observed in the exploratory analyses or to investigate the possibility of mutual confounding among PSE syndromes; the statistical power of some analyses was low. This led to reliance upon the discriminant function, a statistical model with more constraining assumptions. Further, survey non-response and sample attrition affected the final composition of the Stage Two sample. Because many of the syndromes under study were found to occur with relatively low frequency, there has been little opportunity to make any direct study of non-response and attrition as potential sources of bias. In consequence, there are untested assumptions about validity and generalizability of the study results.

Notwithstanding these limitations, the results of this study include new information about the distribution of specific psychiatric disturbances and non-specific psychiatric symptom groups in a US community, as well as the relationships between presence of specific psychiatric syndromes and the use of medical and psychiatric services. As summarized above, these results point towards directions for an elaboration of the filter model of the pathway to psychiatric care. Work along these lines should lead to more specific hypotheses about types of psychiatric syndromes associated with entry into care, including hypotheses that might be tested by using latent variable models in mental health services research. Models of this type would clarify whether the type of syndrome is a determinant in the pathway to psychiatric care, independently of a more general factor of clinical severity.

The results amplify a call for public health efforts to remove obstacles now standing between community residents with psychiatric disturbances and their receipt of health services. Our models for recent general medical services showed no especially large concentration of psychiatric disturbances among persons in recent contact with such services. This result leads us to wonder about the extent to which Baltimore community residents are visiting their primary care doctors and other medical care providers to seek treatment of worrying, depressed mood and other syndromes associated with so-called 'minor' psychiatric illnesses. Indeed, our models showed fairly strong inverse associations between recent medical contact and the presence of some often severe syndromes such as organic impairment and the nuclear and residual syndromes characteristic of schizophrenic and other psychoses. This result leads us to wonder whether community cases with psychiatric disturbances are receiving adequate care, treatment and management of other medical conditions such as hypertension that often compromise their health status (cf. Kramer *et al.*, this volume). From what we know about provision of health services in Baltimore, it seems likely that non-psychiatric medical conditions are often not receiving careful attention among community cases, even when there is regular contact with specialty mental health services.

Finally, our filter model showed many types of psychiatric syndrome to be present in greater concentration among patients in contact with specialty mental health services than among patients in contact with general medical services only. As expected, there were especially strong associations involving the syndromes potentially indicative of schizophrenic and other psychoses. None the less, there is some cause for concern about the untreated cases, including those with syndromes of anxiety and depression. As indicated by our prevalence analyses, the latter sometimes were in contact with providers of general medical care, perhaps seeking a remedy for psychological symptoms, possibly with medical complaints embellished or coloured by active psychiatric disturbances. Yet these syndromes of anxiety and depression were not especially concentrated among patients treated by specialists in psychiatry and mental health care, nor among patients being seen by general providers. The implication is that the mental disorders underlying syndromes of anxiety and depression are not potent determinants of either psychiatric or general medical care in this community. We hope for future research to investigate whether this is in fact a continuing situation, to identify what might account for it, and to determine how organization and delivery of services might enhance possibilities for effective treatment and control of these mental disorders.

ACKNOWLEDGEMENTS

This work was supported in part by research and training grants from the National Institute of Mental Health (MH33870, MH41908, MH14592) and by a Fulbright Senior Scholar award to JCA. In addition, Professor A.S. Henderson and the Social Psychiatry Research Unit of the Australian National University provided resources and Paul Duncan-Jones (now deceased) provided consultation and computing assistance with respect to PSE-Catego computing during the Fulbright award period in Canberra. Dr Paul Bebbington provided consultation and training in the use of the PSE, while Professors E. M. Gruenberg and M.F. Folstein led and directed the Clinical Reappraisal Working Group that was responsible for Stage Two examinations in the Eastern Baltimore survey. Other members of the working group were Drs Raman Chahal and Altaf Merchant, Michael R. von Korff, C. Hendricks Brown, and authors AJR, GN and JCA.

REFERENCES

American Public Health Association, Program Area Committee on Mental Health (1962) *Mental Disorders: a Guide to Control Methods*, New York: APHA.
Anthony, J.C., Folstein, M., Romanoski, A.J., Korff, M.R. von, Nestadt, G., Chahal, R., Merchant, A., Brown, C.H., Shapiro, S., Kramer, M., and Gruenberg, E.M. (1985) 'Comparison of the Lay Diagnostic Interview Schedule and a standardized psychiatric diagnosis: experience in Eastern Baltimore', *Archives of General Psychiatry* 42:667–75.
Cooper, B. (1966) 'Psychiatric disorder in hospital and general practice', *Social Psychiatry* 1:7–10.
Eaton, W.W., Holzer, C.E., Korff, M.R. von, Anthony, J.C., Helzer, J.E., George, L.K., Burnam, M.A., Boyd, J.H., Kessler, L.G., and Locke, B.Z.

(1984) 'The design of the Epidemiologic Catchment Area surveys: the control and measurement of error', *Archives of General Psychiatry* 41:942–8.

Fink, R., Shapiro, S., Goldensohn, S., and Daily, E. (1969) 'The filter-down process to psychotherapy in a group practice medical care program', *American Journal of Public Health* 59:245–60.

Folstein, M.F., Romanoski, A.J., Chahal, R., Anthony, J., Korff, M.R. von, Nestadt, G., Merchant, A., Gruenberg, E.M., and Kramer, M. (1985) 'Eastern Baltimore Mental Health Survey clinical reappraisal', in W.W. Eaton and L.G. Kessler (eds) *Epidemiologic Field Methods in Psychiatry: the NIMH Epidemiologic Catchment Area Program*, New York: Academic Press, pp. 253–84.

Ford, D.E., Anthony, J.C., Nestadt, G.R., and Romanoski, A.J. (1989) 'The General Health Questionnaire by interview: performance in relation to recent use of health services', *Medical Care* 27:367–75.

German, P.S., Shapiro, S., and Skinner, E.A. (1985) 'Mental health of the elderly: use of health and mental health services', *Journal of the American Geriatric Society* 33:246–52.

Goldberg, D. and Huxley, P. (1980) *Mental Illness in the Community: the Pathway to Psychiatric Care*, London and New York: Tavistock.

Helgason, T. (1964) 'Epidemiology of mental disorders in Iceland', *Acta Psychiatrica Scandinavica*, Supplement 173.

Hollingshead, A.B. and Redlich, F.C. (1958) *Social Class and Mental Illness*, New York: John Wiley & Sons.

Kessler, L.G., Burns, B.J., Shapiro, S., Tischler, G.L., George, L.K., Hough, R.L., Bodison, D., and Miller, R.H. (1987) 'Psychiatric diagnoses of medical service users: evidence from the Epidemiologic Catchment Area Program', *American Journal of Public Health* 77:18–24.

Kleinbaum, D.G. and Kupper, L.L. (1978) *Applied Regression Analysis and Other Multivariable Methods*, Boston: Duxbury.

Kramer, M., German, P.S., Anthony, J.C., Korff, M.R. von, and Skinner, E.A. (1985) 'Patterns of mental disorders among the elderly residents of eastern Baltimore', *Journal of the American Geriatric Society* 33:236–42.

Leaf, P.J., Livingston, M.M., Tischler, G.L., Weissman, M.M., Holzer, C.E., and Myers, J.K. (1985) 'Contact with health professionals for the treatment of psychiatric and emotional problems', *Medical Care* 23:1322–37.

Press, S.J. and Wilson, S. (1978) 'Choosing between logistic regression and discriminant analysis', *Journal of the American Statistical Association* 73:699–705.

Romanoski, A.J., Nestadt, G.N., Chahal, R., Merchant, A., Folstein, M.F., Gruenberg, E.M., and McHugh, P.R. (1988) 'Inter-observer reliability of a "Standardized Psychiatric Examination (SPE)" for case-ascertainment', *Journal of Nervous and Mental Disease* 176:63–71.

Shapiro, S., Skinner, E.A., German, P.S., Kramer, M., and Romanoski, A. (1986) 'Need and demand for mental health services in an urban community: an exploration based on household interviews', in J. Barrett and R.M. Rose (eds) *Mental Disorders in the Community: Progress and Challenge*, New York: Guilford Press, pp. 307–20.

Shapiro, S., Skinner, E.A., Kessler, L.G., Korff, M.R von, German, P.S., Tischler, G.L., Leaf, P.J., Benham, L., Cottler, L., and Regier, D.A. (1984) 'Utilization of health and mental health services: three Epidemiologic Catchment Area sites', *Archives of General Psychiatry* 41:971–8.

Shepherd, M., Cooper, B., Brown, A.C., and Kalton, G.W. (1966) *Psychiatric Illness in General Practice*, London: Oxford University Press.

Shepherd, M. and Wilkinson, G. (1988) 'Primary care as the middle ground for psychiatric epidemiology', *Psychological Medicine* 18:263–7.

Tessler, R., Mechanic, D., and Dimond, M. (1976) 'The effect of psychological distress on physician utilization: a prospective study', *Journal of Health and Social Behavior* 17:353–64.

Wing, J.K., Cooper, J.E., and Sartorius, N. (1974) *Measurement and Classification of Psychiatric Symptoms: an Instruction Manual for the PSE and Catego Program*, Cambridge, London, and New York: Cambridge University Press.

Wing, J.K., Bebbington, P., Hurry, J., and Tennant, C. (1981) 'The prevalence in the general population of disorders familiar to psychiatrists in hospital practice', in J.K. Wing, P. Bebbington, and L.N. Robins (eds) *What Is a Case? The Problem of Definition in Psychiatric Community Surveys*, London: Grant McIntyre, pp. 45–61.

Chapter 23

Somatization in primary health care

Prevalence and determinants

Keith W. Bridges and David P. Goldberg

Although the majority of psychiatric illnesses seen in primary care are disorders of mood (Goldberg and Huxley 1980; Hoeper *et al*. 1979; Goldberg and Bridges 1987) and usually consist of a combination of anxiety-related and depression-related symptoms (Goldberg *et al*. 1987), studies on consecutive attenders have shown that the majority of patients present somatic complaints to their doctor rather than affective or cognitive symptoms (Shepherd *et al*. 1966; Goldberg and Blackwell 1970; Goldberg 1979). These patients fall into two main groups: those primarily consulting their doctor about a coexisting physical disorder and those who present somatic manifestations of their psychiatric illness. The presentation of somatic symptoms can distract the attention of a doctor away from considering a psychiatric illness (Goldberg and Blackwell 1970; Goldberg 1979) and may lead to an unnecessary utilization of non-psychiatric health-care services (Clancy and Noyes 1976; Katon 1984; Lipowski 1988; Smith *et al*. 1986).

Many patients who present somatic manifestations of their psychiatric illness do not consider themselves as suffering from a psychiatric illness and attribute their complaints to a physical disorder. This mode of presentation is known as somatization and has been defined as 'the expression of personal and social distress in an idiom of bodily complaints with medical help seeking' (Kleinman and Kleinman 1985). It is a world-wide phenomenon (Katon *et al*. 1982a; Kirmayer 1984) and has been categorized in terms of its course: acute, sub-acute and chronic forms (Rosen *et al*. 1982).

This chapter will present some of the results of our research in Manchester concerned with an assessment of the following three factors:

1 the prevalence of sub-acute somatization in patients aged over 15 years consulting their family doctor with a new illness;
2 the extent to which this mode of presentation accounts for 'hidden psychiatric morbidity' in primary care;
3 the potential determinants of this form of somatization.

Both preliminary and more detailed results of this study have been reported elsewhere (Bridges and Goldberg 1985; Bridges and Goldberg 1987; Bridges *et al*. 1991).

A new illness was defined as any complaint for which medical attention had not been sought in the previous 12 months. Somatization was defined by using the following criteria (Bridges and Goldberg 1985):

1 *Consulting behaviour* – the patient must seek medical help for somatic manifestations of psychiatric illness and does not present overt psychological symptoms.
2 *Attribution* – the patient must consider at the time of consultation that these somatic manifestations are caused by a physical illness.
3 *Presence of a psychiatric illness* – the patient must report symptoms which justify a psychiatric diagnosis when standard research criteria are applied.
4 *Expected response to treatment* – in the opinion of the research psychiatrist, treatment of the psychiatric disorder would cause the somatic manifestations either to disappear or to revert to their level before the episode of psychiatric disorder.

Strictly speaking, a patient had to satisfy all these four criteria. Some patients when interviewed did not attribute their somatic complaints to a physical disorder but believed them to be due to psychological disturbance. However, when seeking help from their family doctor they had expressed concern that their symptoms could indeed have an organic basis. As these patients did not fulfil all the above requirements, we categorized them as 'facultative somatizers' on the basis of their illness behaviour at the time of their consultation with the general practitioner. Psychiatric 'caseness' was determined by DSM-III diagnostic criteria (APA 1980). However, patients with a diagnosis of Adjustment Disorders alone have not been included in this analysis.

In assessing possible determinants of somatization, we considered various hypotheses put forward in published studies of the chronic forms of this phenomenon. These are concerned with: (a) demographic and intellectual factors; (b) psychodynamic defence mechanisms; (c) stigma of mental illness; (d) personality factors; (e) early life experiences; (f) social factors in adult life; and (g) medical factors in adult life (Bridges *et al*. 1991).

MATERIAL AND METHOD

The study took place in fifteen general practices in Greater Manchester, situated in a wide variety of social settings. In each practice a research assistant invited consecutive attenders to complete the twenty-eight-item GHQ (Goldberg and Hillier 1979) and the State Anxiety Inventory (Spielberger *et al*. 1970), and collected these before the patient was seen by the doctor. The general practitioner then completed a short encounter form for every patient seen during the study who had a new illness, defined as any complaint for which help had not been sought in the previous 12 months. On the encounter form the doctor recorded the patient's presenting complaints and classified the illness on a five-point scale of various combinations of physical and psychiatric illness (Table 23.1). The study continued for approximately three weeks in each participating practice.

At the second stage, a stratified sampling procedure was used to select for interview patients identified by the doctor as having a psychiatric illness, or who had high GHQ scores, and these were asked to agree to an interview with a research psychiatrist. The twenty-eight-item GHQ has been reported to have a sensitivity of 84 per cent (Goldberg and Williams 1988). To check for missed cases in this study, a sample of low scorers whose illnesses were classified as entirely physical illness by their doctors were also interviewed.

With this sampling procedure it became evident during the fieldwork that 'somatizers' were substantially more numerous than 'psychologizers' (Bridges and Goldberg 1985; Bridges and Goldberg 1987). Doctors were therefore asked to continue to refer psychologizers to the study after the three-week recording period, so that we should have comparably sized groups of patients to compare for our assessment of the possible determinants of somatization.

Patients were interviewed in their homes soon after their consultation with their doctor and then again 6 months later. They were assessed on a range of standardized inventories, including the Psychiatric Assessment Schedule (Dean et al. 1983), Social Stress and Support Inventory (Jenkins et al. 1981), and the Social Interview Schedule (Clare and Cairns 1978). They were also asked to complete a questionnaire in their own time and to return this using a stamped addressed envelope. This questionnaire consisted of several standardized inventories, including the Whitely Index for Hypochondriasis (Pilowsky and Spence 1976), the Social Desirability Questionnaire (Crowne and Marlowe 1960), the Parental Bonding Instrument (Parker et al. 1979), and MacLean's questionnaire on attitudes towards mental illness (MacLean 1968). Other questions, specifically designed for the study, were also included, such as those relating to the patients' past illness-related experiences and their attitudes towards discussing psychological problems with doctors (Bridges et al. 1991).

RESEARCH FINDINGS

1 Prevalence of somatization

The data, corrected for the sampling procedure used (Goldberg and Williams 1988), are summarized in Table 23.1 in terms of how patients were classified by the general practitioners and their mode of presentation.

Of 590 consecutive patients with new episodes of illness, 195 patients (33.1 per cent) were judged to have a psychiatric illness according to DSM-III criteria. Generalized Anxiety Disorder, Major Depressive Episode and a small proportion with Dysthymic Disorders together accounted for over 95 per cent of the psychiatric diagnoses. The majority of patients who only presented physical symptoms fell into two groups. First, there were those who were consulting their doctor primarily for a physical disorder, to which the coexisting psychiatric illness was either unrelated or secondary. Table 23.1 shows that this group accounted for only 23 per cent of all patients with psychiatric illnesses and represented less than 8 per cent of all new illnesses. Second, there were the patients whose psychiatric disorders were expressed in the form of somatic complaints. The table shows that 57 per cent of patients with a psychiatric illness fulfilled our criteria for either pure or 'facultative' somatization and accounted for over 18 per cent of all new illnesses.

Table 23.2 summarizes the weighted data on patients with a psychiatric illness, in terms of mode of presentation and the presence of a coexisting physical disorder. Of these patients 68 per cent had a coexisting physical disorder and less than 20 per cent had presented affective or cognitive symptoms to their doctors. It is also important to note that somatization occurred in the presence of coexisting physical disorders.

2 Hidden psychiatric morbidity

Because the design of our study required the family doctor to give his opinion on whether or not the patient had a psychiatric illness, we were able to assess the proportion of patients with undetected psychiatric illnesses. It can be seen from Table 23.1 that more than 50 per cent of DSM-III cases were undetected and classified by the general practitioners as 'entirely physical illnesses'. Table 23.3 summarizes the weighted data on this hidden morbidity in terms of mode of presentation and the presence of a coexisting physical disorder. From this it can be seen that hidden morbidity is explained in part by patients consulting their doctor primarily for a physical disorder. However, when somatization occurred, less than 50 per cent of the psychiatric illnesses were detected by the doctors. When patients did report psychological symptoms, the underlying psychiatric illness was detected in the majority of cases.

3 Assessment of potential determinants

Recruitment for this part of the study continued until we had obtained forty-seven 'somatizers' and fifty-five 'psychologizers'; we also recruited ninety-one patients with physical illnesses who were not psychiatrically ill but whose somatic complaints were similar to those of the somatizers.

Table 23.1 Weighted data on a consecutive series of patients with DSM-III psychiatric illness (excluding Adjustment Disorder) in terms of how these were classified by the general practitioners and by mode of presentation (for weighting procedure, see Goldberg and Williams 1988)

General practitioners' classification	No. of patients in consecutive sample	No. of patients with DMS-III disorder (weighted)	Physical illness only	Mode of presentation		
				Somatization		Psychological
				Pure	Facultative	
Entirely physical illnesses	434	100.1	40.2	34.0	24.3	1.6
Unrelated physical and psychiatric illnesses	29	17.8	5.2	6.1	2.6	3.9
Physical illness with secondary psychiatric illness	44	23.1	–	13.9	5.8	3.4
Psychiatric illness with somatic complaints	52	33.3	–	13.1	10.1	10.1
Entirely psychiatric illness	31	20.7	–	1.1	–	19.6
Total	590	195.0	45.4	68.2	42.8	38.6

Table 23.2 Weighted data on patients with DSM-III illnesses in terms of mode of presentation and presence of coexisting physical disorder

	Unrelated physical illness only	Related physical illness only	Mode of presentation Somatization		Psycho-logical
			Pure	Facultative	
Coexisting physical illness	43.7	1.6	49.6	30.1	8.4
No coexisting physical illness	–	–	18.6	12.7	30.2
Total	43.7	1.6	68.2	42.8	38.6

Some demographic features are summarized in Table 23.4. The results of our assessments have been reported in greater detail elsewhere (Bridges *et al.* 1991). In essence we found that somatizers did not constitute a narrowly defined group. This mode of presentation occurred in all age-groups, in both sexes, in all social classes, at all intellectual levels and in patients suffering from different kinds of psychiatric illness. This was also true for the psychological mode of presentation.

The somatizers and psychologizers were also similar in other respects, including features of their personality and upbringing, their responses to the Parental Bonding Instrument, and their memories of childhood, illness-related experiences. Furthermore, they were similar in respect

Table 23.3 Weighted data on 'hidden psychiatric morbidity' in terms of mode of presentation and presence of coexisting physical disorder

	Unrelated physical illness only	Related physical illness only	Mode of presentation Somatization		Psycho-logical
			Pure	Facultative	
Coexisting physical illness	38.6	1.6	30.8	22.7	–
No coexisting physical illness	–	–	3.2	1.6	1.6
Total	38.6	1.6	34.0	24.3	1.6

Table 23.4 Demographic characteristics of patients in study of potential determinants of somatization

Patient groups	Controls (N = 91)	Somatizers (N = 47)	Psychologizers (N = 55)
Male	44	19	14
Female	47	28	41
Mean age (yrs)	44.3	45.6	40.2
(SD)	(19.1)	(16.3)	(15.8)
Social class:			
I	8	4	2
II (non-manual)	33	21	17
III (non-manual)	22	12	16
III (manual)	20	6	14
IV	5	3	5
V	3	1	1
Marital status:			
Single	20	3	7
Married/cohabiting	58	37	41
Divorced/separated	6	3	2
Widowed	7	4	5
Employment:			
Working	56	30	30
Unemployed	6	2	6
Housewife	5	6	12
Retired	19	6	5
Student	5	3	2

Note: 'Facultative' somatizers are not included

of current social factors which might be associated with adoption of the sick role, in their marital relationships and in the attitudes of their partners towards mental illness. The two groups of patients had a similar, basically positive, attitude towards the role of their doctors in dealing with psychological illnesses.

The study found, however, that the somatizers did differ from the psychologizers in at least four main respects. First, they were not as depressed as the psychologizers, according to the results of the latent trait analysis, and had significantly lower GHQ, PSE and STAI scores. Second, the psychologizers reported significantly greater degrees of social dysfunction, dissatisfaction and stress, and were more dependent on their relatives. Third, the somatizers were more likely to have an unsympathetic attitude towards mental illness, as assessed by MacLean's (1968) questionnaire, and, when asked to imagine themselves with symptoms of depression, neurasthenia or panic, they were less likely to consult a doctor about these or, if they did see a doctor, to mention such symptoms to him. Fourth, the somatizers were more likely to have received medical in-patient care in adult life, before consulting their doctors for the current illnesses.

DISCUSSION

The epidemiological data presented here show that a substantial proportion of patients with psychiatric illnesses, which meet research diagnostic criteria, present to their doctors with somatic complaints, and that only a minority of such patients present with overt psychological symptoms. The data also show that much of the 'hidden' psychiatric morbidity in primary-care settings goes unrecognized by the doctors because of this somatic mode of presentation. From our assessment of the possible determinants, it appears that the doctors' responses in their earlier encounters with these patients may have been an important factor.

Although somatic complaints may distract the attention of a doctor from considering a psychiatric diagnosis, our study suggests that somatization may have an adaptive function, in two main ways. First, it appears to serve as a defence mechanism which helps the patient to cope with life's vicissitudes: an explanation which has also been suggested by other researchers (Mayou 1976; Pilowsky 1978; Katon *et al*. 1982b; Lipowski 1988; Barsky 1979; Barsky and Klerman 1983). In attributing his somatic complaints and distress to an underlying organic disorder, the patient may in effect be seeking to absolve himself from responsibility for his present predicament. One consequence of this blame-avoiding function may be that it prevents patients from becoming as depressed as they might otherwise do. Second, the findings also suggest that somatization is a mechanism which enables people who are unsympathetic to psychological illness none the less to adopt the sick role when they themselves become psychologically distressed.

Though not enough is yet known about the consequences of failing to detect psychiatric illness in such cases, it seems likely that its recognition and treatment could benefit both the patient and the health services. Furthermore, many conditions which present in this way tend to become chronic and increasingly difficult to treat successfully if their true nature goes unrecognized. It therefore seems important that family doctors should improve their skills in detecting and managing somatization disorders and in overcoming the patients' typical resistance to the idea that their somatic complaints are due to psychological conflicts (Gask *et al*. 1989).

ACKNOWLEDGEMENT

This research was supported by a grant from the Sir Jules Thorn Charitable Trust.

REFERENCES

American Psychiatric Association (APA) (1980) *Diagnostic and Statistical Manual*, third edn, DSM-III, Washington, DC: APA.

Barsky, A.J. (1979) 'Patients who amplify bodily sensations', *Annals of Internal Medicine* 91:63–73.

Barsky, A. and Klerman, G.L. (1983) 'Overview: hypochondriasis, bodily complaints and somatic styles', *American Journal of Psychiatry* 140:273–83.

Bridges, K.W. and Goldberg, D.P. (1985) 'Somatic presentation of DSM-III psychiatric disorders in primary care', *Journal of Psychosomatic Research* 29:653–69.

Bridges, K.W. and Goldberg, D.P. (1987) 'Somatic presentation of depressive illness in primary care', in P. Freeling, L.J. Downey, and J.C. Malkin (eds) *The Presentation of Depression: Current Approaches*, Occasional Paper No. 36, London: Royal College of General Practitioners.

Bridges, K.W., Goldberg, D.P., Evans, B., and Sharpe, T. (1991) 'Determinants of somatisation in primary care', *Psychological Medicine* 21:473–83.

Clancy, J. and Noyes, R. (1976) 'Anxiety neurosis: a disease for the medical model', *Psychosomatics* 17:90–3.

Clare, A.W. and Cairns, V.E. (1978) 'Design, development and use of a standardized interview to assess social maladjustment and dysfunction in community studies', *Psychological Medicine* 8:589–604.

Crowne, D.P. and Marlowe, D. (1960) 'A new scale of social desirability independent of psychopathology', *Journal of Consulting Psychology* 24:349–54.

Dean, C., Surtees, P., and Sashidharan, S. (1983) 'Comparisons of research diagnostic systems in an Edinburgh community sample', *British Journal of Psychiatry* 142:247–56.

Gask, L., Goldberg, D., Porter, R., and Creed, F. (1989) 'The treatment of somatization: evaluation of a teaching package with general practice trainees', *Journal of Psychosomatic Research* 33:697–703.

Goldberg, D.P. (1979) 'Detection and assessment of emotional disorders in primary care settings', *International Journal of Mental Health* 8:30–48.

Goldberg, D.P. and Blackwell, B. (1970) 'Psychiatric illness in general practice: a detailed study using a new method of case identification', *British Medical Journal* 2:439–43.

Goldberg, D.P. and Bridges, K.W. (1987) 'Screening for psychiatric illness in general practice: the general practitioner vs. the screening questionnaire', *Journal of the Royal College of General Practitioners* 37:15–18.

Goldberg, D.P., Bridges, K.W., Duncan-Jones, P., and Grayson, D. (1987) 'Dimensions of neurosis seen in primary care settings', *Psychological Medicine* 17:461–70.

Goldberg, D.P. and Hillier, V. (1979) 'A scaled version of the General Health Questionnaire', *Psychological Medicine* 9:139–45.

Goldberg, D.P. and Huxley, P. (1980) *Mental Illness in the Community: the Pathway to Psychiatric Care*, London: Tavistock.

Goldberg, D.P. and Williams, P. (1988) *The User's Guide to the General Health Questionnaire*, Slough, UK: NFER/Nelson.

Hoeper, E.W., Nycz, G.P., Cleary, P., Regier, D., and Goldberg, I. (1979) 'Estimated prevalence of RDC mental disorders in primary care', *International Journal of Mental Health* 8:6–15.

Jenkins, R., Mann, A.H., and Belsey, E. (1981) 'The background, design and use of a short interview to assess social stress and support in research and clinical settings', *Social Science and Medicine* 15:195–203.

Katon, W. (1984) 'Panic disorder and somatization: a review of 55 cases', *American Journal of Medicine* 77:101–6.

Katon, W., Kleinman, A., and Rosen, G. (1982a) 'Depression and somatization: a review. Part I', *American Journal of Medicine* 72:127–35.

Katon, W., Kleinman, A., and Rosen, G. (1982b) 'Depression and somatization: a review. Part II', *American Journal of Medicine* 72:241–7.

Kirmayer, L.T. (1984) 'Culture, affect and somatization, Part I', *Transcultural Psychiatric Research Review* 21:159–87.

Kleinman, A. and Kleinman, J. (1985) 'Somatization: the interconnections in Chinese society between culture, depressive experiences and meaning of pain', in A. Kleinman and B. Good (eds) *Culture and Depression. Studies in the Anthropology and Cross-Cultural Psychiatry of Affective Disorder*, London: University of California Press, pp. 429–90.

Lipowski, Z.J. (1988) 'Somatization: the concept and its clinical application', *American Journal of Psychiatry* 145:1358–68.

MacLean, U. (1968) 'The 1966 Edinburgh survey of community attitudes to mental illness', *Health Bulletin* 26:23–7.

Mayou, R. (1976) 'The nature of bodily symptoms', *British Journal of Psychiatry* 129:55–60.

Parker, G., Tupling, H., and Brown, L.B. (1979) 'A parental bonding instrument', *British Journal of Medical Psychology* 52:1–10.

Pilowsky, I. (1978) 'Psychodynamic aspects of pain experience', in R.A. Sternbach (ed.) *The Psychology of Pain*, New York: Raven Press, pp. 203–17.

Pilowsky, I. and Spence, N.D. (1976) 'Patterns of illness behaviour in patients with intractable pain', *Journal of Psychosomatic Research* 19:279–87.

Rosen, G., Kleinman, A., and Katon, W. (1982) 'Somatization in female patients: a biopsychosocial approach', *Journal of Family Practice* 14:493–502.

Shepherd, M., Cooper, B., Brown, A.C., and Kalton, G. (1966) *Psychiatric Illness in General Practice*, London: Oxford University Press.

Smith, R.G., Monson, R.A., and Ray, D.C. (1986) 'Patients with multiple unexplained symptoms', *Archives of Internal Medicine* 146:69–72.

Spielberger, C.D., Gorsuch, R.L., and Lushene, R.E. (1970) *Manual for the State-Trait Anxiety Inventory*, Palo Alto, CA: Consulting Psychological Press.

Index

Abbreviated Mental Test 247
affective disorders in general practice
20, 36; presenting with somatic
complaints 51–2
AGECAT computer diagnosis 246
Agency for Health Care Policy
and Research, US Public Health
Service 95, 96
age-sex registers in general practice 27,
45
alcohol abuse, detection by GPs 217
Alzheimer-type dementia (Alzheimer's
Disease) 246, 249, 253, 277; Patient
Registries in USA 277
ambulatory *see* out-patient
anatomical, chemical and therapeutic
classification system (ACT) 199
antidepressants in general practice 48;
efficacy in mild cases 9
anxiety, latent structure in populations
307–18
anxiety states, consulting rates in
general practice 118

Baehr, G. 32, 33
Balint groups 104
Baltimore City Hospital 69
Baltimore ECA catchment area 74–6,
164–71, 279; mental health survey in
256, 309, 319–40
Balzac, H. de 14
Benzodiazepine prescribing in general
practice 105, 190–1, 206–7
Berger, J. 28
'black lung' in miners 8
Bond, H. 32
British National Health Service xx, 16,
19, 24, 33
British national morbidity surveys 19,
33, 38–40, 102

Budd, W., on typhoid fever 15

Cambridge Examination for
Mental Disorders of the Elderly
(CAMDEX) 214–16, 235–46
passim, 258, 259, 268
Cancer Ward 14, 15
case detection in general practice
217–8; evaluative studies 47
case-identification in primary care
settings (see also detection, GP
recognition, screening) 293–5, 302–4
'case' of sickness: definition 33
case registers, area psychiatric 17,
59, 191–2
CATEGO program *see* Present State
Examination
Center for Epidemiological Studies
Depression Scale 109
Chadwick Report on sanitary
conditions in Victorian England
6, 9, 11
changing disciplines in medicine 26–8
changing the agenda in doctor-patient
transactions 52
Chekhov, A. 14
Clare, A. 3
Clarke Institute of Psychiatry,
Toronto xix
classification of psychiatric lines in
general practice 22, 36–8
Clifton Assessment Procedure for the
Elderly (CAPE) 214; information-
orientation scale 247
Clinical Dementia Rating (CDR) 243,
246, 283
Clinical Interview Schedule (CIS) 36,
133, 189
Coal Mine Health and Safety Act,
USA 8

cognitive impairment: definition of
282; screening for 217–8, 236–8,
257–9, 263, 281–2; *see also* dementia
collaboration between psychiatrists and
GPs 52–4
Colleges of General Practitioners 16
community care 15
community health centres 133, 150
community mental health centres
151, 165
Comprehensive Assessment and
Referral Evaluation (CARE) 246
computerized records in general
practice 27, 101, 136
Consortium to Establish a Registry
for Alzheimer's Disease (CERAD)
279, 281
Cooper, B. 3
cost ratio of screening to diagnosis
302–4
counsellors in general practice
102–6 *passim*
crisis accommodation centres 143

Declaration of Alma-Ata xx, 213
Defined Daily Dose (DDD) 199–208
dementia: assessment procedures
247–8; diagnostic criteria 248–9;
early detection and mortality
rates 238; prevalence in New York
and London 247; rating scales
254; recognition by GPs 218–20;
reversible cases 253; stages of
severity 253, 255, 256; *see also*
cognitive impairment
Department of Health and Social
Security (DHSS) 38, 105
depression: consulting rate for 118;
latent structure in populations
307–18; recognition by general
practitioners 220; *see also* affective
disorders
detection of psychiatric illness by GPs
21, 24, 217–8; efficiency of 21; in
elderly patients 218–20; usefulness
of 47–8
Diagnostic and Statistical Manual,
third revision (DSM-III) 22, 66,
70, 91; criteria for dementia 249;
diagnostic criteria 70, 91, 165,
342, 344
diagnostic guidelines in classification
manuals 45, 70, 91

Diagnostic Interview Schedule (DIS)
70, 165, 309, 321, 336; diagnostic
categories 309
DIS/DSM-III classification system 70,
71, 165, 307–9
doctor-patient interviews: management
skills in 50; videotapes of 48, 49
Duncan-Jones, P. 38
Durham, North Carolina, mental
health survey 164–7 *passim*
Dutch National Study of Morbidity
and Interventions in General
Practice: methods 110–11; findings
111–17

early detection: of dementia 253, 254,
256, 271; of mental disorders in the
elderly 217–20
Eastern Baltimore Mental Health
Survey 69–96, 256, 320; methods
69–72, 321–3; demographic findings
72–4; prevalence estimates 74–83,
323–8; *see also* PSE syndromes
Eastwood, M.R. 3
Eliot, G. 14
emergency room medical care
165–8 *passim*
enzyme-linked immunosorbent assays
(ELISA) for HIV infection 293
epidemiological survey methods in
psychiatry 34–5
Epidemiologic Catchment Area (ECA)
surveys in USA 59, 69, 118, 155,
164–76, 216, 256, 279, 308–10, 311,
321, 336
epidemiology: in general practice 16;
and public health action 3–11, 96;
uses of 5–6, 11
European Research Workshop 16
European Symposium on Social
Psychiatry 34

family care-givers 223–4
Family Practitioner Committee
(FPC) 214
Farr, W. 6, 11
follow-up studies 40–1, 238–40, 246
Frost, W.H. 5, 6
Fry, J. 40

General Health Questionnaire (GHQ)
20, 49–50, 109, 118, 126–9, 133,

217; 60-item version 125; 30-item version (in Italian) 189–90, 193; 20-item version 321; 28-item version 343

general practice: attachment schemes in UK 107; as basis for epidemiological research 16–17, 21–7; early research in 15–16; as 'middle ground' of psychiatric epidemiology 41, 213

general practice patients: categories of presentation 115–17

general practice psychiatric surveys: Cambridge, UK 218–20, 235–47, 256; Greater Manchester, UK 342–8; London, UK 19; Mannheim, Germany 218–20, 256–64; the Netherlands 110–17; North America 45; observation periods in 20

General Practice Research unit 3, 34, 36, 40

general practice surveys in the Netherlands 118

general practitioners: advantages in detection of psychiatric illness 17–18; agreement on psychiatric diagnosis 94–5; awareness of mental health problems 92, 94; as 'gatekeepers' of services 224; public image of 14–15; recognition of psychiatric disorders 9, 48–51, 65–6, 139, 190, 307

General Practitioner Recording Schedule (GPRS) 189

geriatric homes, medication in 221–2

geriatric screening programmes 217

GLIM program package 126

Goldberg, D. 3

Goldberg-Huxley model see pathway to psychiatric care

Greater Manchester, general practice study in 342–8

Griscom, J.C., on sanitary conditions in New York 6–7

Grotjahn, A. 16

Halo effect in morbidity surveys 19

Hamilton, A., on 'importation' of epidemic disease 7

health care systems: in a Brazilian district 134; in Finland 178; in Germany 260; in Italy 188–9; in the UK 99–100; in the USA 163, 278–9

'Health for All 2000' campaign 213

Health Insurance Plan of New York 32

'hidden' psychiatric morbidity 21, 119, 190, 341–8 passim

Hierarchic Dementia Scale (HDS): characteristics 257–9; profiles among elderly patients 264–7; and severity of dementia 268–70

homelessness and onset of mental disorder 156–7

homeless persons: in Australia 143; in Edinburgh 142, 157; foreign-born among 147; in Great Britain 142–3; in Los Angeles 156–7; mental health problems of 142–4; in Sydney 153–7; in USA 142; use of medical services 149–52; patterns of living 153–5

Iceland, cohort study in 319–20

identification see case identification in primary care settings

'identification index': ability to detect mental disorder 48

illness behaviour 36

inception cases in a longitudinal survey 62

inception rates, age-specific 63

informant interviews 237, 249

Institute of Medicine, US National Academy of Sciences 95

Institute of Psychiatry, London xx, 3

International Classification of Diseases (ICD) 22–3, 37, 66, 102, 111, 136; criteria for dementia 249

International Classification of Health Problems in Primary Care (ICHPPC) 22–3, 37, 111

International Classification in Primary Care (ICPC) 111

International Society of General Practice 16

Itapagipe Health District (Bahia), survey in 134–40

Jablensky, A. 3

Jefferson, T., on 'localism' of disease epidemics 7

Johns Hopkins University Hospital, Baltimore 217

Koch, R. 15

Kraepelin, E. 38
Kruskal-Wallis rank variance analysis
 266

Latent class analysis 310; application
 to ECA survey data 311–17
letter to *The Times* on London
 sanitation 10–11
Levin's 'attributable risk' index 124
life-charts and lifelines in longitudinal
 studies 146, 154–6
life expectancy: among males
 in Harlem, New York, and in
 Bangladesh 10; gap between blacks
 and whites in USA 9–10
'lifetime' psychotic disorder 148
linear logistic modelling 126–8, 130
Lisson Grove Health Centre 100–1
local health units in Italy 188, 190
Los Angeles, mental health survey in
 164–71 *passim*, 310

Mackenzie, Sir James, and general
 practice 16, 32, 41
Maclean's questionnaire on attitudes
 to mental illness 343, 347
major depressive disorder 311, 317
Mann, A.H. 3
Mannheim, general practice study of
 dementia in 256–73
Marriage Guidance Council 104
Maudsley Hospital *see* Institute of
 Psychiatry, London
measurement of morbidity, report
 of Registrar General's Advisory
 Committee 33
Medical Practices Committee (UK) 99
'Medicare' and 'Medicaid' programmes
 in USA 15, 277–8
Medizinische Reform, Die (medical
 journal) 6
Melbourne survey of homeless persons
 144–58
memory functions in dementia 255
mental health problems in general
 practice: modes of treatment 100
mental health service utilization in
 ECA communities 171–3
Mental Health Services in General
 Health Care, conference on 95
mental health services in health
 centres 105–7

mental health surveys: in Brazil
 133–9; in Cantabria, Spain 124–9;
 in Finland 180–4; in Third World
 countries 140; *see also* general
 practice psychiatric surveys
mental illness consultation rates 105
Mental Status Questionnaire (MSQ)
 218, 247
Meyer, A. 156
Microcomputers *see* computerized
 records
Milbank Memorial Fund 32
'mild dementia' 218, 234, 239, 242–3,
 253–5, 261, 271; definition of 248–9
'minimal dementia' 237–8, 246
Mini Mental Status Examination
 (MMSE) 70, 144, 216–8, 254,
 257, 235–45 *passim*, 321; cut-off
 point 244
'minor' psychiatric morbidity 213
Monongahela Valley Independent
 Elderly Survey (MoVIES) 279–88
Morris, J.N. 6
mortality among the elderly, in
 relation to dementia 238

National Academy of Sciences,
 USA 95
National Health Insurance in Iceland
 199
National Health Services 188; *see also*
 British National Health Service
National Institutes *see* US
needs and demand in primary health
 care 110, 121
neurasthenia as diagnostic category in
 Netherlands 113
neuropsychological testing 254
New Brunswick, Canada, psychiatric
 services 60–2
New Haven, mental health survey in
 164–7 *passim*
NINCDS-ADRA Work Group 282; *see*
 also dementia
nurses, practice-attached 26, 222

observer variation in diagnosis 36–7
odds ratio estimates: Mantel-Haenszel
 estimators 136, 323; of mental
 disorders in Baltimore survey
 population 84–6, 90
Office of Population Censuses and
 Surveys, London 38

old-age mental disorders, frequency in general practice 226–7
oral contraception, survey of health consequences 16
out-patient psychiatric services: in the USA 174–6; utilization of 324–5

Parental Bonding Instrument 343, 346
Parkinson, J., on the 'shaking palsy' 15
pathway to psychiatric care, level-and-filter model (Goldberg-Huxley model) 24, 44, 109–10, 112, 119–21, 123, 188–95 *passim*, 319, 325; American bypass 334; in Groningen 44; in Manchester 45; in New Brunswick 66; in Verona 44
Pharmacotherapy in primary health care 221–2
physical and psychiatric illness: association between distributions 23, 69, 74–96, 119, 123; in the elderly 221
Pickles, W., on epidemiology in country practice 16
Piedmont, North Carolina, ECA survey 309
Poor Law Amendment Act of 1834 (England) 6
pre-paid health-care plans 163; users in New Haven 164–8
Prescribed Daily Dose (PDD) 199–208
prescribing habits in general practice 190–1, 221–2
Present State Examination (PSE): computer algorithm (Catego) 322; Index of Definition 35
PSE syndromes 322–38; discriminant function analysis 333, 335; prevalence of 325–8; association with medical care 328–33
President Carter's Mental Health Commission xx
prevalence of alcoholism in Brazilian survey 138, 140
prevalence of dementia 214–5, 240–4; in Cambridge, UK 234–8; in pooled data 240; in New Zealand 242
prevalence of illness in general practice populations 295–6
prevalence of mental disorders 76–7;

among homeless persons 148–9, 155–6; among physically ill persons in Baltimore survey 78, 79–80; in New Haven 168–70; sex ratio in 129
prevalence of physical illness in East Baltimore 76, 91; among mentally ill persons 78–9
prevalence of psychotropic drug use, one-month 200–1
prevention in primary health care 26–7
primary care physicians *see* general practitioners
primary health care: and the elderly 256; in Finland 180; in Italy 188; locus in general medical practice 214; in modern industrial society 26; in the UK 99; utilization by homeless 142–3; *see also* general practice, teamwork
primary health care team 26, 99
private psychiatric practice, users in ECA communities 164–76
proactive patient care 27, 28
Psychiatric Assessment Schedule 343, 347
psychiatric care system in Italy 188–9
psychiatric case: criteria 34, 54; definition of 34, 35
Psychiatric Community Nurses (CPNs) 102–5 *passim*
psychiatric diagnoses as proportion of consultations 117
psychiatric diagnostic distribution: in East Baltimore survey 78–80, 325–8; among homeless persons in Melbourne 148–53; in Salvador, Bahia 138–40
psychiatric epidemiology: early development 32–3; in primary health care 3; strategies and sources of data 17; *see also* epidemiology, prevalence
psychiatric hospital admission rates 106
psychiatric hospitals, duration of stay 99
psychiatric illness in general practice: categories according to need for intervention 120; longitudinal study 40–1; and sociodemographic characteristics 126–7
psychiatric illness rates: at different levels of care 18

psychiatric liaison in general practice 52–4; modes of 25–6
psychiatric morbidity, conspicuous *see also* psychiatric illness 51, 190;
psychiatric out-patient clinics, users in ECA communities 165–8
psychiatric specialist referral by general practitioners 23–6, 99, 102, 103, 191–3, 224–5
psychiatric syndromes 319–38; in East Baltimore population 325–8; and use of health services 320, 328–32, 337
psychogeriatric services, integrated model 226–7
'psychological' reasons for general practice consultation 111–12
psychotherapy, supportive 207
psychotropic drug prescribing by general practitioners: for elderly patients 221–2; in Iceland 198–208; in Norway 198; in Scandinavia 198; in S. Verona, Italy 190–1; by telephone 202, 207; in USA 198, 206
psychotropic drug sales 198–9

randomized controlled trials in general practice 221–3
'reason for encounter' in survey recording 110–11
referral to psychiatric specialist agencies 23–6; modes of 225; rates of 224–5; in Verona 191–3
Research Diagnostic Criteria 118
research in general practice: tradition of 15–16; and psychiatric epidemiology 17–18
Rockefeller Foundation 22
Royal College of General Practitioners 38

St Louis, Missouri, mental health survey in 164–7
Sartorius, N. 3
scale of morbidity, from somatic to psychiatric 109–13 *passim*
Schedule of Affective Disorders and Schizophrenia (SADS) 118
Science, moral un-neutrality of 11
screening survey designs: one-phase 300–1; two-phase 235–8, 293–305, 321–2

screening tests: applications 293, 295; false positives 294; relative costs 296–301; sensitivity and specificity 303–5; types of 217; *see also* cognitive impairment
Self-Report Questionnaire 133
segregation in US metropolitan areas, indices of 10
severe mental disorder, definition 144
Shepherd, M. xx, 3
'Skid Row' alcoholics 142
Snow, C.P. 11
Snow, J., on cholera 5, 6, 15
socio-demographic characteristics in survey-data analysis 125–6
Social Desirability Questionnaire 343
Social disadvantage and psychiatric disorder 23
Social Interview Schedule 343
Social Problems Schedule 36
Social Stress and Support Inventory 343
Solzhenitsyn, A. 14, 15
somatization: as adaptive function 348; criteria for 51, 342; definition of 341; in general practice patients 341–8; subacute 51
'somatizers' and 'psychologizers' among general practice patients 343–7
South-Verona: Community Psychiatric Service (CPS) 191–3; Psychiatric Case Register 191–3
special accommodation houses (SAHs) 145
special function of the primary-care physician 27
specialty mental health agencies 72
spectrum of cognitive decline 266
spectrum of psychiatric morbidity 193–5
State Anxiety Inventory 342, 347
Statistical Analysis System Procedures 323
Structured Clinical Interview for DSM-III-R (SCID-R) 144, 148, 154
surveys of mental disorder in elderly populations: in Pennsylvania 280–7; prevalence estimates 240–2; in the UK 214–7; *see also* general practice surveys
'Symptom diagnosis' in survey recording 128

Tansella, M. 3
teaching package for general
    practitioners 51–2, 54
teamwork in primary health
    care 222
Third World countries, old-age mental
    disorders in 228
Thomson, Sir William (Lord Kelvin),
    dictum of 4–5
Training of GPs in diagnostic
    techniques 24
Tudor Hart, J. 26–7

United Mine Workers' Health and
    Welfare Fund 8
University of Pittsburgh 277;
    Alzheimer's Disease Research
    Center 279, 283
US Bureau of the Census 73
US mental health services, *de facto* 3
US National Institute on Aging 277
US National Institute of Mental
    Health (NIMH) 19, 22, 321
usual source of medical care 163–76;
    categories of 164–5;
    in ECA survey areas 166–8
utilization of health and mental health
    services: and cognitive impairment
    284–7; in East Baltimore 86–9,
    91–2; by homeless persons 149–52;
    by specialty 92–4

Verona, services in 189; *see also* South-
    Verona
Veteran Administration hospitals 165
Victorian Council to Homeless
    Persons 143
Victorian Office of Psychiatric
    Services 158
Victoria Psychiatric Case Register
    145, 148
Viner, J., on Kelvin's dictum 5
Virchow, R. 6, 7, 11

Wechsler Memory Scale, 'logical
    memory' sub-test 255–8
Whitely Index for Hypochondriasis 343
Withering, W., and foxglove extract 15
World Health Organization 44, 213;
    'Health for All 2000' campaign xx;
    Mental Health Division 22; study
    of patterns of mental health care in
    Europe 62, 66
World Psychiatric Association, Section
    of Epidemiology and Community
    Psychiatry xix, 3, 35
World Organization of National
    Colleges of General Practice
    (WONCA) 16

yellow fever epidemic in Philadelphia
    7–8
youth crisis centre 145